S0-ECN-801

TURNER'S
School health
and health education

TURNER'S
School health
and health education

Frank H. Jenne, Ph.D.

Associate Professor,
Department of Health Education,
Temple University, Philadelphia, Pennsylvania

Walter H. Greene, Ed.D.

Professor, Health Education,
Temple University, Philadelphia, Pennsylvania

Illustrated

Seventh edition

LB
3405
.T83
1976
west

The C. V. Mosby Company

Saint Louis   1976

Oversize
LB 3405
T 83
1976

Seventh edition

Copyright © 1976 by The C. V. Mosby Company

All rights reserved. No part of this book may be reproduced
in any manner without written permission of the publisher.

Previous editions copyrighted 1947, 1952, 1957, 1961, 1966, 1970

Printed in the United States of America

Distributed in Great Britain by Henry Kimpton, London

Library of Congress Cataloging in Publication Data

Turner, Clair Elsmere, 1890-1974.
Turner's School health and health education, by - and -.
357 p.
Includes Bibliography: p.
Includes index.
1. Health education. I. Jenne, Frank H., 1920-
II. Greene, Walter H. III. Title. IV. Title: School
health and health education. [DNLM: 1. Health
education. 2. School health. WA350 T945]
LB3405.T83 1976   371.7'1   75-43985
ISBN 0-8016-5134-4

1976 (7th ed)

CB/CB/B 9 8 7 6 5 4 3 2 1

8/23/76 - $11.50

Clair E. Turner

1890-1974

Professor Turner's career spanned more than 60 active years. This book and *Personal and Community Health* are his best-known written works. Through the previous six editions of this text and the fourteen editions of the other, thousands of students have obtained health information and attitudes relevant to their personal lives, and many were motivated to enter careers in school or community health education.

Dr. Turner was a distinguished teacher, researcher, and doer as well as a writer. At MIT he taught the first course in health education ever offered in a school of public health and originated the first program leading to the Master of Public Health degree in health education. His studies and demonstrations in the Malden, Massachusetts schools during the 1920's laid the foundation for much of what is done in the field of school health and health education today. During and after World War II much of his effort was directed to the improvement of international health, primarily through his work with the World Health Organization and UNESCO. He was the first president and chief advisor of the International Union for Health Education, as well as the honorary president of that organization from 1968 to 1974, and was active in and honored by a host of other health-related organizations.

It was therefore with some sense of awe that we undertook the task of rewriting and revising *School Health and Health Education*. Our trepidation was not lessened by the social context in which we write, a time of rapid social change, much of which is of a discouraging nature. We were deprived of the benefit of Professor Turner's wisdom and criticism by his death. Any deficiencies are to be charged to us, not to him.

Preface

In this edition we have provided new and updated information. In addition, we have tried to relate the principles and practices of school health and health education to conditions prevailing in American schools and society. Pursuit of this goal has resulted in content less didactic and more issue oriented than that presented in other and earlier school health program texts. The new emphasis on the individuality of children and youth led us to depart from the style of writing characterized by the phrase "the child is." We have also tried to avoid sex role stereotyping. We hope instructors and students who use this text will be more comfortable in doing so as a result.

Rejection of the notion that school professionals should accept without question the dictates of restrictive school and health laws, the orders handed down from on high by authoritative administrators, and the demands of vocal but unrepresentative citizen groups led to the inclusion of two chapters dealing with law, public relations, and administration. Recognition of the importance of school social climate to mental health resulted in a separate chapter devoted to the subject. Affective education has been given greater prominence in this edition, since it is now increasingly practiced in schools.

At the cost of some repetitions, we have attempted to write the book in such a way that instructors may omit selected chapters or sections or may assign chapters in varying sequence at little risk of failing to cover essential principles.

We wish to thank the thinkers and researchers whose work has contributed to the book, our families, and typists Frances Greene and Allan Older.

Frank H. Jenne
Walter H. Greene

Contents

PART SEVEN

Appraising school health and health education

PART ONE

Nature and development of school health and health education

CHAPTER 1

🌱 Place of health in today's schools

School health and health education is at once rewarding and frustrating work. It is rewarding to watch a child or young person improve in health, appearance, and behavior as a result of your efforts as a teacher, nurse, dental hygienist, or other school professional. It is frustrating to view the collapse of your work and plans as a result of your own failure or the apathy, prejudice, or ignorance of some parents, community leaders, or school administrators. The broad purpose of this book is to increase your likelihood of professional success in improving both the health of children and youth and your own job satisfaction.

WHY SCHOOL HEALTH AND HEALTH EDUCATION?

Schools exist for several reasons. First among them is to transmit the culture to the young through organized learning experiences. But schools also serve as agents of cultural change by changing the content of instruction in line with changing knowledge, social needs, and values. Another purpose of schools today is to serve as surrogate homes, with teachers as parents. This function keeps young people out of the job market and permits both legal parents to work or to perform other social roles. School health and health education are intimately involved with and essential to both of these purposes.

Health, schools, and learning. Health is an important part of our culture. Unlike the Christians of ancient Rome who despised the body, we care for it through an elaborate system of health products, information, and services. We recognize and have names for many different kinds of illnesses, just as the Eskimos are said to recognize and have names for many different kinds of snow. By the World Health Organization's definition we have gone beyond the idea of health as the mere absence of disease or infirmity and have embraced the notion of health as a state of positive and total well-being.

School health and health education serve to perpetuate both the system and the ideal. One of their objectives is to assist children and young people in entering the health care system for care related to health promotion as well as for the diagnosis and treatment of health problems. Another is to teach the value of positive health and the known means of promoting it as well as to develop skills in the choice and use of health products and services.

A classic statement of the objectives of general education is to be found in *A Design for General Education,* which says with reference to health that general education should lead a student "to improve and maintain his own health and take his share of responsibility for protecting the health of others." In further elaboration of this primary health objective, the report states:

In order to accomplish this purpose the student should acquire the following:
A. Knowledge and understanding
  1. Of normal body functions in relation to sound health practice
  2. Of the major health hazards, their prevention, and control
  3. Of the interrelation of mental and physical processes in health
  4. Of reliable sources of information on health
  5. Of scientific methods in evaluating health concepts
  6. Of the effect of socio-economic conditions on health
  7. Of community health problems, such as problems related to sanitation, industrial hygiene and school hygiene
  8. Of community organization and services for health maintenance and improvement

3

B. Skills and abilities
   1. The ability to organize time to include planning for food, work, recreation, rest and sleep
   2. The ability to improve and maintain good nutrition
   3. The ability to attain and maintain good emotional adjustment
   4. The ability to select and engage in recreational activities and healthful exercises suitable to individual needs
   5. The ability to avoid unnecessary exposure to disease and infection
   6. The ability to utilize medical and dental services intelligently
   7. The ability to participate in measures for the protection and improvement of community health
   8. The ability to evaluate health beliefs critically
C. Attitudes and appreciations
   1. Desire to maintain optimum health
   2. Personal satisfaction in carrying out sound health practices
   3. Acceptance of responsibility for his own health and for the health of others
   4. Willingness to make personal sacrifices for the health of others
   5. Willingness to comply with health regulations and to work for their improvement*

The source of these statements indicates that school health and health education serve the general education purpose of the schools. Thoughtful consideration shows that the objectives are as valid today as they were three decades ago when they were written. Their interpretation, however, varies in the 1970's from their interpretation in the 1940's. At that time newly discovered antibiotics, pesticides, and other medical and environmental control materials and techniques were ready to be applied to combat disease and premature death. Today we are confronted by problems of overpopulation, food and other resource shortages, and overproduction of economic goods and their resulting pollutants, as well as by personal psychosocial problems related to drug use and sexual behavior. These problems threaten both the quality and continued existence of human life on this planet within the foreseeable future.†

Other and older aspects of health affect learning, and practices of both individuals and schools affect health. Acute hearing, for example, facilitates learning. An undetected, untreated ear infection can damage hearing, and the school health education program can facilitate early detection and treatment of ear infections. Location of a school within a mile of a busy jet airport can also damage hearing, but such a location is preventable by knowledge of the hazard and intelligent school-community planning.

The reports of the Project on Instruction of the National Education Association* published during the 1960's suggest that the school should be directing its educational efforts toward using rational processes, developing social responsibility, making more intelligent consumer choices, building international competence, increasing understanding of complicated issues confronting voters and taxpayers today, learning through discovery, developing self-direction and self-responsibility, and analyzing mass communication and propaganda.

One important implication of this list is that more attention should be paid to learning to learn and to value. Such learning may be more important than learning today's facts, which may turn out to be tomorrow's fallacies. Irrational laws relating to drug use and sexual behavior can be overcome only by rational thinking, social and individual responsibility, and increased voter understanding of issues. Overreliance on what self-appointed authorities tell us has resulted in dangerous self-medication and needless anxiety about our physical and emotional normality. We have accepted monstrous school buildings and intense pressures to learn more faster in the name of quality education, because we have not learned to analyze propaganda and practice self-direction.

Thus, school health and health education

---

*A design for general education, Washington, D.C., 1944, American Council on Education.
†Meadows, D. H., and others: The limits to growth: a report for the Club of Rome's project on the predicament of mankind, Washington, D.C., 1972, Potomac Associates.

---

*National Education Association, Project on the Instructional Program of the Public Schools: Schools for the sixties, a report, New York, 1963, McGraw-Hill, Inc., p. 9.

(as they should be practiced) not only contribute to the transmission and modification of the culture but are in themselves aspects of general education. In addition, by helping to promote, protect, and maintain the health of children and young people, they facilitate development as well as learning. In a classic investigation Turner* showed by a controlled experiment that the introduction of health education without any other changes in school procedure can improve health practices and physical growth rates.

A schoolhouse is a home. Not so long ago the stereotypical American mother aroused herself and her family each morning. She saw to it that her husband and children were fed, supplied with clean clothes, and left the house on time for work or school. After serving as family chauffeur and shopper, she returned home to wash, clean, and cook. If a telephone call came from school about a sick, injured, or misbehaving child, she immediately reassumed responsibility. After school she welcomed her brood home, entertained them, provided moral education, fed them, and saw to it that they bathed and got to bed. Her spare time was spent in PTA, church, and other social and community activities. Home was one thing, school another, and mother was the coordinator.

Such mothers and the homes they make are increasingly rare. The 1970 U.S. census showed that jobs outside the home are held by half of all mothers with children in school. In addition, the increasing number of divorces leaves many children in homes with a single parent who must serve as both provider and homemaker. American mobility leaves the nuclear family unextended by the presence of aunts or grandmothers who might serve as surrogates. Few families can afford household help. And even the availability of work-saving appliances, no-iron clothes, and the prepackaged meals are not sufficient aids to per-

mit mothers to perform all their other traditional functions and to hold down jobs as well.

One clear result of these trends, whether one approves of them or not, is that schools are becoming second homes, and teachers and other school workers must either do more parenting or let children go inadequately parented. The development of prekindergarten programs and child care centers, some of which are school related, is a clear indication that the trend is toward assumption of greater parental responsibility by schools, at least for young children.

Good teachers have always been concerned with the health and welfare of their students. They view health promotion, including parenting, as a privilege as well as a responsibility. It enriches teacher-pupil relationships. It is part of good professional practice. It is an activity for which professional teacher preparation provides essential skills and understandings, and it is clearly becoming a social necessity.

The assumption that children and young people come to school with adequate breakfasts in their stomachs—if it was ever true—is no longer valid; no one works, learns, or relates to others well whose blood glucose level is too low. Thus, the inhabitants of the school-as-home need food, often including breakfast and snacks as well as the now traditional lunch. The school must also be prepared to provide extended temporary care for ill or injured students and perhaps even obtain definitive medical care on behalf of those parents whose work makes them unavailable. However, primary responsibility for obtaining health care still rests with the home, and what schools do in this regard must be done with the advice and consent of the parent. These new responsibilities are modifications of old ones, which can be met by adjustment of existing school feeding and emergency care programs.

In requiring school attendance, the state assumes an obligation to protect the health of students during school activities as well as on their way to and from school. Provision of a safe and healthful school environment, safe passage, and an adequate program of

*Turner, C. E.: Malden studies in health education and growth, Am. J. Public Health **18:**1217-1230, 1928.

communicable disease control are clear-cut responsibilities of the school in collaboration with community health authorities and the police.

Both good schools and good parents maintain surveillance over the health of children and young people. Where health defects or departures from normal health are found, both the school and the parent must be interested in definitive diagnosis and, if indicated, treatment and/or rehabilitation.

WHAT SCHOOL HEALTH AND HEALTH EDUCATION CAN AND CANNOT ACCOMPLISH

Health care, the environment, and the school. As an educational agency, the school has neither the responsibility nor the legal right (at this time) to provide medical treatment to school children. The rights and responsibilities of schools include appraisal of pupil health status, provision of emergency care, guidance in obtaining medical attention, and the control of communicable disease.* Schools also play an important role in rehabilitation, which is in large part an educative activity, through special education and vocational training programs.

That many Americans, adults as well as children, are denied access to medical care by economic, geographic, and racial barriers has been well documented in a recent study. Programs such as Medicaid, designed to overcome these barriers, have been less effective than they might be, partly because of bureaucratic red tape and callous insensitivity.† Legalization of full-scale medical care by the school would be wasteful of manpower and money because the needed facilities and personnel would be idle much of the time and would only duplicate those needed by the total community. The proper role of the school is largely educational; it

can effectively call attention to the problem and explore solutions in health education classes as well as in community forums.

Although schools can provide a safe and healthful physical and social school environment, their ability to do so is limited by the quality of the environment of the entire community. A well-planned and equipped outdoor activity area is useless when the ambient air is seriously polluted. The hazards of walking to school are multiplied for students who must cross the boundaries of a gang to which they do not belong or for any students living in an area with a high crime rate.

Christopher Jencks and associates* argue that achievement of social and economic equality depends much more on changes in our social and economic systems than on educational reform. But equality may not be all that desirable as a goal. A more realistic and attainable aim for schools may be to help individuals achieve whatever potential they come to school with, sensitize them to human problems, and provide them with problem-solving skills.

Behavior modification. Most authorities in health education hold that the central purpose of the subject is to improve both individual and group human health behavior. The present state of the art is such that our success in doing so is best described as mixed. There is much evidence that health education can induce people to utilize available health services. A voluntary topical application fluoride program, for example, was offered to pupils in the Dearborn, Michigan schools at no charge for many years. A continuous dental health education program among both pupils and parents kept participation at about 80%. When a fee representing full cost was instituted by the school board for the service, participation declined only to 75%. With continued education, participation increased to its former higher level in less than 2 years.

With the assistance of other social forces,

*Miller, D. F.: *School health programs: their basis in law,* Cranbury, N.J., 1972, A. S. Branes & Co., Inc., pp. 51-52, 65.
†Citizens Board of Inquiry into Health Services for Americans: *Heal yourself,* Washington, D.C., 1972, The American Public Health Association.

*Jencks, C., and others: *Inequality: a reassessment of the effect of family and schooling in America,* New York, 1972, Basic Books, Inc., Publishers.

health education has succeeded in nearly eliminating the once popular common drinking cup. A few other partial successes include popularized milk drinking, the pap test, hand washing, and the use of birth control methods.

Health education also has its share of conspicuous failures. It has had little impact on tobacco or marijuana smoking, obesity, or the sexual behavior of young people. A hundred years of temperance education, together with over a decade of national prohibition, failed to solve the problems of acute and chronic alcoholism.

Certain general principles that underlie health education may account, at least in part, for both the successes and the failures.

1. *Health status is determined by one's heredity and mode of living as well as by health education and services.* A child with three number 21 chromosomes is born a mongoloid; there is no known curative treatment. Children can be taught how to brush their teeth, but they cannot practice brushing without access to the necessary equipment and facilities. Correction of myopia requires the services of vision specialists. School health and health education alone should not be expected to produce uniform good health among all children. A health-educated individual, however, is more likely to have better health and greater efficiency than one who is not, given the same heredity, home environment, and access to health services.

2. *Health education is acquired from many sources: home, school, and community.* Reported research leads us to believe that parent and peer behavior (or modeling and social pressure) are more effective than formal school or community health education in determining smoking behavior. As a result of health education most of us know that cigarette smoking causes lung cancer, emphysema, and heart disease. However, these dire effects are 20 to 40 years away for the young novice, and the rewards of emulating those he or she admires and wishes to impress are here and now. The history of cigarette smoking in the United States suggests that the practice was masculinized, glamorized, and finally bisexualized and legitimized over a period of 2 or 3 decades by means of advertising, popular songs, and the movies—all forms of health education, albeit negative ones in this case.

3. *Health habits are created by operant conditioning, usually at an early age.* Most of us learn to brush our teeth at home while very young. We do so because we are praised for doing it, yelled at for not doing it, and because we come to realize that doing it makes our mouths feel good, not because it improves dental health. Habits can be taught at school, but only if the desired behavior can be consistently practiced at school and only if rewards and punishments are consistently given during the period of habit formation. Health educators can possibly strengthen good health habits once the habits are learned by pointing out their benefits and by showing how techniques can be improved.

4. *Accentuate the positive.* The immediate effect of telling someone *not* to do something is usually to make him or her want to do it. Health instruction by parents and teachers has too often set forth a long list of "don'ts" as objectives. The student who tries a forbidden behavior and finds it rewarding is likely to question future guidance from the same source.

5. *Much health-related behavior is practiced for nonhealth reasons.* Most of us cover coughs and sneezes not to protect others but because it is polite to do so. We choose foods not for nutritional value but for taste. Athletes observe training rules not for health reasons but to win. The reason behind this principle is that health is not a primary goal in our culture but a means to other ends. One key to success in health education is to help students discover how health or a particular health practice contributes to their own primary goals or values, whatever they are.

6. *Behavior modification requires a controlled environment.* Teachers and other school workers serve as models and conditioning agents, just as parents do. They and the practices and policies of the school should therefore be consistent with the goals

of health education. Every adult in the school, for example, should not only wash his or her hands before lunch, but encourage students to do so. Time must be made available for this practice. Facilities that are clean, pleasant, well equipped, and convenient must clearly be provided for hand-washing. However, in many schools, necessary environmental changes may be difficult or impossible to achieve.

Alternatives to behavior modification. Behavior modification may seem too closely related to brainwashing to suit the philosophies of some schools, teachers, and parents. If this is the case, several alternative approaches can be substituted for it. For example, health education can be taught as any other academic subject; it need not dictate student behavior but instead encourage students to select their own behavior.

Mike Douse* states that health taught as health philosophy would help students develop powers of analysis and criticism. The subject matter would probably be much the same, but the sexual or smoking behavior of students and teachers would be irrelevant. Behavioral changes might be an outcome, but students and teachers would be free to decide the desirability of any particular behavior for themselves as individuals. Value clarification strategies through which students examine, clarify, state, and commit themselves to their unique value systems provide another alternative to behavior modification.

Needs and interests. One difficulty shared by health education with other school subjects is its tendency to bore students. Part of the solution to this problem is to focus instruction on topics in which students express interest. Lussier† found that student interests vary from time to time, and it is reasonable to assume that they may also vary from age to age and place to place.

They should therefore be determined locally and periodically.

Student interests and perceptions of student needs by parents, counselors, and nurses have been shown to be in high agreement.* There is thus no need to teach content that bores students, and there is no need to teach it in a boring and pedantic way.

ECOLOGY OF SCHOOL HEALTH AND HEALTH EDUCATION

The traditional view of school health is that it encompasses three aspects:

1. *Health education,* which seeks to provide and utilize all possible learning experiences contributory to the development of desirable health behavior, attitudes or values, and knowledge.
2. *Health services,* which attempt to appraise health, prevent health defects from occurring, discover health defects and act to obtain definitive diagnosis and treatment as indicated, provide emergency care for injury and sudden illness, and provide health counseling.
3. *Healthful school living,* which aims to provide a safe and healthful physical and social environment.

Within the school all of these aspects are interrelated; they affect and are affected by each other. As has been stated, health education is dependent on the environment for behavior modification. It can improve the environment by influencing the ways students treat the school plant and the ways in which they interact within it. Students can be taught the purposes of school health service procedures, and health service workers provide health education when they do health counseling.

No one of the three aspects is the exclusive domain of any school staff member. Teachers, while mainly responsible for

---

*Douse, M.: Health hints or health philosophy? J. School Health **43:**195-197, March 1973.
†Lussier, R. R.: Health education and student needs, J. Sch. Health **42:**618-620, Dec. 1972.

*Randall, L. C.: An analysis of the health interests and needs of West Virginia high school students —a report, J. Sch. Health **42:**477-480, Oct. 1972.

health education, can be aided or frustrated by those mainly responsible for services or healthful living.

School health is not independent of the larger environment either. The health services offered in schools affect and are affected by the health services available in the community. The presence or absence of ambulance and hospital emergency room service in the community dictates the nature and scope of school emergency care procedures, for example. The purity of the school's water supply depends on the adequacy of the muncipal treatment plant as well as the school's plumbing. The extent and effectiveness of sex education in the school is determined in large part by the prevailing social philosophy of the community.

The only viable view of school health and health education is thus holistic. We utilize the three traditional aspects only as a convenient way of examining things.

QUESTIONS FOR STUDY AND DISCUSSION

1. What reasons for having schools are cited in the text? What other reasons can you give?
2. In your own value system do you consider health to be your primary goal in life or only a means by which you can attain other, more important goals? Explain and defend your answer.
3. Why can school health and health education be considered both part of the general education and supportive of it?
4. Why are schools increasingly becoming second homes?
5. Can and should schools legally provide medical diagnosis and treatment for pupils? What general types of medical services can and do schools legally provide?
6. What reasonable defenses might a parent offer to a legal charge of failing to obtain medical treatment when the child required such service?
7. Is equality in income, social, and health status for all Americans a reasonable goal, and why?
8. What are some of the family, school, and community variables that affect human health and health behavior? To what extent can school health educators modify the health behavior of their students?
9. Which of the specific suggestions of the American Council for Education and the National Education Association for health

education can be best achieved through habit formation? Which can be best achieved through conscious decision making? Does habit formation or conscious decision making seem most relevant to the attainment of the goals listed?
10. Do you favor behavior modification, Douse's suggestion that health be taught as health philosophy, or a combination of those two viewpoints as your guiding philosophy of health education, and why?
11. Do student's needs and interests in health education differ significantly? Are needs and interests likely to change? Why are needs and interests important?
12. What are the aims of health education, health services, and healthful school living? Why and how are they considered to be interrelated rather than separate aspects of the school health program?

REFERENCES

Anderson, C. L.: *School health practice,* ed. 5, St. Louis, 1972, The C. V. Mosby Co.

Citizens Board of Inquiry into Health Services for Americans: *Heal yourself,* ed. 2, Washington, D.C., 1972, American Public Health Association.

Grout, R. E.: *Health teaching in schools,* ed. 5, Philadelphia, 1968, W. B. Saunders Co.

Joint Committee on Health Problems in Education of the National Education Association and the American Medical Association: *School health services,* ed. 2, Washington, D.C. and Chicago, 1964, NEA and AMA.

Joint Committee on Health Problems in Education of the National Education Association and the American Medical Association: *Healthful school environment,* Washington, D.C. and Chicago, 1969, NEA and AMA.

Mayshark, C., and Shaw, D. D.: *Administration of school health programs,* St. Louis, 1967, The C. V. Mosby Co.

Meadows, D. H. and others: *The limits to growth: a report for the Club of Rome's project on the predicament of mankind,* Washington, D.C., 1972, Potomac Associates.

Means, R. K.: *A history of health education in the United States,* Philadelphia, 1962, Lea & Febiger.

Miller, D. F.: *School health programs: their basis in law,* Cranbury, N. J., 1972, A. S. Barnes & Co., Inc.

National Education Association, project on the Instructional Program of the Public Schools: *Schools for the sixties, a report,* New York, 1963, McGraw-Hill, Inc.

National Education Association, Project on the Instructional Program of the Public Schools: *Deciding what to teach, education in a changing society, planning and organizing for teaching,* Washington, D.C., 1964, The Association.

Nemir, A.: *The school health program,* ed. 3, Philadelphia, 1970, W. B. Saunders Co.

CHAPTER 2 ❧ Emergence, development, and future of school health and health education

Health problems exist in every society and vary in nature and severity with time and circumstances. What a society does about its health needs depends on its goals (physical affluence or spiritual development, for example), its social philosophy (humanitarian or repressive), the development of its health knowledge and technology, and its economic and human resources.*

The primary goal in the United States has been economic growth, which has often been inconsistent with the humanitarian and spiritual goals of many people, but which has stimulated the growth of sciences and technologies, including those related to health. Health science and technology have been applied to make possible the existence of large cities and schools in furtherance of the economic goal through the media of public health, school health and health education, and nonpublic health care services. These agencies have largely succeeded in controlling the communicable diseases, but the success of their efforts together with the achievement of affluence has created new health problems.

HUMAN FIGHT FOR LIFE AND HEALTH

To primitive peoples life was a constant struggle for survival. They were inadequately fed, clothed, and sheltered. Their only protection against disease was their isolation from other humans, whatever placebo effect their charms and sacrifices

may have had, and such serendipitous discoveries as the fact that chewing cinchona bark (a source of quinine) helped protect them against malaria. As a result of environmental and health care deficiencies, more than half of their children died before reaching adolescence; but they lived in harmony with this environment because nature, not they, controlled it.

As humans gained supremacy over their physical environment and the other living things within it, their risk of premature death declined to some extent. Until comparatively recent times, however, population growth was controlled by famine and disease. For example, plague swept over Europe in the fourteenth century killing a fourth of the population. Famines depleted the populations of India and China in the nineteenth century.

From the mid 1800's to the mid 1900's human progress toward better health and longer life was spectacular, as shown in Fig. 2-1. Note especially the large proportions of the population that died at school age or preschool age during these two different periods. Note also that in 1850 only 17% of the population reached the age of 50 years, whereas a little over a century later over 85% reached that age.

Of the many factors that led to the dramatic increase in age at death since 1850, the most important has been the reduction in infant and child deaths from communicable diseases. It has been estimated that humanity has lived on earth for more than a million years, and yet the near conquest of microscopic parasites (we still have no effective vaccine or treatment for the common

---

*Goerke, L. S., and Stebbins, E. L.: *Mustard's introduction to public health,* ed. 5, New York, 1968, Macmillan, Inc., p. 2.

10

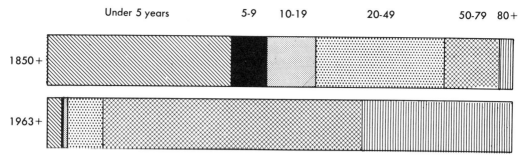

Fig. 2-1. Expectations of life in the United States, 1850 and 1963. In 1850 over half of all deaths occurred in those under 20 years of age. In 1963, about seven eighths of all deaths occurred in people past 50. (Basic data from U. S. Bureau of the Census.)

cold, chicken pox, or many other viral diseases) has taken place only in little more than the last 100 years.

To be sure, certain curative drugs were used in ancient Egypt. The Nigerians, the Turks, and the Chinese successfully used a vaccine prepared from dried smallpox sores to innoculate people against the disease long before Jenner developed his much safer vaccine from cowpox in 1796. The ancient Hebrews developed sound practices of isolating those ill with communicable disease and practiced sanitation in respect to food preparation and human waste disposal. The construction of a safe, sanitary water supply and sewage disposal system made ancient Rome a habitable city. The quarantine of ships from other ports was practiced in Venice and other city states during the fourteenth century. However, these practices were developed and used without scientific knowledge of why they worked and were thus much less effective than the more sophisticated procedures used today. As late as 1793 Benjamin Rush assigned coffee rotting on a wharf as the cause of a Philadelphia yellow fever epidemic.

In the 1860's Pasteur's work with microscopic organisms opened the way for the development of modern communicable disease control techniques, including sanitation and immunization. By 1900 the cause and effective prevention of a number of bacterial and protozoan diseases were known and began to be applied on a wide scale. The rapid development of food and water sani-

tation, sanitary techniques for sewage disposal, and immunology after 1890 made it possible to control such diseases as diphtheria and typhoid.

During the 1890's European scientists demonstrated the existence of viruses, which could not be seen through the light microscopes then in use. In spite of the inability of scientists to see or culture viruses (they replicate only in living cells), effective vaccines had been prepared against smallpox and rabies. However, Reed's elucidation of the viral cause of mosquito-borne yellow fever and its control in 1901 were facilitated by the work of these earlier scientists. The development of DDT and other new insecticides in the 1940's facilitated the control of malaria, another mosquito-borne disease, and of lice and louse-borne diseases, but it also endangered the environment. The development of the electron microscope and techniques of tissue culture in the 1930's and 1940's led to the conquest of poliomyelitis and several other viral diseases via vaccines.

In the 1930's the development of the sulfa drugs permitted effective treatment of streptococcal and certain other infections for the first time. Antibiotics such as penicillin, which permitted the effective treatment of meningococcic meningitis, gonorrhea, syphilis, and other diseases, began to appear in the 1940's.

We can see what has happened to death rates in this country by examining data from Boston that extend back over a longer period than data for the whole United States.

Table 2-1 illustrates the reduction of crude death rates from communicable diseases that affected mainly children and young adults and the consequent increase in deaths from cancer and heart disease that occur largely at older age levels. However, these data do not take into account the change in the age makeup of Boston's population from younger to older and thus exaggerate the increase in cancer and heart disease mortality.

With the effects of changing age composition statistically controlled, Fig. 2-2 shows three stages in the history of death in the whole United States since 1900. First, there was the gradual downward trend from 1900 to 1937 as the then known techniques of immunization and sanitation were applied. This stage was broken in 1918 by the great influenza pandemic; no effective means for preventing influenza were then available. Second, a more dramatic decline occurred between 1938 and 1954 as effective chemotherapeutic and antibiotic treatment agents were developed and applied. Finally, a relative plateau was reached in the 1950's. This represents an apparent end of progress in control of death by way of communicable disease control.

Although the control of communicable diseases, especially those of childhood, represented the most striking development, there were many others of great importance. The development of open heart surgery not only saved the lives of many young victims of congenital and rheumatic heart disease but improved the quality of their lives as

Table 2-1. Changes in Boston death rates in a century

	1865	1905	1965
Deaths per 1,000 population	23.6	18.4	13.3
Births per 1,000 population	—	26.8	18.8
Infant deaths per 1,000 live births	—	136.5	24.1
Maternal deaths per 1,000 live births	—	6.7	0.2
Pulmonary tuberculosis death rates*	422.7	204.7	9.9
Diphtheria death rate*	69.7	22.1	0.0
Typhoid fever death rate*	65.0	19.6	0.0
Scarlet fever death rate*	26.0	7.4	0.0
Measles death rate*	7.8	9.0	0.0
Smallpox death rate*	59.8	0.2	0.0
Pneumonia death rate*	162.3	213.1	56.7
Cancer death rate*	29.6	105.0	231.0
Heart disease death rate*	65.0	181.0	573.6

*Per 100,000 population.

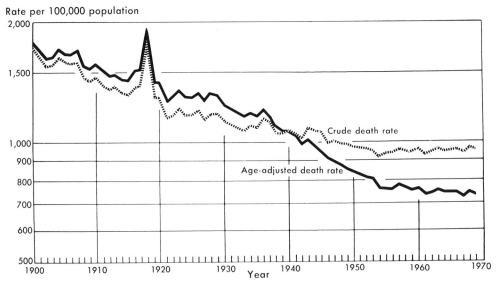

Fig. 2-2. Crude and age-adjusted death rates: death registration for states, 1900-1932, and United States, 1933-1969. (Data from National Center for Health Statistics.)

well. Anticonvulsive drugs have enabled many victims of epilepsy to lead essentially normal lives. Insulin has permitted juvenile diabetics to survive childhood and reproduce (thus increasing the prevalence of this disorder). Current research results give hope that an effective treatment for the acute leukemia of childhood may be on the horizon.

Researchers in physical growth and development have observed that children increase in height and weight and that girls experience menarche at earlier ages with each succeeding generation in civilized countries. Krogman* attributes these trends primarily to improved health and nutrition and socioeconomic conditions, rather than to genetic or evolutionary factors.

BIRTH, GROWTH, AND DEVELOPMENT OF SCHOOL HEALTH AND HEALTH EDUCATION

The Constitution of the United States makes no specific mention of either public education or public health. Both public health and education thus developed in this country as functions of the individual states, because the Tenth Amendment reserves to the states all powers that are not specifically reserved to the federal government. Several broad powers of the federal government, such as the general welfare provision, are construed to justify national activities in health and education, however.

Community health activities and schools can be traced back to colonial times in America and to the Old World before then. The beginning of modern public health, public schools, and school health and health education in the United States, however, can be said to have originated in the work of Horace Mann and Lemuel Shattuck in Massachusetts in the years between 1830 and 1850.

Mann was a social reformer concerned with temperance, the abolition of slavery, and the curbing of the excesses of unbridled

capitalism. As a state legislator he promoted the free public school as a means of solution to these and other social problems. As secretary of the Massachusetts Board of Education from 1837 to 1848 he popularized and developed common school education and teacher education. His own ill health, together with his interest in temperance and his acceptance of the pseudoscience of phrenology, led him to promote health education, or hygiene as it was then called, as a school subject.*

Shattuck was an elementary schoolteacher, book dealer, statistician, and, like Mann, a Massachusetts state legislator. He was appointed to a legislative committee to study the public health problems of the Commonwealth, because he had already compiled vital statistics of the city of Boston. His famous *Report of the Sanitary Commission of Massachusetts* provided about fifty recommendations, most of which are accepted public health practices today.† These included health education in the schools and health surveys by committees of pupils under the direction of their teachers.‡ In the 1850's when tax-supported schools were new, schoolhouses were primitive by modern standards and remained so for many years. Plumbing was usually limited to a hand pump and earth-pit privies. Lighting was inadequate. Windows and woodburning stoves provided ventilation and heat, and teachers doubled as janitors. The curriculum was usually limited to reading, writing, arithmetic, geography, and history. Learning and good behavior were largely motivated by corporal punishment, despite the protests of Horace Mann and other humanitarian educators. A very small proportion went to high school, and the high schools were mainly devoted to pre-

---

*Krogman, W. M.: *Child growth*, Ann Arbor, 1972, The University of Michigan Press, pp. 36-42.

---

*Curti, M.: *The social ideas of American educators*, Patterson, N.J., 1961, Littlefield, Adams & Co., pp. 101-138.
†Goerke, L. S.: *Mustard's introduction to public health*, pp. 27-28.
‡Shattuck, L.: *Report of the Sanitary Commission of Massachusetts* (Boston, 1850, facsimile edition), Cambridge, 1950, Harvard University Press.

paring students for college. Even elementary education was far from universal, especially in the South.

Still, under the influence of Mann and others who were influenced in turn by the more precocious development of education in Europe, public education made remarkable progress until the Civil War. This event impeded the development of education in the South but also introduced an era of economic and industrial development and urbanization that later led to the rapid expansions of both educational opportunity and the curriculum. World Wars I and II gave further impetus to the development of the economy and the schools. The depression of the 1930's stimulated school and college attendance (there was little else for young people to do), as did the earlier abolition of child labor and slavery. However, what goes on in schools is influenced by changing ideas of the importance and content of learning. At various times intellectual and moral discipline, vocational training, and individual development have been thought to be of greatest importance. In the 1950's and early 1960's there was a resurgence of emphasis on mental discipline and scientific training related to our "cold war" competition with Russia in putting satellites into orbit, for example, with a concomitant deemphasis on health education.

Public health developed more slowly than education. Only since 1885 has each state enacted legislation creating a state board of health or its equivalent. Early state and local health departments were primarily concerned with the control of communicable diseases through sanitation, immunization, isolation, and quarantine. Maternal and child health activities were first stimulated by the establishment of the U.S. Children's Bureau in 1912. In 1921 federal funds for maternal and child health work by local and state health departments were first provided by the Bureau through the Shepard-Towner Act, which lapsed in 1929. The depression again stimulated appropriations of funds for this purpose, this time through the passage of the Social Security Act of 1935.

After World War II a national movement led by Haven Emerson sought to promote local health departments throughout the nation and was partially successful in achieving its goal. As envisioned by Emerson, public health would focus on the promotion of health and disease prevention. It would avoid involvement in medical care, a role left to private medical practice and charitable clinics.

Congressional enactment of the Medicare and Medicaid provisions of the Social Security Act in 1965 introduced medical care as an accepted welfare–public health function of government.

State and local public health services in the United States today typically include personal health services of both preventive and treatment nature, as well as environmental health services. Laboratory, health education, nursing, and other services are provided to support personal and environmental health services. But the extent of services varies, and some counties still have no public health services. Furthermore, important aspects of public health are shared with other agencies at all levels of government. The Environmental Protection Agency created in 1970 at the federal level and the roles of the federal and state agriculture departments in food sanitation serve as examples.*

During the 1960's a host of new federal programs were undertaken to equalize opportunity for better education and improved health. These included civil rights legislation, provisions of the Economic Opportunities Act such as Operation Head Start, federal aid to expand educational opportunities for disadvantaged children, and the establishment of community mental health centers. These and other programs were based on the philosophy that federal funding should be used to solve specific and compelling national problems through programs primarily controlled at the national level. A trend

---

*Wilner, D. M., Walkley, R. P., and Goerke, L. S.: *Introduction to public health,* ed. 6, New York, 1973, Macmillan, Inc.

toward curtailment of such categorical programs and a general reduction of federal spending for health and education appeared in 1972. This trend represented a change in philosophy to one that holds that the superior taxing powers of the federal government should be utilized to supplement local funds for purposes locally determined. At its inception the effect of the new policy appeared to be that less federal money with fewer strings attached would be available.

School health education. Largely through Mann's influence, school courses in physiology and hygiene were introduced prior to 1880. Between 1880 and 1890, as a result of lobbying activities by the temperance movement, every state in the union passed laws requiring instruction concerning the effects of alcohol and narcotics. Some 40 states required broader health instruction as well.

Physical education, with which health education was closely associated during much of its history, had been introduced in Massachusetts as early as 1825. The German-American gymnastic societies known as Turnvereine (groups devoted to political, social, and religious reform as well as physical activity) greatly stimulated the development of physical education. The professionalization of physical education began with the formation of the American Physical Education Association in 1885. This group joined the National Education Association in 1937 and grew into the present American Alliance for Health, Physical Education, and Recreation. A movement toward separation of physical education from health education during the 1960's resulted in the separation of structures and journals within the Alliance.

From the turn of the century health authorities began to realize the need to inform the public concerning its role in the promotion of health. Mass media and community organization techniques were developed and used and are still used today. Today public health education also attempts to achieve its goals by influencing the decisions and actions of political and social groups through

direct work with their leaders. School and public health educators now work together for professional improvement through the School Health and Public Health Education Sections of the American Public Health Association.

In 1914 the Health Department of New York City became the first official organization to establish a bureau of health education. In 1915 a voluntary agency, the National Tuberculosis Association as it was then called, introduced the "Modern Health Crusade" as a device for promoting the health of school children. It was based upon an extrinsic reward ("knighthood") for following specified health habits. The development of school and public health education is thus interrelated.

World Wars I and II facilitated the development of health education. Draft rejection statistics were used to argue the cause with some success, despite the fact that medical examinations vary in quality and standards for rejection also vary during any given war with the need for draftees. The same questionable data were used to promote health services and physical education.

Health education practice was influenced during the 1920's and through the 1940's by a number of research and demonstration projects. The Malden, Massachusetts project conducted by Turner beginning in 1921 with the cooperation of the Department of Biology and Public Health of the Massachusetts Institute of Technology has been mentioned. Others were sponsored in various parts of the country by such organizations and foundations as the American Red Cross, the Commonwealth Fund, the Milbank Memorial Fund, and the Kellogg Foundation. One of the assumptions of such sponsors was that the demonstration projects they supported would be continued with tax funds, if successful. This was not generally the case, but the projects did in fact stimulate local and state health curriculum development.

The Joint Committee on Health Problems in Education of the National Education Association and the American Medical

Association issued its first report, *Health Education,* in 1924. This and later reports of the Committee provided at any point in time the best current thinking of the several disciplines involved in school health and health education as to what objectives and practices in the field should be. These reports have perhaps been as influential as any other force in upgrading and standardizing goals for health education practice across the United States.

During the 1960's two attempts to develop national curriculum projects in health education were undertaken. The Health Education Division (now the Association for the Advancement of Health Education) of the American Association (now Alliance) for Health, Physical Education, and Recreation identified crucial health problems and their significance, formulated broad concepts or generalizations related to each problem area, and prepared supporting material for school use. The School Health Study, sponsored first by the Samuel Bronfman Foundation and later by the 3M Company, included studies of the status of health education in U.S. schools and of reported research in the field. The study culminated with curriculum experimentation and full-scale curriculum development also based on a conceptual approach. The stated purpose of both studies was to provide a beginning point for further curriculum development at the local and state levels rather than a single curriculum for nationwide use.*

During the 1950's and 1960's school community health education received increased international attention. In 1949 the World Health Organization (WHO) established a section on Health Education of the Public. In 1951 the International Union for Health Education, a nongovernment organization, was established to promote both public and school health education. Health education activities have also been conducted by the United Nations Educational, Scientific and Cultural Organization (UNESCO), the Food and Agricultural Organization (FAO), and the United Nations Children's Fund (UNICEF). The Agency for International Development (AID) of the United States promoted health education in its program of health assistance to developing countries. Current political developments in the United States, however, indicate a possibility that this country may be entering a period of relative isolationism and withdrawal from such activities.

In 1968 a meeting of the Joint Committee of the National School Boards Association and the American Association of School Administrators unanimously recommended "a comprehensive program of health education in grades K through 12."

Gradually there has developed a degree of acceptance of health education as an important school subject. Throughout its history there have been efforts to define and redefine its philosophy, to state and restate objectives in line with current problems, and to improve and update content and methods of instruction. Why then is health not as widely taught as English, science, or other school subjects?

Warren Johnson* has suggested that health education is not generally accepted as an academic discipline and will not be until it divests itself of the magic-morals aura that still clings to it from times past. Another reason may be that health education is not viewed as a discrete discipline such as mathematics, but as one that borrows its body of knowledge and methods of investigation from other fields.

Health services. Although health inspections of schools and children by a physician were required by statute in Paris as early as 1842-1843, this activity had only been suggested in the United States at that time. William Alcott, a teacher and physician, urged the appointment of school physicians in his book *Health in Common Schools,* which was published in Boston in

---

*Johns, E. B.: Two national projects in health education, Bulletin of the National Association of Secondary School Principals **52**(326):70-80, March 1968.

*Johnson, W. R.: Magic, morals, and health, School Health Review **1**:5-9, Nov. 1969.

1840. Shattuck repeated the suggestion 10 years later. The first public school physician in the United States was appointed a half-century later by New York City in 1892. Other large cities followed the New York example. By 1900 inspection and exclusion of pupils and supervision of sanitary conditions for the purpose of controlling communicable diseases were common practice.*

It is not surprising that pupils once excluded because they had a communicable disease or lacked a smallpox vaccination scar did not return to school. Schools in those days were not usually pleasant places. In addition, many parents were poor, uneducated with respect to health, and unfamiliar with the English language. In an attempt to counsel and encourage parents to secure needed health care for excluded children and return them to school, Lillian Wald loaned the services of one of the Henry Street Settlement visiting nurses to the New York schools. The attempt succeeded, and school nursing was established as such in 1902.† Its first purpose, that of counseling and assisting parents in obtaining needed health care for children, remains today as perhaps its most important and useful function.

As other health problems of children were recognized and knowledge of child health, growth, and development increased, other school health service functions were added. Examination of pupils for visual defects was required by the state of Connecticut in 1902, and routine medical examinations of all children began to be required by some states at that time. Such examinations, as conducted in most schools, were hurried, assembly-line affairs of little value.‡

In 1903 the first school dentist was appointed in Reading, Pennsylvania. Dental examinations and school treatment clinics were established in other cities within a few years. In 1913 Alfred C. Fones opened the first school for dental hygienists in Bridgeport, Connecticut. From the start hygienists were trained specifically for school health service.* It was not until the 1940's that it became generally recognized that school dental treatment programs were unable to meet the needs with the limited resources of manpower and money available and that school dental health work should therefore concentrate its efforts on primary prevention rather than treatment.

The American Association of School Physicians was founded in 1927 to improve school health service work. In 1934 the organization opened membership to other school health professionals, including educators as well as health service workers, and changed its name to the American School Health Association. This professional organization, like the Joint Committee on Health Problems in Education, the American Association for Health, Physical Education, and Recreation, and the School Health Section of the American Public Health Association, has done much to stimulate and standardize school health service practice.

Recognition of the need of children for medical attention *before* school entrance led National Congress of Parents and Teachers to initiate its "Summer Round-Up" program in 1925.† These programs were perhaps the first to utilize lay volunteers in school health service work. They were successful in stimulating preschool health examinations, immunizations, and correction of health defects. In more recent years the PTA has advocated a program of health supervision beginning before school entrance and continuing throughout school life.

William Alcott in 1840 had proposed

*Wilson, C. C., editor: *School health services,* ed. 2, Washington, D.C. and Chicago, 1964, National Education Association and American Medical Association, pp. 361-364.
†Wilson, C. C., editor: *School health services,* p. 364.
‡Means, R. K.: *A history of health education in the United States,* Philadelphia, 1962, Lea & Febiger, pp. 59-60.

*Wilson, C. C., editor: *School health services,* p. 365.
†Wilson, C. C., editor: *School health services,* p. 380.

that teachers inspect children for possible health problems and refer them to the school physician for attention. It was not until about 1940 that this idea, which was expanded to include specific training of teachers for observation and further evaluation of children jointly in teacher-nurse conference prior to referral, was tested in a demonstration project in the Astoria section of New York City. The idea was proven useful (eight out of ten children thus referred had real medical problems)* and found its way into national practice.

School health services have thus grown and changed to meet perceived needs as philosophy and social viewpoints have changed, and as knowledge has changed. It owes much of its past development to farsighted individuals and organizations. Further change is to be expected as a result of the same kinds of influences.

Healthful school living. In 1829 William Alcott wrote his *Essay on the Construction of Schoolhouses,*† and about that same time Bronson Alcott tried to train children for citizenship by encouraging them to practice the art of self-government in the school.‡ Between them the Alcotts thus recognized the importance of both the physical and social environment of the school and promoted its improvement.

Physical sanitary inspection of school buildings was a recognized responsibility of the early school physicians (or medical inspectors) in the 1890's and early 1900's, because the relation between environment and communicable disease outbreaks was recognized.

Before the discovery of tests to detect tuberculosis and before effective methods of treatment, this disease was a major killer of children and young people. Fresh air, proper diet, and rest were the only recognized means of prevention and treatment.

In 1908 an open-air school was established in Providence, Rhode Island, and other cities took up the idea. Thus began our modern concern with ventilation, temperature, and humidity control. Today, of course, our concern lies in keeping air pollutants out of school buildings and in air cleansing rather than opening windows.

The first publication of the Joint Committee on Health Problems in Education, in 1914, dealt with the subject of physical sanitation in rural schools.* Later publications have covered social as well as physical aspects of the environment.† School environmental health concerns that have arisen more recently include accident prevention, provisions for handicapped children, the organization and conduct of the school as it relates to social and emotional health, and the physical and social aspects of school-feeding programs.

Formal school lunch programs began in New York City in 1910 as a result of earlier demonstrations of their worth. The great depression of the 1930's gave national impetus to school feeding when federal legislation was passed providing for the support of school lunch programs through the U.S. Department of Agriculture. The basic purposes of this initial legislation were to dispose of agricultural surplus and provide work for the unemployed, rather than to improve nutrition. Later, improvement of nutritional intake and social education were added as legitimate goals. As this is written, a worldwide food shortage is apparent, and the latter two goals seem likely to replace entirely the initial ones. Many schools have added breakfast programs since World War II to the benefit of children of working mothers or the poor.

Throughout the history of American education some schools have provided pleasant social environments in which teachers, chil-

---

*Nyswander D. B.: *Solving school health problems,* New York, 1942, Commonwealth Fund.
†Means, R. K.: *A history of health education in the United States,* p. 31.
‡Curti, M.: *The social ideas of American educators,* p. 60.

*Wilson, C. C., editor: *School health services,* pp. 370-371.
†Wilson, C. C., and Wilson, E. A., editors: *Healthful school environment,* Washington, D.C. and Chicago, 1969, National Education Association and American Medical Association.

dren, and young people can and do work and learn. These schools seem to represent in practice John Dewey's progressive education movement, which emphasized the development of responsiveness and sharing in common and pleasurable tasks, the idea of the school as a social center, and treating energy and originality as positive virtues, among other things. Less pleasant schools, at least to this observer, seem to be based in one of two major countermovements. The first of these grew out of the post–World War II cold war with Russia. It emphasized scientific and technical training and the other basic intellectual disciplines. The other was a movement based on behavioristic psychology, which emphasized social conformity and the adjustment of the individual to the environment, and it developed during the decades following World War I.* It may be that the behaviorist philosophy holds the key to human survival, as argued by B. F. Skinner in *Beyond Freedom and Dignity*, but it may also be the case that survival is not worth the price.

TODAY'S HEALTH PROBLEMS

We have seen the tremendous progress in health and education that has taken place. However, many old problems persist, and new ones appear. Let us look at some of the more important health problems that demand attention in shaping today's program of school health and health education. Some of the problems discussed below will be considered in greater detail in later chapters.

Too many people. Our success in controlling death through the application of health science resulted in a tripling of world population from about 1 billion in 1800 to over 3 billion today. Projections indicate that before the end of this century world population will outrun food supply to the extent that present areas of inadequate nutrition will be so expanded as to threaten

both world health and world peace. People consume not only food but fuel and other finite natural resources as well, and as they consume, they produce pollutants that pose added threats to life and health.*

The fact of food shortages became clearly apparent in America in 1973 in terms of high cost and inconvenience. However, the Food and Agricultural Organization of the United Nations estimates that 20% of the inhabitants of the developing areas of the world now have insufficient calories and that 60% have insufficient protein, a deficiency that impedes both physical and mental development in newly weaned children. Although some increase in total world food production is now taking place, the supply of arable land and the potential growth of our capabilities in agricultural and food processing technology are limited. There is little likelihood that present dietary standards can be maintained unless there is a sharp decline in the world birth rate.

The increased responsibility of the school to provide birth control education and perhaps even access to birth control services seems obvious, but such activities run counter to the values of important segments of our society.

Birth defects. Birth defects are caused by both heredity and environmental factors. Some genetic defects are preventable by means of counseling that is based on examinations of family histories and use of screening tests, which may suggest to a couple that adoption rather than mating is more likely to provide them with healthy offspring. Environmentally caused birth defects may be partially prevented by avoiding known causes. For example, defects caused by occurrence of German measles in mothers can be prevented by childhood immunization.

School health services can provide, perhaps on a group basis, screening tests (such as that for sickle cell anemia) and genetic

---

*Curti, M.: *The social ideas of American educators,* pp. XXV-XLIV, 499-541.

*Meadows, D. H., and associates: *The limits to growth,* New York, 1972, The New American Library Inc.

counseling. The school environment should exclude or control known teratogenic agents, such as the ionizing radiation that may be produced in science laboratories. Health education can profitably include instruction in the means by which future parents can protect and promote the health of their unborn offspring.

Pollution. All large cities are finding it increasingly difficult to secure enough pure water, to control air pollution (caused mainly by automobiles), and to dispose of organic and industrial wastes without producing nuisances and dangers to health. These difficulties increase as both population and economic growth increase. The pesticides and some of the additives that help increase food supply and preserve food for distribution also have negative effects on the environment and human health.

Does school health education help students develop values that permit them to choose responsibly between walking and riding, driving and public transportation, luxury automobiles and small ones that pollute less? Does the school waste paper or conserve and recycle it? Would sweaters worn by teachers and students on cold days enable the school to turn down its thermostats a little?

Affluence, disease, and survival. The leading causes of death in the United States are heart and circulatory diseases (including strokes) and cancer. These are diseases that primarily kill older people, but some of them (such as leukemia and congenital heart diseases) still kill in childhood, youth, and young adulthood. These and others are among the diseases of affluence. Asbestos and radioactive materials used in modern industry, as well as cigarettes and other pollutants, cause cancer. Lack of physical activity and the dietary patterns of the affluent produce certain diseases of the heart and blood vessels.

Perhaps children and young people can consider the advantages and disadvantages of individual and social behaviors that will tend to postpone these diseases and the fatalities that result from them until old age. Perhaps also we can revise the values of our culture and the state of individual mental health to accept a more modest living standard and death in later life as the inevitable and welcome final stage of human development.

Personal health services. Modern scientific medicine has a previously undreamed-of capacity for the prevention of disease, its cure when it does occur, and the rehabilitation of its victims when it is not cured. Yet the complexity of its specialties, its tendency to hold the diagnosis rather than the individual in view, its concentration in urban medical centers, and its high cost raise barriers between it and those it could serve.

Part of the solution to the problem lies in reform of the structure of personal health services and of the means by which they are financed. A second part of the solution is to teach people how to choose and use health products and services to their best advantage.

Through its health services the school utilizes preventive procedures (such as immunizations) and detects departures from normal health in vision, hearing, nutrition, and many other areas. It moves those with problems toward appropriate personal health services that may be available to them and that include habilitative special education programs within the school. School health services are educational by example, as when children are given prophylaxis by dental hygienists. Counseling by the school nurse and education by the teacher help children and youth to prevent health problems, select and utilize health services, and adjust to residual difficulties. Recent developments and proposals relative to the restructuring of health services and their financing are important topics in consumer health education.

Mental health and mental retardation. While the proportion of the U.S. population believed to be in need of care for emotional disturbances or mental illness varies with definitions of mental health and mental illness, sample surveys indicate that about one in ten of us needs care at any given time, and almost all of us may need help at some time or other. By IQ definition about 3% of the U.S. population is classified as mentally retarded. Many cases of emotional and social illnesses are believed to result from the inability to cope with life's stresses. Such cases might be prevented by direct instruction of children and young people in techniques of coping with anger, disappointment, sexual tension, and other sources of stress. Some cases of mental retardation may be prevented by environmental actions such as community programs to remove and control the use of lead base paint in locations where infants and children might ingest it.

Community mental health centers exist in some areas of the United States. These centers were designed to replace large state hospitals with treatment and rehabilitation services centered in the patients' own communities. Some of the centers are well staffed and supported and offer a full range of services to the mentally ill, the retarded, and narcotic and alcohol addicts. Insufficient funding by the federal and state governments, lack of trained professionals, and bureaucratic practices have prevented the full development of other centers.

By observing behavior in light of their training in psychology and child development, teachers are better able to detect mental health problems in children and young people than most parents. They often help students cope with minor crises, but either the school or the community must provide some sort of treatment service. Some

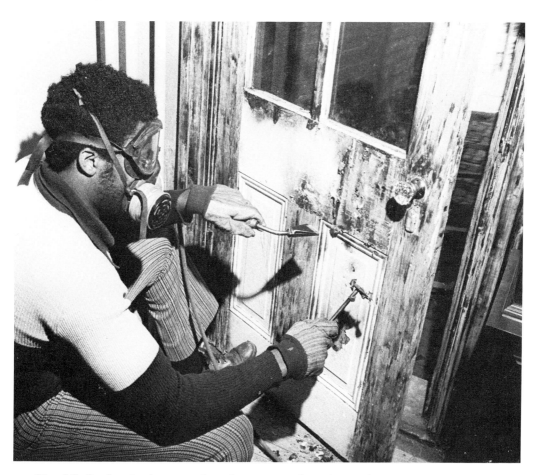

Fig. 2-3. Lead poisoning control worker removes hazardous paint from a home interior. (Courtesy Philadelphia Department of Health.)

schools and school systems provide special education services that help many mentally ill and mentally retarded children and young people become socially self-sufficient. Even when a full range of services is available, however, present treatment and rehabilitation modalities are not altogether successful. Research in mental health and mental retardation is a pressing need.

Psychoactive drugs. Use, misuse and abuse, and dependence on psychoactive drugs including caffeine, alcohol, tobacco, other stimulants and depressants, and hallucinogens by children and young people as well as adults stem from and contribute to emotional and social problems.

Moralistic tirades against use of psychoactive drugs, propaganda techniques, and legal prohibitions have failed to control the problem in the past and are unlikely to control it in the future. One approach that seems likely to be more effective is the provision and evaluation of experiences that offer the desirable effects of drugs without their use, such as religious or meditative experiences, listening to music, and interactions with others. Another approach is consideration by each individual of the consistency or inconsistency of the use of various specific drugs with his or her own life goals, whatever they may be, based on honest information about consequences, good as well as bad. Drug education, however, is not the only role of the school. Each teacher and school must face the issue of what to do when a case of drug use is discovered.

Sex, youth, and school-age mothers. Sex is something we are as well as something we do. Sex roles begin to be taught at birth by both modeling and conditioning administered by both adults and peers. What is and what is not appropriate sexual behavior in any society is taught the same way. But we are undergoing a sexual evolution. Role and behavior standards are ill defined, and neither young people nor society has yet adapted well to change.

All this is not new. Older generations have been distressed at sexuality in their offspring. Young people in the past have worried about their sexuality, and as long as girls have gone to school there have been pregnant schoolgirls.

The sexual evolution seems to be ushering in an age when schools and teachers can substitute assistance to young people in defining their own roles and behavior for moral preachments and punishments. We begin to recognize that young people make their own values; they do not accept completely those we try to hand them ready made. We can, however, help them think through and clarify their values, let them express commitment to their values freely, and then live by them. Schools, teachers, and school nurses have always been quick to identify pregnency at an early stage. But instead of excluding the girl from school and turning her over to a not necessarily sympathetic parent and/or social agency, we are now able to continue her schooling, help her realize the many other courses of action she might take, and allow her to make her own informed choices of action.

VD and other reemergent plagues. The intimate personal contact of children and youth both in and out of school facilitates the spread of communicable diseases, especially those that are most difficult to control. Infectious mononucleosis and the common cold, which are major causes of illness and school absence, are not susceptible to available preventive or treatment methods. The occasional neglect of sanitation still permits the spread of intestinal disease. Inadequate school-community immunization programs still result in occasional outbreaks of such preventable personal contact diseases as diphtheria, poliomyelitis, and measles. Gonorrhea is completely out of control in the United States at this time even though it is treatable and partially preventable.

It is obviously a responsibility of the school system, the health department, and other community agencies to protect students against the spread of communicable diseases through well-planned, coordinated, and implemented programs of health education, immunization, early detection and treatment, and sanitation.

Violence. Accidents rank first among the leading causes of death of children and young people from kindergarden through high school. Accidental death rates are highest during the high school years and are much higher for boys than girls. Malignant neoplasms (mainly leukemia) rank second, but the rate is only a fraction of that for accidents. In the 15- to 19-year age group (where accidents account for more than half of all deaths) deaths from suicide and homicide combined exceed those for malignant neoplasms. Despite the fact that a majority of accidental deaths involved automobiles, violent deaths among school-age children in the United States have decreased markedly since 1930.* Still, violent death is too common.

About three out of ten school-age children and youth are nonfatally injured each year to an extent that requires either medical attention or at least 1 day of restricted activity.†

Accident control in schools, of course, involves environmental controls and education. An adequate school-community program of emergency care in some cases prevents aggravation of injury or even death.

Jan Fawcett postulates that the presence of hope is a deterrent to violence and that hopefulness (that one's goals can be achieved) can be attained by such means as improving society in general and by individually setting short-range goals for ourselves that represent attainable stages in reaching our long-range goals.‡ It is reasonable to suppose that this applies to at least some accidents as well as to suicides or homicides. Accidents often occur as a result of conscious or unconscious intent, and in-

vestigators undoubtedly wrongly assign violent death in some instances to one of the three causes—usually accidental which is socially acceptable.

FRAMEWORK AND FUTURE OF SCHOOL HEALTH AND HEALTH EDUCATION

The traditional framework of the school health program was described briefly in Chapter 1. Although crystal-ball gazing is a hazardous occupation, it seems reasonable to believe that healthful school living, health services, and health instruction will continue to be useful concepts in describing and organizing the subject. The point has already been made, however, that none of the three parts can be considered independent of each other or of what goes on in the community. School health and health education follow Barry Commoner's first law of ecology: "Everything is connected to everything else."

School, home, and community relationships are all involved. These have traditionally included contacts of teachers and other school employees with parents, parent observation and participation in school health activities, and relationships with community health education, health services, and social and physical aspects of the community environment. In some places such contacts have tended toward one-way communication as when the school merely informs a parent of a health problem. They clearly should be construed to include intercommunication and joint efforts to recognize and solve problems. Assumptions that schools, homes, or communities exist or behave in accordance with stereotypes are not valid in our rapidly changing society.

School health and health education have traditionally and properly focused primarily on children and young people, but the health and health problems of school employees are important, too. Teacher health affects teacher effectiveness and teaching, and the school environment affects teacher health and teaching.

Healthful school living. Healthful school living depends on (1) *environmental sanitation* to guarantee: safe and efficient water

---

*National Center for Health Statistics: *The change in mortality trend in the United States,* Public Health Service Publication No. 1000, Series 3, No. 1, Washington, D.C., 1964, U.S. Government Printing Office.
†National Center for Health Statistics: *Children and youth, selected characteristics,* Public Health Service Publication No. 1000, Series 10, No. 62, Washington, D.C., 1971, U.S. Government Printing Office.
‡Fawcett, J., editor: *Dynamics of violence,* Chicago, 1972, American Medical Association.

supply, water use, and sewage disposal systems; attractive and sanitary facilities and practices for food service, health service, and other auxiliary activities; sanitary and nonpolluting disposal of solid waste; adequate climate control and lighting systems that conserve energy resources; a safe and attractive school building and site that provide space and facilities for physical activity, recreation, socialization, and learning for school staff and the community as well as for students. It also requires (2) *school schedules, organization, and operating policies and procedures* that are consistent with general home and community standards and with the physical and mental health needs of school staff and students. These considerations will include the length and timing of the school day and provision of a variation of the kind of activity in the schedule, selection, and sequence of subjects, the amount and timing of homework, class size, examination and grading procedures, rules of conduct and discipline, selection of learning materials, provision for conduct of health services and practices, extra-class activities, feeding, and the like. Finally, it includes (3) *the maintainance of a healthful emotional environment* through good teacher-pupil and intergroup relationships, recognition and acceptance of individual differences, and curriculum adaptation. This third category is perhaps the most difficult to achieve, for it depends on the selection and training of administrators and staff, the nature of homes and the community, and physical facilities and school policies, practices, and procedures as well.

Health services. In the school, health services are limited to exclude *definitive* diagnosis and treatment, and this limitation will probably remain more or less constant for reasons presented elsewhere. The purposes of health services for both students and staff include (1) *health appraisal* to determine the health assets and limitations of individuals and to establish a *working* diagnosis. Services also include (2) *health counseling and follow-up* based on the health appraisal and the situation of the family. This

aspect includes guidance to appropriate sources of definitive diagnosis and treatment, liaison between that source and the school, counseling with the individual and/or family, appropriate modification of in-school activities pending and following a report of definitive diagnosis and treatment, and assistance to the individual in obtaining continuing treatment and other needed community services. This aspect also includes counseling with respect to individual concerns of students, staff, and parents, which may reveal either a need for assurance that all is well ("this is normal and healthy at your age") or a more complex problem that requires extensive service. Health services are also involved with (3) *disease prevention and health promotion.* This means recognition and action to obtain correction of the physical and social environmental conditions that threaten health, safety, comfort, or working efficiency. It means the provision of appropriate immunizations directly or indirectly through the use of community resources. It implies the use of health education and health counseling and of other school and community resources to improve nutrition, to control both obesity and the use of hazardous substances, and to foster positive physical and mental health. Perhaps the most obvious aspect of health services is that of (4) *emergency care of injuries and sudden illness.* This involves a planned school-community program of first aid, transportation and definitive care in some cases, and no more than a bandage or a place to rest under observation in other cases. Finally, health services include (5) *the maintenance of students and staff health records,* which provide factual information to assist in the administration of any of the other four functions of school health services.

Health instruction. Health teaching and learning should include not only the formal classroom health education of students, but also education of students through involvement in the planning and conduct of healthful school living and health services and in the planning of the health curriculum as well. Health instruction programs should also be designed and provided for parents and school staff members, either directly by the school or indirectly by use of the resources offered by other community agencies.

Legitimizing innovation. New approaches to school health and health education are required to solve today's health problems. New ways of doing things are often resisted by those involved who are comfortable in the old ways. When new ways run counter to old cultural values, they are resisted by those who cling to old values whether the new ways require action by them or not.

In one Michigan town a few years ago the schools and the health department jointly developed and put into effect a program to help meet the health and educational needs of pregnant schoolgirls. The program was conducted in a nonschool location. The girls continued their regular coursework, were instructed in maternal health and child care, and received medical care and sympathetic counseling aimed at helping them solve the problems presented by their pregnancy. The program was carefully planned by those who would be carrying it out (teachers, counselors, nurses, physicians, and others) with the advice of outside experts. The old cultural way of handling such problems included exclusion from school and usually forced marriage. The new program functioned successfully and to the satisfaction of both the girls and the involved professionals.

When the existence of the program became generally known in the community, there resulted a flood of angry sermons from church pulpits, editorials and letters in the local newspaper, and adverse criticism from citizens who generally felt that the program condoned and encouraged immoral behavior. This viewpoint was so widely held and vociferously stated that it forced discontinuation of the program.

The professionals had been involved in planning the new program, so they accepted and supported the change; but other community leaders had not been involved. Had the newspaper editor, clergymen, and other influential persons been involved from the start—that is, at the point where the existence of the problem was recognized and before planning was even begun—the program might have continued in existence with broadly based community support.

QUESTIONS FOR STUDY AND DISCUSSION

1. Identify an important specific health problem in the United States at present. What is our society doing about the problem? How are our actions with regard to it influenced by our present national goals, social philosophy, health knowledge, and health manpower and spending?
2. What have been the basic changes in health status in the United States since 1850? What have been the causes of these changes?
3. Which level of government in the United States has the greatest direct responsibility for public health and education, and why?
4. What were the main contributions of Shattuck, Mann, and William and Bronson Alcott to school health and health education?
5. How have national events such as wars, the temperance movement, and the depression of the 1930's, as well as scientific developments, influenced public health and health education in the United States?
6. What is the nature and scope of public health services in the United States at present?
7. What major changes have occurred in school health and health education in the United States since 1850, and why?
8. To what specific national organizations might any school health professional (such as teacher, nurse, dental hygienist) belong today? What are the advantages of membership in each of these organizations?
9. What arguments can you offer for and against a behaviorist philosophy of health education?
10. Which of today's health problems may be said to be by-products of progress? Which ones may be better classified as old problems that we have not yet been able to solve?
11. What changes would be helpful in the elementary and high schools you attended in dealing with today's health problems? Can you cite examples of such changes that you have heard or read about?
12. What is the broad scope and nature of (a) healthful school living, (b) health services, and (c) health instruction?
13. Why and how is everything in the school health program "connected to everything else?" Why and how are school health and health education related to home and community and to teacher health?
14. What sources of opposition to innovative programs exist? What technique for legitimizing new programs is suggested in the text? Can you think of other techniques that might be used?

REFERENCES

Anderson, C. L.: *School health practice,* ed. 5, St. Louis, 1972, The C. V. Mosby Co.

Curti, M.: *The social ideas of American educators,* Patterson, N.J., 1961, Littlefield, Adams & Co.

Edwards, N., and Richey, H. G.: *The school in the American social order,* ed. 2, Boston, 1963, Houghton Mifflin Co.

Goerke, L. S., and Stebbins, E. L.: *Mustard's introduction to public health,* ed. 5, New York, 1968, Macmillan, Inc.

Meadows, D. H., and others: *The limits to growth,* New York, 1972, The New American Library Inc.

Means, R. K.: *A history of health education in the United States,* Philadelphia, 1962, Lea & Febiger.

National Committee on School Health Policies: *Suggested school health policies,* ed. 4, Washington, D.C. and Chicago, 1966, Joint Committee on Health Problems in Education of the National Education Association and the American Medical Association.

Nemir, A.: *The school health program,* ed. 3, Philadelphia, 1970, W. B. Saunders Co.

Schmidt, W. M.: The development of health services for mothers and children in the United States, Am. J. Public Health **63:**419-427, June 1973.

Shattuck, L.: *Report of the Sanitary Commission of Massachusetts* (Boston, 1850, facsimile edition), Cambridge, Mass., 1950, Harvard University Press.

Turner, C. E.: *Planning for health education in schools,* Geneva, Switzerland, 1966, UNESCO and WHO.

Wheatley, G. M., and Hallock, G. T.: *Health observation of school children,* ed. 3, New York, 1968, McGraw-Hill, Inc.

Wilner, D. M., Walkley, R. P., and Goerke, L. S.: *Introduction to public health,* ed. 6, New York, 1973, Macmillan, Inc.

Wilson, C. C., editor: *School health services,* ed. 2, Washington, D.C. and Chicago, 1964, National Education Association and American Medical Association.

Wilson, C. C., and Wilson, E. A., editors: *Healthful school environment,* Washington, D.C. and Chicago, 1969, National Education Association and American Medical Association.

PART TWO

Organization and administration of school health and health education

CHAPTER 3 ❧ School health: its laws, governments, and publics

People acting as individuals or groups, as professionals, or as elected or appointed officers of government determine how school health and health education in a given community are organized and administered, what school health and health education professionals do, and how they do it. People sometimes act through their governments by influencing legislation, election or appointment of officials, and tax levies. At other times they act directly to exert pressure on the decisions of teachers, other school health professionals, and the administrators of schools and other related community agencies. People tend to get what they want and are willing to pay for, and the options available to professionals are thus somewhat limited. To the extent that professionals earn the trust and respect of the people—their several publics—their freedom to act in the best interests of school health and health education is increased.

This chapter is a description of how various kinds of laws and other actions emanating from various levels and branches of government operate to influence school health and health education. The various publics that influence school health and health education will also be identified and discussed.

NATURE OF LAW

Any given law may be classified as either *permissive* or *mandatory*. Permissive legislation allows a specified act to be performed but does not require performance. For example, a Michigan law (Michigan, P.A. 1968, No. 44) permits but does not require school districts to teach sex education. A mandatory law either requires or prohibits the performance of a given act. For example, many states require certain vaccinations as

a condition of admission to school, and one (North Dakota) prohibits vaccination as a prerequisite to admission.*

In addition, laws may be categorized by four broad categories: constitutional law, statutory law, administrative law, and common law.†

Constitutional law. This type of law is that written into the United States Constitution and its Bill of Rights, and the constitutions of the fifty states. These documents describe the general form and functions of our federal and state governments and define the relationship of these governments to the people.

It was noted in Chapter 2 that nowhere in the United States Constitution do the words "health" or "education" appear. For this reason, public health and education are considered state functions, since all powers not specifically delegated to the federal government or prohibited to the states are reserved to the states or to the people (Article X). You will probably find in your own state constitution one or more provisions concerning health and education. The United States Constitution is supreme; no state or local government may contravene it, and no law in conflict with it is valid.

The federal and state constitutions contain their own provisions for amending them. Thus like other bodies of law, what they say may change with time and public pressure. What constitutional and other legal provisions mean also changes with time as a

---

*Miller, D. F., *School health programs: their basis in law,* Cranbury, N.J., 1972, A. S. Barnes & Co., Inc., pp. 35-36, 103.
†Mayshark, C., and Shaw, D. D.: *Administration of school health programs: its theory and practice,* St. Louis, 1967, The C. V. Mosby Co., pp. 382-384.

result of court decisions, official opinions expressed by the attorneys general, government applications, and unchallenged statutory laws. For example, federal support of public education may be justified on the constitutional grounds that the Preamble to the U.S. Constitution requires the federal government to "promote the general welfare." Although minors have not in the past been considered to enjoy the full protection of the Bill of Rights, recent court decisions have increasingly extended those rights to them and prohibited school officials from contravention of those rights.

Statutory law. Statutes are laws written under constitutional authority by the legislative branches of governments. The examples of both permissive and mandatory legislation cited earlier serve also as examples of statutory law. Statutory laws may be enacted by the U.S. Congress or by state legislatures.

Administrative law. This type of law consists of rules and regulations written by executive agencies of government rather than the legislative branch. Such agencies must be specifically authorized by legislative action to write administrative law. The rationale for having administrative law is that new knowledge and circumstances may dictate fairly rapid change in the details of laws, and therefore modern legislatures tend to set forth general requirements in statutory law and to authorize executive agencies to write and revise detail as needed. The legislature sets forth procedures, such as prior publication of a proposed administrative law and public hearings on it, which the agency is required to follow. Rules and regulations so passed have the full force and effect of statutory law.

Sources of administrative law important to school health and health education include the state and local boards of education and public health as well as federal agencies that administer relevant programs. State and local boards of health are the sources of specific communicable disease regulations in most states, for example. In some states the nature of the health education curriculum is specified in state statutory law, while in others state or local boards of education specify it in the form of administrative law.

Common law. The primary distinguishing characteristics of common law are that it grows out of long-term social acceptance and custom and that it is unwritten. What constitutes common law is determined largely on the basis of precedents set by court decisions. For many years school districts (as well as other government units) were immune from liability suits for damages a person might suffer as a result of the negligence of members or employees of the board of education. This immunity was based on an old common law doctrine that "the king can do no wrong." Recent court decisions and (in some states) new statutory law have recognized the inherent injustice of this immunity and have thus modified its application so that damage suits arising out of government negligence may now be entertained by the courts under certain conditions.

SCHOOL HEALTH AND THE LAW

Miller* analyzed law pertaining to school health programs in the United States. He found considerable variation among the fifty states, but certain common principles emerged regarding each of the three broad areas of the school health program.

Health instruction. As long as the state's constitution or statutes do not prohibit it, health may be included in the curriculum as a school subject by school boards as a matter of common law. Forty-four of the fifty states require instruction with respect to alcohol and narcotics. Sex education is constitutional and legal, depending on specific state statutes. Common law, however, provides for the exclusion of children from "certain aspects of the school instructional program which are found to be in conflict with one's religious beliefs."†

School health services. Health services are guided by statutes in most states. School districts may employ medical personnel for these purposes: "(1) to appraise the health

---

*Miller, D. F.: *School health programs.*
†Miller, D. F.: *School health programs*, p. 46.

status of the students, (2) to render emergency care, and (3) through consultation to guide the students to the place where the needed medical attention can be received."* Schools may exclude a child suspected of carrying a communicable disease from attendance. Schools should keep student health records, which "should be made available to those who have reason to use the information."† "Overwhelmingly, court precedent has supported statutory requirements, health department regulations, and school board rules and requisitions providing for vaccination and immunization of school children."‡ Such requirements have not been regarded by the courts as an infringement upon religious freedom, and noncompliance may be treated as an instance of child neglect by the parents or cause for excluding a child from school when an epidemic occurs. (In our opinion, the risk of the presence of a relatively few unimmunized individuals in a school is usually outweighed by the cost of litigation in terms of effort, money, and human relations.) Proof of immunization may also be required of teachers.

Healthful school living. School districts are legally as well as morally obliged to provide a safe and healthful environment for children not only on the school site itself but on the way between home and school as well. Schools are also obligated not to produce a more dangerous environmental condition in the process of alleviating a hazard. All school personnel are personally legally responsible for the safety of school grounds and facilities. Schools may organize voluntary school safety patrols but are not usually required to do so. In so doing, parental permission should be secured, and patrol members should be given proper instruction. Schools may operate nonprofit school-feeding programs and require students to remain at school during the lunch period.§

What's wrong with school health law? The few and rather general commonalities cited above affect school health and health education throughout the United States. In any given school district additional guidelines of state constitutional law, state and local statutory law, and state and local administrative law may apply. These laws sometimes require interpretation and are always subject to change. Fortunately, most school districts employ one or more attorneys on a full or parttime basis whose roles include the search for and interpretation of legal guidelines for the board and administrative staff. Some states publish useful school law manuals for the benefit of professionals. In addition, there is published for each state a constantly updated reference entitled *Statutes Annotated,* which is cross-indexed and contains not only state statutes but relevant historical, judicial, and attorney general interpretations of them as well.

Based on a review of school health law in California, McNamara and his co-workers* concluded that current law is outdated in its focus on communicable disease. While provision is often made for school liability (thus scandal-proofing school safety), it mandates no concrete plans for emergency care. There is a lack of legal emphasis on prevention of such current problems as obesity and smoking. Laws fail to capitalize on the potential of schools as sites for screening for other than vision or hearing problems. They fail to recognize the relationship between health problems and school problems. Other critics have frequently observed that school health laws seem to set forth minimal requirements but fail to encourage program improvement.

These defects exist, but their presence has not prevented schools from improving their programs and pioneering new ones when and usually as they desire to do so.† Laws

---

*Miller, D. F.: *School health programs,* p. 65.
†Miller, D. F.: *School health programs,* p. 65.
‡Miller, D. F.: *School health programs,* p. 104.
§Miller, D. F.: *School health programs,* pp. 111-137.

*McNamara, J. J., Conheim, R., and Meyerhoff, P.: Toward a model school health law, J. Sch. Health **43:**507-509, Oct. 1973.
†Hughes, S. K.: Sixty years of school nursing in Reading, Pennsylvania, unpublished master's thesis, Temple University, 1972.

that serve as barriers can be amended or repealed. Professionals can and should be more active than they are in this process. Their most effective vehicles for legal change are their professional organizations, many of which maintain national and state lobbies.

SCHOOL HEALTH AND ITS GOVERNMENTS

We in the United States live under three traditional levels of government: federal, state, and local. Each level is composed of three coequal branches: legislative, judicial, and administrative or executive. These branches make, interpret, and apply law, and collect and distribute taxes, and thereby have profound effects on the nature of school health and health education.

People and the health problems they create, however, do not confine themselves to these geopolitical subdivisions. Some of us live in one state or county and work or go to school in another. Air pollution created by industry may be blown across a city, county, state, or even national boundary. For this reason, a new level of government, entitled regional government or authority, has emerged in recent years. These governments are primarily administrative or executive in nature and cross local, state, and even national boundaries.*

State government. The state is the level of government most germane to school health and health education. Although patterns vary with the state, there are within each state departments or divisions that are devoted to education and health. Typically, there are state boards of education and public health that enact administrative law and determine statewide education and public health policy. There are chief state executive officers for public health and education whose specific titles vary with the state. These officers and the members of their boards are usually elected or politically ap-

pointed to office and are usually not civil service employees. Most of them are thus subject to political pressures and influences. In some states the health and education executives are required to meet stated educational qualifications.

Other state departments and divisions may directly or indirectly affect school health and health education. The department of agriculture, for example, may be concerned with school feeding and nutrition education activities. In some states mental health and medical care programs are considered welfare rather than public health functions.

Local boards of education are classified as quasi-state agencies rather than as local governments, and city or county governments have no control over local school districts unless the state specifically delegates such control. This principle has been reiterated in many court decisions. For example, the Michigan Supreme Court in 1908 held that "the Constitution of Michigan turns the whole subject of education over to the legislature and the subject is no part of the local self-government inherent in townships and municipalities except so far as the legislature may choose to make it such." States vary in the extent of power delegated to local boards. One state, Hawaii, has no local boards of education, but operates as a single statewide school district.

The crazy-quilt nature of the organization of governments for health and education has led to both formal and informal interagency groups of officials who meet for the purpose of coordinating their functions. Such groups and the need for them exist at all levels of government. They sometimes grow to include representation from related professional and voluntary organizations.

Local government. City, township, and county government impinges on school health and health education in many ways. In some localities boards of education have the power to levy their own school taxes. In others education must compete for funds directly with such other essential local ser-

---

*Mayshark, C., and Shaw, D. D.: *Administration of school health programs*, pp. 384-386.

vices as those of the police, fire, and public health departments. In any community the nature of school health and health education is partially determined by the scope and quality of such locally available public services as water supply, traffic safety, clinics, and hospitals. These may or may not be well funded, managed, and staffed, and free of pernicious political influence. Whether they are or not, maximum interagency cooperation and coordination are essential.

Although they are state agencies, local school districts are usually governed by a locally elected board of education, which employs a superintendent of schools as its chief executive officer. Theoretically, the board is an administrative agency that sets policy (administrative law) to the extent permitted by the state. The board of education also usually serves in a quasi-judicial capacity; for example, it may adjudicate cases in which the administration seeks to discharge a teacher. The superintendent administers the schools under board policy. In fact, some superintendents may function with considerable independence and may directly influence the board in its policy-making and judicial roles if they have the support and tacit concent of the board in doing so.

Local health departments are organized and operate in much the same way. The board is usually appointed (which in turn usually appoints its chief health officer) and serves as an administrative agency.

With respect to both health and education the major difference between the local and state levels is that local boards are primarily concerned with the direct delivery of services to people, while state boards are more involved with making policy, promoting local effort and quality of service, and providing central services to the local agencies. Most states retain the power to discharge and to assume the functions of local boards of health and education, although this power is seldom used.

Other local government services are generally more subject than health and education to the direct control of such legislative bodies as city councils, county commissions, and local executive officers such as mayors or managers. Even so, it seems fair to say that the scope and quality of all local services, including health and education, vary with both the financial resources available and the integrity of local officials.

Federal government. National health and education functions have traditionally been largely confined to research and development and to financial support of local and state effort. The federal government has attempted to avoid regulation of local and state functions except in support of such constitutionally oriented goals as the promotion of civil rights and the regulation of interstate and foreign commerce.

Most federal health and health education –related activities are concentrated in the Education Division and the Public Health Service, which together with the Social and Rehabilitation Service, the Office of Human Development, and the Social Security Administration comprise the agencies of the U.S. Department of Health, Education, and Welfare. This gargantuan department was created in 1953 in an attempt to coordinate all the federal functions named in its title by linking them in a single administrative department. Even so, some functions were left outside for historical and political reasons (such as the school feeding program of the U.S. Department of Agriculture). One important new unit, the Environmental Protection Agency, was created in 1970. Its chief administrator reports directly to the President.

The operating units of the Public Health Service are the Food and Drug Administration (consumer protection), the National Institutes of Health (research), the Center for Disease Control, and the Health Services and Mental Health Administration. This last-mentioned unit is the most directly relevant to school health and health education. It includes subdivisions devoted to the development and delivery of such services as disease control, community environmental management, maternal and child health, and mental health.

In recent years there has been a tendency for federal financial support to move away from categorical grants for specific services toward block grants that provide for increased state and local options as to how they are spent. Formerly, federal funds were routinely passed on to local governments via specified state agencies. Today, direct federal funding of local programs is not uncommon, and general revenue sharing is in effect.

Regional governments. Regionalism in government can and does exist at the international, interstate, and/or intercounty and intercity levels. At the international level, regionalism is exemplified by the World Health Organization, which functions in such areas as international quarantine and the worldwide standardization of drugs and vaccines, and which provides technical assistance to member nations. In addition, WHO maintains six regional offices, one of which serves the American countries. About 25 years ago the states bordering the Ohio River formed a regional administrative government to control pollution of the river. Less populous communities within a single state frequently participate in regional school or health districts. A more extensive school curriculum or public health program can be provided by such local regional governments.

A rationale for regionalization for health was proposed by the National Commission on Community Health Services in 1967. The Commission suggested that any given community naturally belongs to a number of different "communities of solution," each of which contains a health problem, and its solution and may cross city, county, or state boundary lines. The same rationale can be applied to many school health problems, such as the need of children with a given rare handicap for special education. A sufficiently large population of such children to justify support of special services may be brought together through a regional organization of several small school districts. Development of logical "community of solu-

tion" regions, however, is often inhibited by fear of loss of local control or identity.*

POLITICKING FOR SCHOOL HEALTH AND HEALTH EDUCATION

Compliant acceptance of adverse laws and court decisions and inadequate budgets for school health and health education is neither necessary nor desirable. A combination of group and individual effort by health and education professionals can improve the laws and budgets under which we operate. The first step is group and individual cognizance of the legislative and administrative structures and procedures outlined above, supplemented by detailed knowledge of the relevant governments in your own state, county, and city or town.

Until very recently most professional health and education organizations have avoided endorsement of individual candidates for elective and appointive power positions. Now some are beginning to probe the positions of candidates and to support actively those with favorable atitudes toward health and education. Once elected, such individuals are in a position to introduce and support adoption of desirable changes in constitutional, statutory, and administrative law. They are unlikely to do so on their own, however. A request by an organized group, supplemented by letters (perferably individualized) and phone calls from group members and sympathizers, is essential.

Professional organizations are rightly categorized as "special interest groups," and their political activities are therefore often suspect. For this reason it is helpful to enlist the support of civic groups. One effective means of obtaining such support is to utilize the good offices of professional group members who also happen to be members of civic groups.

Once desired legislation is introduced, it is usually subject to a process of committee

---

*National Commission on Community Health Services: *Health is a community affair,* Cambridge, Mass., 1967, Harvard University Press, pp. 2-6.

study, public hearings, and revision. Chances of passage are enhanced by introduction early in a given legislative session, by professional and citizen testimony in support of the legislation at hearings, by the willingness of the sponsors to agree to reasonable compromise with those opposed to the legislation, and by floods of communication of all kinds to key legislators at crucial times. It is well to be aware of the attitudes of individual legislators and to keep them in mind in the course of contacts. A public health bill was once lost in a state legislature committee through ignorance of the anti-feminist attitude of the swing-vote legislator. The bill had nothing to do with women's rights, but several women's groups had been recruited to testify in its favor.

Court decisions are rarely, and then only illegally and unethically, influenced by political intervention. However, in one major city a judge easily won an election over powerful opposition partly because she was well known as an effective advocate of the welfare of children. Laws and administrative decisions adverse to school health and health education can be challenged in court, and adverse court decisions can be appealed. The high cost of pursuing a court case and the inclination of many persons to avoid involvement in litigation tend to inhibit such action in many justified cases. Here again, powerful and affluent professional organizations are in a position to act where individuals are often not. The American Civil Liberties Union is an effective agent in cases that involve violations of fundamental liberties. The role of the individual health and education professional is to bring the need for court action to the attention of an appropriate organization.

SCHOOL HEALTH AND ITS PUBLICS

Research by the Joint Committee on Health Problems in Education of the National Education Association and the American Medical Association has resulted in a number of projections for 1985. Projections concerned with politics and values include:

1. An expansion in participatory democracy with greater youth involvement
2. Expansion in the legal rights and responsibility of youth
3. Increased use of violence as a political tactic
4. Greater attention to domestic concerns
5. Greater resistance to authority
6. Increased anti-intellectualism
7. Less dictation of personal conduct*

The validity of futuristic predictions can be established only by future events. If valid, one clear implication of these projections is that school health and health education must base decisions more on the felt needs of people, particularly the young, and correspondingly less on the dictates of authorities.

Students, then, make up the most important of the publics of school health and health education not only because their power is increasing but also because school health and health education exist to serve them. Parents and other adult citizens represent an important public because they can give or withhold social, political, and financial support. Health and education professionals and paraprofessionals are important because they are the health and health education program providers both in and out of school as well as useful resources in program planning. Members of all these publics may function either as individuals or in organized groups. A given individual may be a member of more than one public, and the obvious roles of the several publics may overlap.

Students. A statewide survey of Connecticut youngsters in grades kindergarten through twelve revealed high interest in health education and the precise health interests typical at each grade level. Elementary grade children were most interested in their bodies, junior high youngsters in their physical, social, and emotional development, and senior high students in mental health,

*Joint Committee on Health Problems in Education of the National Education Association and American Medical Association: School health 1985, School Health Review **3:**3, 2-10, May-June 1972.

sex, and drugs. The findings are useful (and are used) in teacher education, curriculum development, and counseling.*

Students can be involved in school health and health education in many ways. School nurses have long used student assistants in the health service program. Student safety patrols contribute to safety and safety education. However, too often student involvement is limited to the performance of mundane tasks conceived by adults. When students do become involved in program planning, their suggestions are often ignored or rejected with no adequate reason given.

In many schools students have reacted to rejection by resorting to violent protest. In one city students developed a bill of rights that included statements of student responsibilities as well as of due process requirements to be used in cases of student misconduct. The code was adopted by the local board of education over teacher and administrator opposition.

Experience suggests several conditions that may be necessary for useful and effective student involvement.

1. Students will perform routine tasks willingly if they are rewarded for doing them and if the reasons why the tasks are important make sense to them.
2. It is valuable to listen to students. They *do* know their own needs, and their ideas are sometimes better than those of adults.
3. Students will reject those who routinely reject or ignore them or their ideas. They will recognize and react negatively to those who give only lip service to student involvement.
4. Students will accept occasional rejection or modification of their ideas if honest, sensible, and acceptable reasons are given.
5. Given needed training and guidance,

students are capable of high levels of planning and task performance.

Parents and other adult citizens. A 1973 Gallup poll revealed that parents of public school children are becoming more favorable in their attitudes toward the schools, while nonparents were becoming less favorable. Parents tend to rely on their children for information about schools, while nonparents rely on newspapers. Adults generally agree that schools are getting too large and that small classes facilitate achievement. Majorities favor more emphasis on career education and the establishment of alternative schools and disapprove of lowering the school entry age to 4 years.*

Systematic sampling of public opinion is perhaps the best means of determining public attitudes, because highly vocal minorities exist who loudly espouse viewpoints in direct opposition to some of those cited above. The difference in attitudes of parents and nonparents supports the idea that students themselves and school contacts are probably the most effective public relations media for schools.

A survey of Albuquerque elementary school parents revealed that parents endorse the idea that parents and students be used as assistants to school nurses and, surprisingly, that middle and lower class parents do *not* consider health information about their children to be highly confidential, although upper class parents do. Upper class parents were more supportive of sex education than were lower class parents. Parents of all classes desired expansion of school health services.† Such findings, which might well differ at other times or in other geographic locations, have significant implications for program planning and implementation. They suggest that more planning and

---

*Byler, R. V.: *Teach us what we want to know,* New York, 1969, Mental Health Materials Center. See also Byler, R. V.: Teach us what we want to know, J. Sch. Health **40:**252-255, May 1970.

*Gallup, G. H.: Fifth annual poll of public attitudes toward education, Phi Delta Kappan **55:** 38-51, Sept. 1973.
†Pelizza, J. J.: A comparative study of how parents from different social classes perceive school health services, J. Sch. Health **43:**176-180, March 1973.

decision making take place at the building level, for example.

Volunteer adults have been successfully trained and utilized to perform such tasks as initial hearing screening with subsequent professional review.* In one school multi-lingual adults served as translators and communicators between the school nurse and foreign-born parents. Others assisted in the planning and conduct of health-screen-ing programs and served as members of health education curriculum committees and planning committees for new school build-ings. Adults who serve in such ways become health educated themselves and become supportive of school programs. Through contact with them, school health profes-sionals grow in awareness of parent's needs, interests, and attitudes.

Parental volunteerism presents several problems. As noted in Chapter 1, families in which both parents are employed are now in the majority, and time for volunteer service is thus not as available as it once was. Volunteer service is costly in terms of lunch and transportation money as well as in time, and some who might volunteer are therefore unable to do so. Training volun-teers may consume more time than the re-sulting volunteer effort is worth. Finally, volunteers are not always reliable. One trend that may be of value in solving some of these problems is the employment of community adults for service as paid para-professionals. Whether workers are volun-teers or paid, costs to the school and the worker should be compared to benefits re-ceived to determine whether a given activity is worthy.

Some citizens, like some professionals and students, may be classified as militants who stress involvement in schools for its own sake. One study of the attitudes of parents, teachers, administrators, and paraprofes-sionals led the researcher to conclude that militant citizens who become involved are

likely to find themselves confronted by equally militant teachers and that involve-ment is likely to broaden the viewpoints of all those involved.*

Other means of home-school interaction and communication include conferences be-tween parents and school staff members at home or at school. Both of these kinds of individual personal contacts provide op-portunity to establish friendly relationships as well as mutual understanding of the child and the interaction of the youngster's two most important environments. Such confer-ences are also the most effective means of counseling and follow-up with respect to a child's health problem. Whether or not a conference is effective depends on the con-ferees' mutual acceptance of each other as worthy persons. The process is facilitated by focusing on the subject of mutual interest and concern—the child and the problem rather than whatever deficiencies may beset the home or the school. Possibilities for solutions are affected by the environment, which therefore is a matter of which con-ferees need to be aware. Recriminations about "your lousy home" or "your lousy school" are of no assistance.

Telephone conferences are a fair substi-tute for face-to-face conferences; they are personal, provide opportunity for interac-tion, and save time. Most local telephone companies offer literature, and some even provide staff training in techniques of friendly and effective telephone communi-cation. However, telephone conferences do not provide opportunity to become aware of environmental limitations. Additional time saving is the one advantage of imper-sonal written or printed communications. Modern office equipment makes possible the personalization of form letters.

In any form of personal communication school representatives should assume that the parent is intelligent (remembering that lack of education does *not* imply lack of

---

*Berlin, C. J., and others: Auditory screening of school children by volunteer mothers, J. Sch. Health **39**:95-101, Feb. 1969.

*Gottesfeld, H.: Educational issues in a low-in-come area as seen by community people and edu-cators, Phi Delta Kappan **52**:366-368, Feb. 1971.

intelligence) and well motivated. These assumptions may be false, but the danger of insulting the parent is lessened, and good intentions may thus be motivated if they do not already exist.

Professionals and paraprofessionals. A paraprofessional may be defined as one who works alongside a professional in a capacity that resembles that of the professional. The designation has received common use in health and education in recent years to describe teachers' and nurses' aides, among others, who usually come from the community and who receive informal or formal on-the-job training to relieve the teacher or nurse of tasks that do not require full professional competence. On the other hand the professional is one who has competence in his or her field, usually acquired through formal education and sometimes assured through legal certification or license. Both are identified with an institution such as a school, health department, or other agency. Both may also be citizens of the community in which they serve, but this may be more likely to be true of paraprofessionals.

Professionals tend to take a somewhat elitest view of their training, their jobs, and themselves. Their professional preparation is unlikely to include the development of supervisory skills. Conflicts are likely to develop for both these reasons. Bryan stressed the importance of clear task assignments and job descriptions, careful selection and training of personnel, continual supervision of a paraprofessional by a professional who is trained to supervise, preparation of the professionals to accept and utilize the paraprofessionals, and continuing evaluation of the effectiveness of paraprofessional assistance.* Thus assured of a pleasant and useful work life, both the paraprofessional and the professional are likely to represent the institution in the community in a positive and effective way.

Internal dissension, which is likely to

affect both performance effectiveness and community relations, may arise between one group of professionals and another within a school or other institution. Causative factors may include the attitude that "my profession is better than your profession" as well as salary or job benefit inequities. Interprofessional animosity may be negated in the process of working together toward a common goal. Collective bargaining can remove inequities if teachers and nurses, for example, belong to a common union.

Effective school health and health education depend on cooperation between school professionals and paraprofessionals and their counterparts in the community. Examples of such cooperation include communications between the school and a child's personal physician, advice to the school about environmental problems from public health and industrial safety engineers, and coordination of school health education content and objectives with those of community health agencies. Mutually agreed task and role definitions between the school and outside professionals as well as acceptance by each of the others' importance are essentials. In one city cooperation and mutual acceptance were fostered when the public health nurses invited the school nurses to attend inservice lectures of interest to both groups. The school nurses, in turn, invited the public health nurses to use school facilities for telephone calls and conferences.

Use of publicity. Personal contacts and school-community organization and cooperation have been emphasized in this discussion as perhaps the most effective means of achieving and maintaining good relationships between school health and health education and their publics. Other useful means include the use of printed and audiovisual media, which should be viewed as adjuncts to organization and cooperation rather than as substitutes for them.

Most large school districts maintain public relations offices whose role includes the

---

*Bryan, D. S.: *School nursing in transition,* St. Louis, 1973, The C. V. Mosby Co., p. 23.

collection and dissemination of information about school problems and programs through press, radio, and television outlets. Knowledge of the existence of such an office, acquaintance with those who staff it, and the ability to recognize an unusual and therefore newsworthy event when it occurs combine to provide for effective utilization of mass media. In smaller districts where everyone knows everyone else, a public relations office is not needed to bridge the gap between school and media. In either case, local policy (or one's own good sense of self-preservation) usually dictates that a potential story be cleared through a given administrator before its release.

Choice of medium is related to intended target groups. The school newspaper is read by most students and some faculty members and parents. Most faculty members and parents are better reached through community press, radio and television, or through bulletins addressed directly to them. A communication to local physicians is likely to be received when it appears in the local medical society journal or is announced at a society meeting.

Parent-teacher associations (or their local equivalent) are primarily attended by parents who are interested in what is going on at school. In our experience, speeches and lectures designed to teach the art of parenthood are unlikely to be well attended. Curriculum fairs or other kinds of demonstrations of what the children are doing tend to be well attended. Parents are more interested in audiovisual presentations produced by their children than in those concocted by school professionals.

Conclusion. A school health and health education administration or program that ignores or caters exclusively to the needs or desires of any one of its publics is headed for trouble, as is one that attempts to be all things to all people. Then comes the complex and never-ending task of defining common needs and goals, devising methods and approving roles for meeting them, and evaluating and revising programs and policies.

QUESTIONS FOR STUDY AND DISCUSSION

1. What is the difference between permissive and mandatory legislation? Cite an example of each that applies to you personally, for example as a driver.
2. How do constitutional law, statutory law, administrative law, and common law differ?
3. What does the U.S. Constitution have to say about health and education? Why do you think this is so?
4. What does your own state constitution say about health and education? Who is given the power to direct public health and education in your state?
5. What general legal guidelines are set forth for health instruction, school health services, and healthful school living in most states?
6. Research the annotated statutes for your state to determine legal guidelines with respect to a specific aspect of school health and health education selected by you. Report your findings to the class.
7. A legal issue not discussed in the text is selective law enforcement. For example, a policeman tickets one person for a given traffic offense and fails to ticket another for an identical offense. Should such discretion be permitted, and why? Should school health laws (such as requiring vaccination or health instruction) be rigidly or selectively enforced against objecting parents, and why?
8. A committee in a local school district decides that a program to screen high school students for VD should be instituted. The superintendent rejects the proposal, saying, "That would be illegal!" Other than dropping the proposal, what steps, if any, can the committee take?
9. What criticisms of school health law are offered by McNamara and his associates? Is the best answer to these criticisms new legislation, and why?
10. What characteristics are shared by federal, state, and local governments? How do they differ in respect to their roles in school health and health education?
11. Which level of government has the most power with respect to school health and health education? What advantages and disadvantages might accompany a constitutional shift in power to any of the other levels?
12. Can any one branch of government (executive, legislative, judicial) be said to be superior to other branches in its influence on school health and health education, and why?
13. How are state departments of health and education *usually* organized and administered? How are these departments organized and administered in your state?
14. What is the usual legal status of local boards of education?
15. How are your own boards of health and education and their chief administrative officers chosen? What advantages and disadvantages do you see in this plan?

16. In what ways are your own local schools dependent on or independent of city or county government? What advantages and disadvantages stem from dependencies and independencies?
17. What generalizations can be made with respect to federal, state, and local roles in health and health education?
18. What department at the federal level is most involved with school health and health education? What are some of the specific federal agencies involved?
19. What is the rationale for regional governments? What are the general characteristics of regional governments?
20. Can you name and describe the purpose of a regional government in which your home is located?
21. Looking back to your own high school experience, describe one or more ways in which you were involved in the planning and conduct of school health and health education programs. Which, if any, of these experiences would you consider to be useful and meaningful to you, and which would you describe as "lip service" attempts at involvement?
22. Make your own list (not limited to those cited in the text) of:
    a. Reasons why students, adults, citizens, and professionals are important publics of school health
    b. Ways in which each of these publics can be involved in the planning or conducting of school health programs
    c. Guidelines that might help school health professionals relate to each of these publics in meaningful ways
23. How can the school best deal with militant students, professionals, and citizens?

24. A century or a century and a half ago, there were no school or health professionals in the school except the teacher, who usually filled the role of janitor as well. Why do schools today have so many different professionals and paraprofessionals on their staffs?

REFERENCES

Mayshark, C., and Shaw, D. D.: *Administration of school health programs: its theory and practice,* St. Louis, 1967, The C. V. Mosby Co.

Miller, D. F.: *School health programs: their basis in law,* Cranbury, N.J., 1972, A. S. Barnes & Co.

National Commission on Community Health Services: *Health is a community affair,* Cambridge, Mass., 1967, Harvard University Press.

National Committee on School Health Policies: *Suggested school health policies,* ed. 4, Washington, D.C. and Chicago, 1966, The Joint Committee on Health Problems in Education of the National Education Association and the American Medical Association.

Nemir, A.: *The school health program,* ed. 3, Philadelphia, 1970, W. B. Saunders Co.

Wilner, D. M., Walkley, R. P., and Goerke, L. S.: *Introduction to public health,* ed. 6, New York, 1973, Macmillan, Inc.

Wilson, C. C., editor: *School health services,* ed. 2, Washington, D.C. and Chicago, 1964, National Education Association and American Medical Association.

Wilson, C. C. and Wilson, E. A., editors: *Healthful school environment,* Washington, D.C. and Chicago, 1969, National Education Association and American Medical Association.

CHAPTER 4 ❧ Styles of organization and administration

"Organization of a school or other institution refers to the structure or formal relationships through which people operate to achieve the common goals of the institution."* "Administration" has been defined as "a complex, fluid set of processes carried out by people" referred to as administrators, supervisors, directors, or other descriptive titles.† It is these two aspects of school health and health education with which this chapter is concerned. Achievement of professional goals and satisfaction is closely affected by both structure and process.

PATTERNS OF ORGANIZATION

School health and health education vary from most school functions in that they are closely allied with community health, as well as with every other operational task or administrative area of the public schools. For these reasons the school health program in some cities and states has organizational and administrative relationships that extend both inside and outside the school system.

External organization. At the state level it is not unusual for certain school health functions to be placed in whole or in part outside the state department of education. One Florida statute, for example, places medical examinations of school children under the control of the state board of health, while others provide for joint state board of education and health regulation of school sanitation.‡ The logic behind such arrange-

ments is that board of health professionals are generally better qualified than board of education professionals in medicine and sanitation and have direct access to important support services such as those of the state public health laboratory. On the other hand, it can be argued that it is easier to work for one boss than for two who might be in disagreement and that the state school system is large enough to support its own experts and services. A cynic might be inclined to suspect that whichever set of arrangements prevails is more the result of empire building by an administrator than of logical thinking.

In a minority of local districts, school health services are organized either under the jurisdiction of the health department or under the joint jurisdiction of both the board of education and the health department.* Either of these plans is based on the concept of best use of human resources and expertise. Medical and environmental consultation and resources are available through the health department. Instead of two nurses contacting the same home for two agencies, one nurse does the job for both of them. If the services are under joint jurisdiction, that nurse has direct access to the resources of both agencies. Joint or health department administration does *not* necessarily imply economy in field staff operation, however. It is unreasonable to expect one nurse to do the work of two.

In the context of another program, community education, which of necessity also involves both the school and other community agencies, Moore has this to say:

*Campbell, R. F., and others: *Introduction to educational administration,* Boston, 1971, Allyn & Bacon, Inc., pp. 172-173.
†Mayshark, C., and Shaw, D. D.: *Administration of school health programs: its theory and practice,* St. Louis, 1967, The C. V. Mosby Co., p. 52.
‡Mayshark, C., and Shaw, D. D.: *Administration of school health programs,* p. 395.

*Wolf, J. M., and Pritham, H. C.: *Administrative patterns of school health services,* J.A.M.A. **193:** 195-199, July 1966.

Line control of many aspects of the community education program is difficult to establish. This has advantages and disadvantages, the chief advantage being that strong human and cooperative relationships have to be developed and the principal disadvantages being that such relationships can disintegrate rapidly, lack stability, and lack an accountability plan.*

The reason cited by most school superintendents for favoring board of education control is that school administrators and teachers are more likely to cooperate with the health program if it is staffed by school employees rather than by health department employees.† Luby‡ and Jenne§ observed that board of health–employed nurses tended to report feeling like "lone workers" in the schools that they serve. Patterson‖ concluded that there was no difference in the effectiveness of follow-up services associated with board of education or health department organization, although he found follow-up services to take less time under board of education organization.

In considering the subject, the Council of Chief State School Officers and the Association of State and Territorial Health Officers¶ concluded that whichever type of organization is chosen, school health services should be jointly planned by all appropriate agencies and interested citizens and professional groups and that it is essential that school superintendents and health officers recognize each other's authority and responsibility and work closely together.

Whether joint or board of health jurisdiction is wise is a question probably best left to a representative local planning group equipped to evaluate local needs and resources and guided by sound principles of organization and applicable state statutes. Situational factors must also be considered in deciding the issue. For example, a local school district may have boundaries that cross those of two or more local health departments, or either the school or health department may be in danger of undesirable political intervention.

Internal organization. Within a school or school district, organization may be viewed in many different ways, two of which are particularly salient here. The first has to do with line of authority, or who one's boss is and how one communicates with others. The second has to do with how the school district is organized to achieve its tasks, or who works in the same department or division and who works elsewhere. Theoretically, these organizational patterns reflect the philosophy of the school district, either past or present. Practically, the ability of any school professional to accomplish his or her work and survive in a hierarchy depends to a large extent on a knowledge of these two aspects of the organization of the school or school district.

Lines and authority. The first definition of the word authority according to the *American Heritage Dictionary* is "the right and power to command, enforce laws, exact obedience, and judge." It is also defined as "power delegated to others." The same source defines the word power as "the ability or capacity to perform effectively" and as "the ability or official capacity to exercise control." Thus the two words are often used synonymously, but the authority one has is largely given by others, while power emphasizes the idea of individual ability or capacity. Some individuals are officially placed in positions of authority but lack the internal power to exercise that authority. In such cases, the "power behind the throne" may be exercised by individuals or groups who lack officially appointed authority but

*Moore, H. E.: Organizational and administrative and other problems and practice, Phi Delta Kappan **54:**168-170, Nov. 1972.
†Wolf, J. M., and Pritham, H. C.: Administrative patterns of school health services, p. 198.
‡Luby, R. R.: *The nurse in the school health services program,* unpublished doctor's dissertation, Wayne State University, 1957.
§Jenne, F. H.: Variations in nursing service characteristics and teachers' health observation practices, J. Sch. Health **40:**248-250, May 1970.
‖Patterson, J.: Effectiveness of the follow-up of health referrals under two different administrative patterns, J. Sch. Health **39:**687-692, Dec. 1965.
¶Council of Chief State School Officers and Association of State and Territorial Health Officers: *Responsibilities of state departments of education and health for school health services,* Washington, D.C., 1959, The Council, pp. 5-8.

who possess intrinsic power. In an authoritarian administration, power and authority tend to be vested in the same individual. In a democratic administration, authority is still officially delegated, but considerable power is retained by the people. Almost all modern administrators give lip service to democracy, and some of them actually practice it.

In most U.S. school districts, delegated authority is organized on a "line and staff" plan or one of its main variants. A board of education receives authority, usually by vote of the people, to manage a school district as provided by state law. The board appoints a superintendent and grants part of its authority to him or her. Following an organization plan, part of the superintendent's authority is next delegated to a school building principal (who used to be called the principal teacher because the duties included both teaching and administration), and part of the principal's authority is delegated to each classroom teacher, who may in turn democratically delegate some authority to the students. In large, complex schools and school systems the line of authority may pass through subcategories of superintendents (such as deputy, associate, or area superintendents) before it reaches the principal, and through an assistant or vice-principal before it reaches the teacher and the students. Intervening authorities are justified on the grounds that no one administrator can reasonably be expected to interact with a large number of subordinates. Thus, the superintendent may be far removed from the classroom in a district that is too large.

What is described above is the typical *line* authority of a school district. In theory, the line of communication follows the line of authority. A teacher who wishes to communicate with the superintendent is not supposed to do so directly but is to communicate by way of all of the authorities up the line, any of whom may read and comment on the communication. The process almost invariably affects the candor of the communication, the importance attached to it by the superintendent, and the time lapse between transmission and receipt. Violations are expected or tolerated in some school systems but not in others. The prevailing guidelines for communication may or may not appear in written policy, but they are known by experienced professionals.

Pure line organization originated in the military and was borrowed by schools. It served both the military and the schools reasonably well until the advent of specialization. Generals were well acquainted with command, muskets, cannons, and horses; and superintendents knew all about administration, schoolhouses, and the teaching of the three R's. As the technologies of killing and teaching became more complex, neither generals nor superintendents could continue to be masters of their professions. They needed specialists to help, people who knew much about part of their respective professions. Thus the staff specialist developed.

In a pure form of *line and staff* organization a central office specialist in school health, who may in turn have a team of subspecialists in health education, health services, and environmental health on his or her staff, *advises* the superintendent with respect to the administration of the school health program. The specialist has no authority to give orders; his or her advice to the superintendent may be taken directly or modified before it is passed down the line through the principal to the teacher, nurse, or other staff members involved in the school. Communications from building level specialists to central office specialists also follow the line (or alternative established) route. The rationale is that the line authority must be kept informed and must also fulfill its responsibilities to coordinate all school programs so that they function well together and to observe legal and policy restrictions. Thus the system requires that communications between a building level teacher and nurse, or either of these and the building custodian, also go through the line (principal).

In some variants of line and staff organization, central office specialists are delegated some degree of authority over the purely professional activities of building level specialists, with the line authorities retaining responsibility for nonprofessional activities. For example, instructions to a nurse about how to do vision screening might come from the central office specialist, while when and where it is done might be determined by the principal or some other authority up the line. Such an arrangement is designated a *functional* plan of organization, not because it describes divisions organized by function, but because it provides the specialist increased opportunity to achieve program goals. One variation of functional organization applies this principle at the lowest levels*: teachers and nurses confer directly and make as many decisions on their own as possible. The implications of this are that functional organization can permit democratic practices and that teachers, nurses, and others must be professionally competent to make decisions on their own. Upper level administrators are also freed to serve more as coordinators and facilitators of school programs and less as authorities. Dangers are that lower level coordination and accountability may suffer and that administrators may know less about what is going on than they do under a pure line and staff form.

Boxes and tasks. Campbell and his co-authors suggest that one possible way of grouping the operational tasks of school administration is:

1. School-community relationships
2. Curriculum and instruction
3. Pupil personnel
4. Staff personnel
5. Physical facilities
6. Finance and business management†

They point out that these same tasks exist at any level of the school structure.

In a larger school system divisions or departments may each be named to suggest placement of staff responsibilities for one or more of these operational areas or for part of one of them. In smaller school systems certain line or staff professionals may be given specific task responsibilities with or without task-related titles. Additional task areas, such as research and data processing or school health and health education, may be defined and staffed in either way.

Campbell* suggests that health services be subsumed under pupil personnel services together with such related operations as counseling, psychological and psychiatric services, speech therapy, and special education. Under such a design, health education would logically fall under the curriculum and instruction task area, and healthful school living might be retained under health services, with management of health and safety aspects of the physical environment possibly made part of the physical facilities task. On the other hand, if the primary goal of school health and health education as a whole is assumed to be educational, it can be argued that all aspects of school health and health education should function under the division of curriculum and instruction.

If considered part of the curriculum and instruction task, school health and health education, or health education alone, can be organized either as a separate subject or combined with another subject or group of subjects. One such combination, based on historical relationships, is with physical education. Other logically possible relationships include ties with the social and behavioral or physical sciences.

Every school specialist tends to view his or her specialty as the most important in the curriculum or in the school service structure, and specialists in school health and health education are no exception. Many would like to see the specialty organized as a separate department or division at the

---

*Mayshark, C., and Shaw, D. D.: *Administration of school health programs,* pp. 88-90.
†Campbell, R. F., and others: *Introduction to educational administration,* pp. 136-137.

*Campbell, R. F., and others: *Introduction to educational administration,* pp. 151-152.

very top of the hierarchical heap. However, it is unreasonable to expect mathematicians or school psychologists to agree that school health is a more worthy specialty than theirs. At best, school health and health education may expect to achieve equal status.

A model for the future? A 1967 Cambridge, Massachusetts city ordinance unified school health and other community well and sick child health services under a combined Department of Health, Hospital and Welfare. Direction of these child health services was delegated to the Cambridge Hospital Department of Pediatrics. Pediatric nurse practitioners now serve as primary medical caretakers in neighborhood health centers as well as in the school and other agencies. Every child is evaluated periodically by a pediatrician. With the assistance of health aides, nurse practitioners give routine physical examinations and screening tests, provide care for minor illnesses and injuries, make home visits, and refer children for care of more complex problems. More complete and effective services are thus provided from birth through the school years at the same cost as that of the previously spent total for preexisting school health services and well child programs.*

THE ADMINISTRATIVE PROCESS

Components. The administrative process of acting to achieve goals has been described as cyclical and made up of five components: "decision making, programming, stimulating, coordinating, and appraising."†

Decision making can be authoritative (done alone) or democratic (done through group involvement). It can be based on logical thinking, which involves definition and analysis of the problem, collection of relevant information, and the selection of one solution as best from among all the available options. Or, it can be based on irrational whim.

Programming is a matter of deciding how to implement the option selected. It involves further decisions about personnel, funds, and facilities. These kinds of decisions also may be made democratically or authoritatively and arrived at logically or illogically.

In *stimulating action* an administrator may give orders, exert other kinds of direct pressure, or, if possible, do so by group process in which those individuals who must act to implement a decision are stimulated to commit themselves to act because of their prior involvement in the decision-making and programming phases.

Coordinating is largely a matter of role and goal assignment, or decision making about who is to do what and for what purpose. The process may involve the use of volunteers and group decision, administrative direction, or a combination of both. Coordination will be discussed in greater detail in the last section of this chapter.

Appraising or evaluating involves determining how well the objectives are being met, how smoothly and efficiently the process of achieving them is functioning, and whether and how a higher level of achievement can be obtained and the process improved. Its end result is a new round of decision making, programming, stimulating action, coordinating, and appraising. Evaluations can be made by administrators alone, outside experts, or by group self-study. Chapter 20 is devoted to a fuller consideration of evaluation.

How effective administrators operate. Mayshark and Shaw offer this definition of administrative ability:

> The ability to state a goal and reach it
>   Through the efforts of other people
> And satisfy those whose judgment must be
>   respected
>   Under conditions of stress
> In a context of accelerating change.*

*Porter, P. J., Avery, E. H., and Fellows, J. T.: A model for the reorganization of child health services within an urban community, Am. J. Public Health **64:**618-619, June 1974.

†Campbell, R. F., and others: *Introduction to educational administration,* p. 189.

*Mayshark, C., and Shaw, D. D.: *Administration of school health programs,* p. 52.

The process of stating a goal and reaching it was described in the preceding section. It was implied in discussing the process that an administrator can, if he or she chooses to do so, either function alone or involve other people at each step. If he or she functions alone, the process is invisible, or nearly so, and therefore not possible to judge. Involvement makes the process visible and tends to satisfy those involved if group consensus is either accepted by the administrator or if rejection of the consensus is explained to the satisfaction of the group.

It is not to be expected that an effective administrator will involve others each time an administrative decision is to be made or that each consecutive step of the process will always be followed. A fair share of administrative decisions and implementations are of no legitimate interest to others or are the kinds of decisions that must be made and implemented quickly. A humane decision to grant an employee a brief leave to deal with an urgent personal problem when no leave time can be strictly justified under policy is one example. In this same instance little or no stimulation, coordination, or appraisal is called for. Thus one of the marks of an effective administrator is the use of good judgment in deciding when to involve others in the process and when the process can justifiably be condensed and how.

Another problem is that of satisfying "those whose judgment must be respected." An effective administrator is aware that no one can either satisfy or "fool all of the people all of the time." Administrative job security depends on satisfying most of the board members and most of the school staff most of the time. But with respect to any particular problem, the administrator must first identify those whose judgment must be respected in regard to that problem. In deciding whether and how to implement a program to screen black students for sickle cell anemia, for example, the judgment of white English teachers is not especially relevant, but the judgments of black students and parents, health service workers, health education professionals, expert professionals in the community, and principals of schools with substantial black populations are relevant. Persons identified as representative of the relevant groups who can also serve as communicators are then brought together and involved in its administrative process. Hopefully, most if not all of the representatives chosen will be willing and able to function as advocates of the young as well as of their adult group positions.

Stressful conditions can be both stimulative of useful and rewarding activity and destructive to individuals. In one city the stress of a period of rapid economic development and population immigration stimulated well-coordinated planning and implementation of school improvements of all kinds, including buildings, curriculum, community and staff relations, and the health program. That so much was accomplished in a few short years can be attributed to wise and democratic use of the administrative process by the superintendent. That those who planned and worked with him grew in self-esteem and commitment to the task attests to how well he understood human relations and motivations and how much he cared for individuals.

Another administrator, newly arrived in a settled, prosperous community attempted to initiate change from a traditional to an open classroom concept of education by administrative edict. The resulting storm of dissension and controversy divided students, staff, and citizens. He left town a failure in less than one semester.

Accelerating change is characteristic of modern society. Content in their roles and environment, some individuals resist change and are disturbed by it. Others seek to foster change out of discontent. Still others are committed to mediation. The effective administrator will usually utilize group processes that involve conservatives, activists, and mediators in an attempt to work out at least a compromise and, better yet, a consensus suitable to all. He or she will often act as a mediator. Only when a situation demands it will the effective administrator act as a referee, whose decision is accompanied by reasons that reflect concern for the feelings and rationales of those the judgment goes against.

The Peter Principle holds that in any hierarchial organization people tend to rise to their level of incompetence. A competent teacher may be promoted to principal. Incompetent teachers remain teachers. Competent principals tend to move further up the hierarchial ladder. Incompetent principals remain principals. In his book *The Peter Prescription* Peter suggests ways in which the mediocracy thus created can be mitigated. One proposal is that individuals can protect their own competence by knowing themselves and their goals, the hierarchy within which they work, and knowing how to defend themselves against promotion to their levels of incompetence. Another suggestion is that administrators attempt to function more competently by stating measurable goals, using rational processes to achieve them, basing prophecies on available hard evidence, and compensating people for goal achievement.*

"It's Not in the Budget." The director of finance of one school district received as a Christmas gift from his colleagues a recording of numerous repetitions of what the donors perceived to be his favorite words, "It's not in the budget!" In an authoritarian administration the implication of this perception is that it might evolve from dictatorial decision making. In the case cited, the director's frequent use of the phrase really represented enforcement of group decisions, because everyone concerned from teachers to the board of education, was involved in budget development and review. Lack of funds in the budget to implement a given administrative decision therefore resulted as much from lack of foresight by the participants in projecting needs as from the need of the board to limit taxes and the role of the director in carrying out board policy.

Staff participation in the development of

---

*Peter, L. J.: *The Peter prescription,* New York, 1972, William Morrow & Co., Inc.

a budget may be limited to estimating material needs required to conduct programs for the ensuing year. In other institutions staff may be requested to estimate both time and materials required to carry out each of the separate program functions in which they are involved. Rarely, estimates of the time and material costs of alternative ways of achieving program objectives may be sought. Each of these types of requests is related to a different basic form of budgeting.

All schools and all forms of budgeting include *line item budgeting.* In this form, separate budget lines (or costs) are developed for salaries and for each of several categories of expendable and nonexpendable equipment, supplies, travel funds, and the like. No differentiation is made as to the specific programs or program segments for which expenditures are intended. Thus, no specific estimate is made of the cost of the vision screening program.

In addition to line item budgeting, some school systems develop *functional or program budgets.* Such budgets break down proposed expenditures not only by object categories (such as salaries, supplies, equipment) but also by the programs for which their expenditure is anticipated (such as vision screening).

A few institutions have further refined budgeting format to include some type of *alternative budgeting.* In this form the costs of several different methods of reaching each program objective are estimated. For example, what is the anticipated cost of individually prescribed instruction in health education versus common group instruction? What benefits are likely to be achieved by each method?

The advantage of a pure line item budget over the other two forms is that it is much simpler to put together. Only one question is asked, "What do we need to conduct our proposed total program next year?" The disadvantage is that when cuts are made in the budget, as they usually are, a line item may be reduced to the extent that funds are insufficient to conduct a vital program segment, such as vision screening. Sufficient staff may be budgeted, but no allowance is made for equipment regarded as essential.

Functional or program budgeting requires additional effort. The proportion of the nurse's time and other line costs devoted to vision screening, for example, must be determined. When cuts are made, however, a single program segment can be deleted without affecting other programs. The line items will remain intact for the estimated costs of other programs that are retained.

Alternative budgeting is extremely difficult. All the analysis involved in line item and functional or program budgeting is still required. In addition, costs are estimated for two or more different ways of fulfilling a given program objective. The advantage is that when cuts are made, essential programs need not be deleted. Instead, a less expensive way of conducting a program can be selected.

Whichever form of budgeting is adopted is likely to be successful only if explicit instructions are given to those involved in the process, if expert consultation and advice are provided for them, and if they are given feedback and opportunity to discuss and approve changes as modifications are made by higher authority.

All groups need to be aware that a budget remains nothing more than a *proposed budget* or *budget request* until it is officially approved by the board of education as well as the superintendent. The reason for this is that these higher authorities are responsible for seeing to it that total expenditures do not exceed income except when a deficit in income is accepted as justified and is itself included in the budget.

Once a budget is adopted, living within it becomes the problem. Some degree of flexibility helps. Flexibility is often built into the budget in the form of a "contingency" line and as regulations that permit the transfer of funds from one specified line to another. Administrators also receive periodic reports that show cumulative expenditures to date against budgeted funds for the period. This information guides the closing off or continuation of expenditures in each line.

In practice, both administrators and staff members tend to overrequest funds on the grounds that their requests will be cut anyway and to expend all the money allotted because failure to do so is likely to result in a lower appropriation the following year. Financial administrators attempt to control these tendencies by requiring explicit justification of requested funds and prior approval of unusual expenditures. Awareness by all concerned that money that is overbudgeted and overspent increases their own tax rates, makes less money available for salary increases, and decreases public confidence in the schools may provide greater incentive than external controls to practice fiscal responsibility.

PUTTING IT ALL TOGETHER

Throughout this chapter the importance of *coordination* in both organization and administration has been stressed. In this section, structures and practice for coordination will be discussed.

Structure for coordination. It has been suggested that possible structures for coordination include informal procedures, ad hoc committees, standing councils or committees, specialized advisory committees, and combination or adaptations of the preceding forms.* Any or all may be utilized at any administrative level.

Informal procedures are unofficial or unplanned contacts between two or more people who share a problem and the resources or means to solve it. The local health officer and superintendent may thus meet regularly for lunch or casually at social events to discuss and solve mutual problems. A nurse and a teacher may meet for the same purpose over coffee in the faculty lounge. Such discussions can lead to direct solution of problems that are limited in

---

*National Conference on Coordination of the School Health Program: *Teamwork in school health,* Washington, D.C., 1972, American Association for Health, Physical Education, and Recreation, pp. 7-14.

scope, such as interpretation of a new health regulation or how to deal with an uncooperative parent. Or, they can lead to the recognition that others should be involved in the decision-making and/or implementation processes. One danger is that informal procedures may lead to decisions in which others should have been involved but were not. An advantage is that useful interpersonal relationships may be developed and strengthened.

Ad hoc committees are formally appointed for specific purposes and discharged when their missions are accomplished or when failure is acknowledged. Such a committee might be formed to coordinate health curriculum development, to plan a coordinated campaign to increase immunization levels, or to propose solutions to the problem of increasing vandalism, for example.

Advantages of ad hoc committees over other forms include their involvement of those who are closest to the specific problem, the saving in time and energy that might otherwise be spent in making numerous informal contacts, and that committee life does not continue beyond its time of usefulness. One limitation is the likelihood that interprofessional or interagency conflict may impede progress. Others are that these committees may tend to overlook the implications of their recommendations for the total school health program and that they may be discharged before their recommendations are implemented and can be evaluated.

Standing councils or committees have been utilized in the continuing coordination of school health and health education for many years. In some localities the appellation "committee" is used to designate a building level group, while "council" indicates a district or systemwide unit. Such councils and committees typically concern themselves with the total school health and health education program and may include in their membership representatives of the school and public health administrations and staffs, other community health agencies and professional groups, parents, students, and

others closely involved in or affected by the total program. They may meet either regularly or on call and may have more or less formal structures, including standing or ad hoc subcommittees.

Specialized advisory committees, as the designation indicates, are designed to provide specialized technical advice. Such a committee, for example, might bring together school and community specialists in law, obstetrics, social work, nursing, and other relevant disciplines to advise school professionals or the school health committee or council regarding proposed policies or programs relating to pregnant students. They reflect specialist opinions, not necessarily those of the community, and therefore may properly be regarded as adjuncts to other coordinating structures rather than as substitutes for them.

Combinations or *adaptations* of the above structures are probably more the rule than the exception. Informal procedures are likely to be stimulated by contacts made in formal settings. In one possible adaptation the school health committee or council functions as part of a larger community health council.

Still another adaptation is an organized group of school and community professionals who conduct case conferences in which the relevant resources of the community are brought to bear on developing and coordinating solutions to individual problems of children and young people.

Practices in coordination. Principles and guidelines that apply regardless of the structures utilized and that are essential to successful democratic coordination have evolved from experience. A number of these are listed below.

1. Any person or group that recognizes a problem can and should call attention to it.
2. That legally vested authority, such as that of the superintendent or health officer, cannot be delegated must be recognized. Therefore, the role of coordinating structures is advisory.
3. For the above reason, the success of

a coordinating group depends on the active involvement and commitment of relevant officials.

4. Without a problem, a coordinating group has nothing to coordinate.
5. Success breeds success, and failure breeds failure. Therefore, new coordinating groups should start with easy problems and tackle hard ones only after success has been achieved.
6. Effectiveness increases with broadness of representation but decreases with size. Solutions to this paradox include selection of representatives of more than one public (a teacher who is also a parent) and the use of subcommittees.
7. Special interest groups should be invited to name their own representatives. This increases the likelihood that the representative will really represent the group and communicate with it.
8. Parliamentary legalizing and complex structures tend to focus on roles and process rather than problems. This tends to result in majority decisions rather than solid consensus. Therefore, keep the structure simple. For further guidance, observe a Quaker meeting.
9. Success depends on stimulating leadership and on logical problem solving. Persons with such qualities will emerge in almost any group if identified and allowed to exercise their capabilities.
10. Coordination is the role of a coordinating group. Defined roles, like good fences, make good neighbors. Therefore, such groups should confine themselves to planning and avoid the actual conduct of programs.

Getting along with administrators. Contrary to the Peter Principle, Cuban found that the average tenure among big city school superintendents had declined to just over 4 years. Those few who had successfully retained their jobs for many years were those he classified as "negotiator-statesmen,"

leaders who tended to practice the principles of democratic administration described above. Ineffective superintendents may therefore not have to be endured for long.

Cuban* classified those who did not last on the job as teacher-scholars and administrative chiefs. Both make the important decisions themselves. They seek to avoid too much involvement of others, and they abhor conflict. Those staff members who obey their directives, respond promptly to their requests for information, and avoid rocking the boat will probably outlast either type.

The negotiator-statesmen demand staff involvement and seem to welcome conflict, because they believe that resolving conflicts breeds change and progress. Individuals whose professional commitment demands that they be involved in change and decision making are most likely to find lasting job satisfaction with a negotiator-statesman administrator.

QUESTIONS FOR STUDY AND DISCUSSION

1. What major characteristics distinguish "organization" from "administration?"
2. Debate the issue of joint or health department control versus board of education control of school health programs, citing other arguments as well as those included in the text.
3. Distinguish between "pure line," "line and staff," and "functional" plans of organization. What are the advantages and disadvantages inherent in each? How would a health teacher or nurse work to accomplish his or her goals under each of these plans?
4. What are the six operational tasks of school administration identified by Campbell and his associates? Which best represents the primary task of the school? Why can school health and health education justifiably be said to be involved in all of them?
5. Under what administrative departments in your school system is responsibility for school health instruction, health services, and healthful environment placed? Where would you prefer them to be placed, and why?
6. List and describe each of the five components of the administrative process identified by Campbell and his associates. What are the implications of the administrative process for

*Cuban, L.: Urban superintendents: vulnerable experts, Phi Delta Kappan **56**:279-282, Dec, 1974.

the behavior of professionals at the building level?

7. State and explain Mayshark and Shaw's definition of administrative ability. How and why does this change or confirm your own perception of how an effective administrator operates?

8. How does an effective administrator institute change, and why does he or she do it that way?

9. Read *The Peter Prescription;* it is brief, inexpensive, funny, and stimulating. How did reading it change or confirm your view of an administrative position as a personal goal, and why? What new tips did you pick up as to how effective administrators operate?

10. Distinguish between and cite the relative advantages and disadvantages of *pure line item, functional or program,* and *alternative* budgeting. Distinguish between a *budget* and a *budget request or proposal.*

11. As a teacher or other school staff professional, how, if at all, would you expect to be involved in budget development? Would you welcome such involvement or not, and why?

12. Some administrators try to present fully justifiable budget requests and to live within their budget allocations. Others pad requests and overspend allocations as a matter of course. Suggest reasons favoring and opposed to each of these types of behavior.

13. List and describe each of the possible structures for coordination cited in the text. What are the advantages and disadvantages of each?

14. What principles and guidelines are cited to guide democratic coordination processes? From your own experiences on committees or other such structures can you present case histories that support or cast doubt on any of these guidelines or that suggest others not cited in the text?

REFERENCES

Campbell, R. F., and others: *Introduction to educational administration,* ed. 4, Boston, 1971, Allyn & Bacon, Inc.

Council of Chief State School Officers and Association of State and Territorial Health Officers: *Responsibilities of state departments of education and health for school health services,* Washington, D.C., 1954, The Council.

Mayshark, C., and Shaw, D. D.: *Administration of school health programs,* St. Louis, 1967, The C. V. Mosby Co.

National Conference on Coordination of the School Health Program: *Teamwork in school health,* Washington, D.C., 1962, American Association for Health, Physical Education, and Recreation.

Peter, L. J.: *The Peter prescription,* New York, 1972, William Morrow & Co., Inc.

PART THREE

School health education

CHAPTER 5 ❧ Planning for health instruction

The success of most human enterprises, including educational programs, is dependent on (1) sound planning and (2) good execution. The relationship between these factors is somewhat analogous to that between the neural and cardiovascular systems of the human body. They both are highly essential to the life and integrity of the total organism, each is dependent on the other, and in many instances their functions are so intertwined as to appear to overlap. To push the comparison a bit further, the planning function, like many of the less visible systems of the body, often fails to receive full credit for the importance of its contribution. The casual observer of a teacher operating within a good program of health education tends to base his or her judgments solely on the teacher's skills of execution, that is, on his or her ability to use various teaching techniques. The teacher's success is credited to speaking ability, to the clever use of role playing, or to the simple capacity of relating well to the students. The teacher's performance in the classroom is somewhat like the tip of an iceberg; one must look beneath the surface to gain an appreciation of the sizable structure that supports it. In the teacher's case the support is provided by an elaborate planning process.

ROLE OF PLANNING

When conducted properly as in an exemplary program of health instruction, the planning process is almost infinitely subtle and complicated, with many persons and factors making their contributions in successive stages as specific aspects of the program move from the drawing board to the classroom. The analysis of this complex phenomenon probably best begins at the end rather than the beginning, that is, with the action in the classroom that comprises the end result of the planning process. Consider, for example, the following description of a single day's experiences of a hypothetical teacher in a better than average program.

A day's health instruction. As we look in on Miss Richards's first period health class, we find that she is preparing her group of high school seniors for the viewing of a film dealing with a regional effort to combat water pollution. In this process she briefly outlines the main points that will be presented and asks the class to make a special effort to identify the persons, groups, or circumstances that made major contributions to the success of the river cleanup campaign that was described in the film. Immediately following the 20-minute film she asks for questions or comments on the film, and a short 5-minute class discussion ensues. At this point she distributes a single page "film reaction sheet" consisting of five provocative questions on the film's contents, together with appropriate spaces for their written answers; she gives the class the balance of the period to work on this assignment.

The events that took place in her second period class were almost identical to first period except perhaps for the fact that the discussion following the film ran a bit longer. Her third period class also began in much the same manner but soon took a quite different course. Immediately following the film some of the students challenged the manner in which many of the main facts were presented and interpreted by the makers of the film. In one sequence the president of a major chemical company voluntarily ordered the purchase and installation of $1.5 million of antipollution equipment in order to render his plant's liquid wastes safe for discharge into the river. This particular group of seniors had just finished a unit on the American corporation in their American problems class, and they generally felt that this corporate president's behavior was unique rather than typical as depicted by the film. As one student put it, "That guy has got to be some sort of ecology 'nut'; those bigwigs don't act that way; why, he'd be torn apart in the next meeting of his board of directors!"

"That might make an interesting scene," concurred Miss Richards, "Let's see how that might go." With this she recruited a "president" and five "directors" and placed them around a table at the front of the room. For the balance of the period the "president" sought to defend his actions to the "board" on the basis of their public relations value and their probable effect of heading off the even more expensive measures that aroused federal agencies might impose. As one might suspect, she never got around to handing out the film reaction guide in this class.

As we observe her fourth and final health class, we might conclude that she has completely abandoned the curriculum plan. The film projector and screen have been removed, and in their place we find a panel of students at the front of the room presenting a series of reports, not on water pollution as a regional problem, but on air pollution in the local community. The first student panelist related the main points she had learned in an interview with the chairman of a local citizen's group that was working in support of a clean environment and embellished her report with playbacks of portions of the actual interview on a tape recorder. The second panel member supported his report both with data on pollution levels provided by the local public health department and by a series of colored slides of billowing factory stacks, burning garbage, and smoky automobiles. The final panelist reported the views of several members of the city council who responded to his letters concerning the proposed new air pollution control ordinance.

Behind the scenes analysis. The obvious differences in the classroom activities of this teacher's various sections make it appear that she was operating basically as a free agent who was improvising the curriculum from day to day and in some cases from minute to minute. Although she had indeed made many adjustments, a deeper analysis of her activities reveals that she was operating within the limits of a fairly tightly organized curricular framework and one that represented the planning efforts of several persons whose influence was exerted over an extended period of time. It would be impossible to identify the genesis of every aspect of any curriculum; however, in this case the sequence probably went something like this.

State legislature. Approximately 10 years prior to this episode the state legislature drafted a law that outlined a health and physical education requirement in general terms and among other things specified that "Instruction shall include material related to nutrition; disease prevention; safety; alcohol, tobacco, and drug abuse; health products and services; community health organizations; mental hygiene and family living." This action established the basic *content area* of community health within which Miss Richards was teaching on the day of our observation.

Local school district. The initial response to this broad and extremely general mandate was a district level curriculum project, which produced a relatively primitive health education guide based primarily on the textbook that was then in current use. This early effort was considerably improved 5 years later by a similar committee, which developed a conceptually based health curriculum within the general framework of the state law. Within the topic of community health they identified four concepts or "big ideas"* to serve as focal points for learning

---

*Fodor, J. T., and Dalis, G. T.: *Health instruction: theory and application,* ed. 2, Philadelphia, 1974, Lea & Febiger, p. 28.

experiences on a kindergarten through grade twelve basis. Among these one was worded, "The actions which a community takes to protect the health of its members are affected by a wide variety of factors." Here we see the origin of the *concept* that provided general guidance to Miss Richards's activities on this particular day. This committee also specified one *behavioral objective* related to this concept for each school level. The one for the senior high level was stated:

> Given a description of a community's efforts to solve a serious health problem, the learner will identify the persons, groups, or circumstances which have major effects on the decision-making process and discuss the nature of these effects.

Although this behavioral objective is not worded as specifically as many of the more zealous proponents of behavioral objectives might wish, it does convey to the teacher the curriculum committee's decision that senior high school students should study a community health problem of some sort and determine who or what in the community was helping solve the problem and perhaps what forces were contributing to its intensity. In support of this task the committee had also incorporated into the district curriculum guide a brief *content outline,* four suggested *learning activities,* suggested *resources* including both references for the teacher and materials for student use, and, finally, suggested techniques for *evaluation.*

Building committee. In this case a formalized health curriculum committee did not exist within Miss Richards's particular school; however, the health instructors did meet during the 2 days that had been alloted during the previous spring for planning and in-service training. They reviewed the district guide and noted that the content outline tended to place heavy emphasis on citizens' protest groups and demonstrations as factors that affect community health decisions. Although such groups had been highly active 5 years earlier when the district guide was written, their watchdog role was now being handled with reasonable effectiveness by special government agencies that their pressure had helped create; conse-

quently, the health education staff members opted for a more balanced emphasis, giving attention to official agencies, business and industrial groups, government agencies, the mass media, and a variety of economic factors and conflicting public needs that were affecting public opinion. This group also at this meeting reviewed their film needs for the coming year and ordered, among others, the film that Miss Richards used in three of her four classes.

Individual instructor. Immediately following the spring meeting, Miss Richards did some additional planning of her own as she made tentative decisions concerning the basic approach she would take to various units of study, giving particular attention to any teacher materials or resources that she would need so that purchase orders, requests to the school's librarian or to the instructional material center director, orders for free materials, and so forth could be made at that time. These plans were "fine-tuned" once the fall term began a week or two prior to the beginning of each unit. By the time the community health unit approached, she had observed that her first three classes seemed to function best in tightly structured learning situations, whereas the fourth was willing and able to take the initiative in pupil-centered activities. Here emphasis was placed on the next stage of the planning process.

Teacher-learner planning. Some degree of student participation took place in all of Miss Richards's classes, ranging in importance from a simple allowance of individual choice of topics for special reports to full cooperative planning of the topic, as was apparently the case in her fourth period class. The degree of class participation depended basically on the readiness of the particular group involved, and in turn this readiness was dependent on many factors such as the previous experience of the class in cooperative planning, their familiarity or lack of familiarity with the topic at hand, and the presence or absence of student leadership within the group. During the planning process Miss Richards had limited the class to options that fell within the concept and behavioral objectives for the community health unit; however, as noted these were broadly stated, thus allowing a broad range of choices. It should also be noted that both teacher and students were represented in the original committee that had specified these components of the curriculum.

Teacher improvisation during class. The adjustments that most experienced teachers occasionally make in their lesson plans in response to conditions that develop during the course of the lesson represent perhaps the most intimate relationship between the

planning and the implementation processes. During this particular day of Miss Richards's teaching the best example of this occurred within her third period class when she abandoned her use of the film reaction guide and organized an impromptu role-playing situation of the ecology-minded executive and his board of directors. This was a departure from the preplanned activities; however, once again this change occurred within the larger framework of the task specified 5 years earlier by the district committee. Both the film guide and the content of the role-playing situation provided students the opportunity to identify and discuss fac-

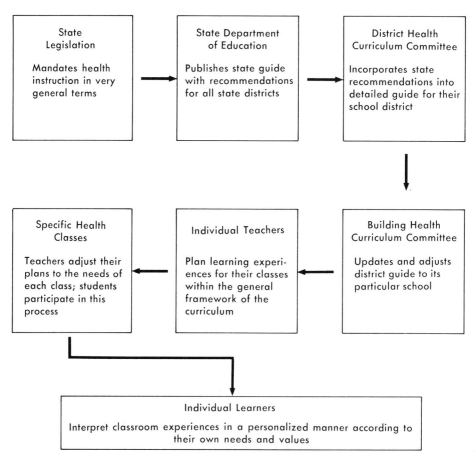

Fig. 5-1. Curriculum planning in school health education. Although no flow chart can incorporate the many subtleties and complexities of the planning process, the health curriculum typically begins as a generalized plan that is devised by persons remote from the actual teaching situation and then undergoes successive modifications and embellishments as it moves closer to each individual instance of application.

tors affecting decision making in community health problems as prescribed by the behavioral objective.

Learner response. Within the course of this hypothetical situation the planning process has been followed from the extremely general form it took as legislation at the state level, through successive changes at the district, building, and individual teacher levels, to its ultimate implementation in a form appropriate to a particular classroom group of students. The final recipient of all this planning is, of course, the individual learner, but this recipient is not simply a receptacle into which the end products of the curriculum are deposited. Individual students each make some final adjustments of their own as the facts, emotional connotations, and other perceptions reach them in the classroom. Some items too alien to a particular learner's interest pattern or value structure will be retained in that portion of the brain labeled "for test purposes only," whereas still other items that are more compatible will be built into his or her permanent conceptual structure and thus carry the potential for affecting future behavior relative to the issue involved, which is in this case community action for health needs. This total planning process is shown graphically in Fig. 5-1.

Importance of the teacher's planning role. Because teachers are the principal implementers of the curriculum, the importance of their role in actualizing or "bringing to life in the classroom" the products of the planning process is obvious. However, despite the fact that the school's curriculum is officially controlled by various laws, regulations, and policies formulated by various agencies and committees operating outside the classroom, teachers typically play a crucial role in the planning as well as the implementing process. This is particularly true as applied to health education. There appear to be two major reasons for this; one is characteristic of good management of the health program, whereas the other represents a by-product of program neglect.

Built-in flexibility. Those persons responsible for the development of state or district level curriculum guides often word the main components of the curriculum in general terms and thus depend on teachers to translate this material into the most effective terms for their particular students. In the example above, the teachers were asked to teach about the factors affecting decisions made in efforts to cope with community health problems; however, the specific problems and factors to be studied were left largely in the hands of the teacher. Another behavioral objective might require that students describe the characteristics of two drugs commonly abused within their community; consequently, one teacher might appropriately discuss amphetamines and barbiturates, whereas another teacher operating within another community might approach this objective by presenting material on alcohol and heroin.

It is neither practical nor efficient to produce detailed curriculum guides each year for each subject within each school district; therefore, the planning of such guides is typically done by persons who are removed by many months of time and sometimes by many miles of space from the actual situations of use. Built-in flexibility is essential under these circumstances, but with these disadvantages go certain compensations. Major planning groups often have far more than individual teachers in terms of material and human resources as well as the time to study student needs, societal trends, and other such foundational factors in depth and thus assemble a sound curricular framework. Ideally, teachers and curriculum planners form a balanced team in the planning process.

Administrative neglect. A second major reason for the teacher's importance, which applies to many school situations, does not reflect favorably on the programs involved. This is the not uncommon tendency for many schools to neglect health education. In some cases all the attention may go to the "academic" subjects. In other instances the program may exist as an unwanted stepchild of physical education or of the health service program.

The reasons for this attitude may vary, but the effects are much the same. There is little support for curriculum planning; there may be no money for hiring consultants or even for providing clerical help for the committee. Once completed, the curriculum guide is seldom revised; consequently, the new teacher may arrive on the scene and be presented with a guide that was written 10 years ago under poor circumstances. It is probably fortunate that in such situations the supervision of health instruction is also lax and teachers are thus spared the frustration of trying to implement such poorly conceived content. Often the entire planning process comes under their control by default. Such blantant examples are rare; however, in virtually all school districts there is a certain degree of administrative lag in the planning process for which teachers must compensate.

PRODUCTS OF PLANNING

A thorough understanding of the planning process as applied to health education requires a consideration of, first, the products of planning and, second, the process by which these products are created. It is difficult to comprehend this relatively complex process without first examining what it is directed toward. Therefore, this discussion will begin with a look at the curriculum guides, courses of study, unit plans, and lesson plans that comprise its visible results. Although the underlying principles, which should guide the development of these necessary items, are logical and simple enough, a relatively complex terminology has developed for describing the various components. This complexity has been compounded by the constant emergence of new terms, by the lack of authoritative definitions of terms, and by failure on the part of many professionals to adhere to accepted definitions. Therefore, those making their first venture into the unique world of curriculum planning may sometimes feel they have blundered into a swamp that contains precious little solid ground. Hopefully this section will provide sufficient landmarks for a safe journey.

Structural components. The visible products of the planning process, whether they be state guides or daily lesson plans, are typically prepared in the form of written documents and, except for lesson plans, are designed to communicate directions or suggestions to teachers who often did not participate in their creation. Although these documents vary greatly in scope and format, depending on their basic purpose and preferences and sometimes on the idiosyncrasies of their sponsoring group, they tend to be very similar in their basic structure. Many of the same components can be found within any guide or unit plan even though different terms may be used to label and describe them. A brief review of the general purpose and function of these basic components can lead to a better understanding and use of these various types of written plans.

Statements of philosophy. Among the most pervasive factors influencing the general tone and content of any planning document are the beliefs of the planner or planners in regard to the basic elements involved in the teaching of their subject. As applied to health education, these are such things as the nature of health, the role of health education, the natural characteristics of children and youth, and the nature of the learning process. One group, for example, might believe very strongly that learning experiences should be directed toward the encouragement of specific types of behavior such as the brushing of teeth, the avoidance of cigarette smoking, and the use of compromise or negotiation in settling conflicts. Another group, however, might view the main task of health education as the promotion of a better understanding of the underlying factors that affect health status and might tend to leave the specific behavioral choices to the learner. The writers of curriculum documents in most cases have an obligation to put these basic beliefs on record (that is, to tell potential users of these products "where they're coming from," so to speak) as an aid to the potential user's interpretation and evaluation of their material.

Although most groups recognized this obligation, many of them find it very difficult to meet. The task of identifying and verbalizing one's salient beliefs is a complex and somewhat unnatural task for most persons. Consequently, many statements of philosophy tend to be meaningless assemblages of clichés, broad generalities, and authoritative definitions. After encountering a few such efforts, one tends to ignore philosophical statements and rely instead on inferences drawn from the main content of the guide as clues to its philosophical thrust. Although this procedure is often necessary, it is well to give the philosophical statement a chance; some of them are well expressed and serve to increase the usefulness of the guide.

Goals. The goals of a total school curriculum or of a major portion of the curriculum should describe the end results that the planner would like to see achieved in terms of increased capabilities, favorable attitudes, or other types of behavioral change as manifested by the learner. For example, a guide developed for the schools of Los Angeles County includes the following goals:

1. Cares for the human body
2. Develops a mature personality
3. Builds a satisfying human relationship
4. Assumes a responsible health role in society
5. Copes with contemporary health problems*

Although these goals are stated in terms of learner behavior, they are expressed in very general terms so that the entire thrust of the program could be incorporated in a manageable list of statements. It is not feasible to word goals in a manner that would make them directly testable. However, when carefully and accurately stated, they provide guidance to the development of the more specific components of the curriculum, such as concepts or behavioral objectives. For example, goals 2 and 3 of this particular group suggest the need for a strong emphasis on mental health, particularly on

normal personality and human relations rather than on pathological aspects.

Content areas. The goals of any curriculum or major subject are, in effect, a further experssion of the basic philosophy of those constructing the curriculum. Therefore the first structural components of the curriculum, which are usually formed by a curriculum committee, are the content areas; these are the major subjects or topics around which learning experiences are formed. Within a well-constructed curriculum the content areas are known technically as *organizing elements* because they extend vertically through all levels of the curriculum from kindergarten to grade twelve. Examples of these components in their traditional form are nutrition, disease, mental health, and family living; however, the current trend is toward more broadly stated areas of study that encompass the increased scope of the subject matter of modern health curricula. The relatively new Maryland state guide for health education organized its content into these six areas:

1. Natural conditions
2. Man-made products and services
3. Social forces
4. Sensory stimulation
5. Assimilated substances
6. Genetic perpetuation*

Each curriculum group will usually devise a different set of content areas in keeping with its particular views; however, almost all versions serve to divide the curriculum into five to ten sections that are relevant to all grade levels. For instance, "disease control" might be a logical content area, whereas "venereal disease" would not since it would have little relevance at the primary level.

Concepts. According to one authoritative definition, a concept is "a relatively complete and meaningful idea in the mind of a person. It is an understanding of something."† As "meaningful ideas," concepts

Project Quest: health instructional guide, Los Angeles, Calif., 1968, Los Angeles County Superintendent of Schools.

Health education: a curricular approach to optimal health, Baltimore, Md., 1973, Maryland State Department of Education.
†Woodruff, A. D.: *Basic concepts of teaching,* San Francisco, 1961, Chandler Publishing Co.

tend to be retained by the learner and affect his or her behavior over extended periods of time, perhaps for a lifetime. Consequently, it is important that concepts be valid and comprehensive if they are to lead the learner into favorable health practices. A young person who views physicians as basically unscrupulous purveyors of pills and needless surgery would probably be unable to function as a good patient because of this concept. A good program of health education might, among many other things, help young people develop a truer concept of the general range of competence and ethical conduct of physicians so as to encourage their development as intelligent and discriminating consumers of health care.

In the process of curriculum development many groups have found it useful to state the main components of their content in conceptual form. The following are examples of conceptual statements.

> The vast majority of disease control is accomplished by "natural defenses," disease-retarding factors contained within the body.
> Water pollution and water uses must often be controlled through joint action at local, regional, state, national, and even international levels.
> Cultural and environmental factors have a considerable influence on the development of personality and behavior.*

Learning experiences designed to help young people develop concepts such as these could be presented at any grade level, provided that the specific content involved was well selected. Consequently, concepts are often used to divide the content areas into smaller, more specific vertical strands that extend throughout the K-12 curriculum. The second grade child, for example, might be taught that "the right foods and sufficient sleep help his body fight disease" by a teacher who is seeking to develop the first concept above pertaining to "natural defenses." This same general idea would reappear periodically in the curriculum in successively more complex forms, culminat-

ing at the senior high level in a relatively sophisticated study of the antigen-antibody response as it applies to immunity, allergies, tissue rejection, and possible defense against cancer.

Behavioral objectives. The development of a concept, such as an understanding of the natural defenses of the body against disease, to the optimal degree of complexity requires many well-ordered learning experiences extending over the learner's total school career. A well-selected and well-stated behavioral objective represents one effective way to describe to a particular teacher the learning experience his or her students need at their present stage of development.

Objectives become "behavioral" objectives when they describe an educational task in terms of observable behavior, that is, in terms of what the learner becomes capable of doing as a result of the learning experience. This characteristic enables behavioral objectives to be used as evaluative tools as well as guides to learning experiences. This is particularly true when behavioral objectives are written in "strict constructionist" style such as that advocated by Robert Mager. He provides the following example:

> Given a human skeleton, the student must be able to correctly identify by labeling at least 40 of the following bones; there will be no penalty for guessing (list of bones inserted here).*

This objective includes the four components of a fully "Magerized" objective: (1) *the conditions* under which the learner is to operate are described in the phrase "given a human skeleton"; (2) *the behavior* the learner is to exhibit is clearly specified as "correctly identifying by labeling"; (3) *the content* is described as "the following bones" together with the inserted list; and (4) *the performance* criterion is provided by the words "at least 40." Although purist would maintain that all four are essential, the behavioral component is commonly regarded as the key to an objective's

Health concepts: guides for health instruction, Washington, D.C., 1967, American Association for Health, Physical Education, and Recreation.

*Mager, R. F.: *Preparing instructional objectives,* Palo Alto, Calif., 1962, Fearon Publishers, p. 49.

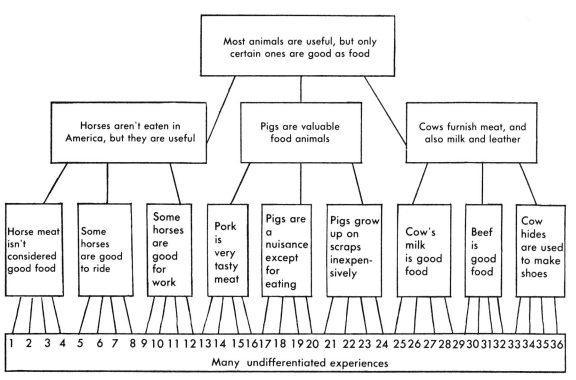

Fig. 5-2. Concept development from undifferentiated experiences to a generalized concept. In the 36 different experiences shown along the bottom of the figure, the child became partly familiar with many things. Among them were the following experiences that helped to produce the concepts shown above them. Numbers in the chart match those below. (From Woodruff, A. D.: *Basic concepts of teaching,* San Francisco, 1961, Chandler Publishing Co.)

1. I had a pet horse.
2. I saw a man feed his cat horse meat.
3. My friends make fun of horse meat.
4. I read a ban on horse meat in the Bible.
5. I saw a man riding a horse.
6. I had a ride on a horse.
7. I rode a work horse, but it was not comfortable.
8. I heard people talk about good riding horses.
9. I saw a high-spirited horse wreck a cart.
10. I saw a strong horse pull a load.
11. A farmer's horse pulled our car.
12. I saw a picture of a horse pulling an ore car.
13. I tasted some bacon.
14. I had some baked ham.
15. I had some barbecued ribs.
16. I had some sausage.
17. I have never seen a pig work.
18. The pigs I saw were dirty.
19. I saw Mr. Black try to catch a pig and he couldn't.
20. Pig squeals hurt my ears.
21. I fed scraps to some pigs.
22. I saw pigs eating weeds.
23. We feed our pigs waste corn husks.
24. We bought a little feed for them.
25. I tasted some cream.
26. We made some butter.
27. We made some ice cream.
28. We ate some hot milk toast.
29. We had a roast.
30. I ate some liver.
31. I had a steak.
32. I saw an ad for beef.
33. I visited a shoe shop.
34. I tanned some hide.
35. I read a news item on leather.
36. My shoe label says "Top grain leather."

value as a facilitator of accountability or evaluation. When such verbs as "lists," "identifies," or "selects" are used, it is relatively easy to determine whether or not the learner has indeed achieved the objective; whereas the use of such verbs as "understands," "appreciates," or "realizes" make evaluation much more difficult.

Critics of behavioral objectives feel that precision is gained at the expense of relevance as classroom experiences are reduced to a series of listing, matching, sorting, and defining while efforts to achieve a true understanding of important concepts are neglected. Proponents, however, point out that the relative balance between relevance and precision can be varied to meet the needs of particular programs and emphasize the value of analyzing learning experiences in terms of their most important result, namely, improvement in the learner's behavioral capabilities. The wisest course probably lies somewhere between the extremes of this controversy; behavioral objectives can be highly useful in communicating the learning outcomes a curriculum planning group feel would be most worthwhile. However, such groups must not allow their real decisions to be distorted by the need to meet unrealistic standards of precision.*

Other critics of behavioral objectives maintain that these objectives are useful only to describe cognitive behaviors such as comprehending, analyzing, and so forth and have little value in identifying affective outcomes such as responding, accepting, and supporting, which lie in the general realm of attitudes and values. In all likelihood this view results from the fact that those curriculum builders who are partial to behavioral objectives do not like the loss in precision and accountability that is often a necessary result of efforts to deal with feelings and emotions in the classroom. But if the

desired outcomes pertain to these types of behaviors, then any curriculum guide or unit plan must communicate them to the classroom teachers. This can be done quite effectively by use of behavioral objectives. Consider the following example:

Given a description of a continuum of drug-taking behavior ranging from the refusal to take drugs under any circumstances to the use of drugs as the central purpose of one's life, the learners will locate their personal positions on this continuum and examine them in comparison to the positions taken by their classmates.

Any teacher familiar with values clarification techniques (see pp. 104-105) would have little trouble devising classroom learning experiences that would provide the learner with an opportunity to meet this objective. In this manner behavioral objectives serve the highly useful function of communicating clear, concise descriptions of the recommendations of a planning group to their professional colleagues who must implement the health education program. The classroom teacher is of course the most important target of this communication process.

Content outlines. In years past the teaching of carefully selected facts and principles was often regarded as an end in itself. This point of view often carried with it a view of teaching as telling and explaining things to the students in which the emphasis was placed on what the teacher did in the classroom rather than on what the students achieved. The primary responsibility of teachers was to "cover" the material, and this could be done effectively by lecturing from an outline of the topics to be covered. Within this general educational approach the content outline became the major component of many curriculum guides. There may have been a statement of philosophy and some general goals at the front of the documents and a resource list at the rear, but the main body of the guide consisted basically of an outline of the material to be covered within various units of study.

Within the modern curriculum or unit guide the content outline still retains an important place, but its role has been re-

*For a useful discussion of the controversy surrounding behavioral objectives see Gagne, R. N.: Behavioral Objectives? Yes! and Kueller, G. F.: Behavioral Objectives? No!, both articles in Educational Leadership **29:**394-416, Feb. 1972.

duced to that of a single component within a coordinated group of components. It has been replaced by the behavioral objective as the immediate end product of classroom learning, and it basically provides the teacher with the information the learners need to attain the objective.

Suggested methods and materials. In the modern view the "medium is often the message"; consequently, part of the traditional function of the content outline has also been usurped by the methods and materials sections of the typical curriculum guide. Often the "how" of teaching (the methods used) is so intimately related to the "what" (the health information) that it is difficult to distinguish between them. Health educators have also come to recognize the fact that learners need the involvement with the subject matter that good methods and good materials can provide if they are to retain and put into practice the things they learn in the classroom. Under the traditional system information often hit the students like a flash flood that built up rapidly for a final examination or unit test then "ran off" equally as fast with little opportunity for absorption. The more modern view maintains that less content should be presented but that it should be presented more effectively; thus suggestions for teaching approaches and specific types of media to use have become increasingly important. The terms used to describe these two types of teacher aids vary considerably with such examples as "learning activities," "learning opportunities," and "teaching-learning activities," which are commonly used for the former, and "learning resources," "learning materials," "teacher-learner resources," and similar terms often used for the latter. Also, it is not uncommon to see these two categories combined in a single section because of their close relationship.

Evaluation. Most health educators support the view that evaluation should be an integral part of the teaching-learning process rather than something that takes the form of a test at the end of a unit of study for purposes of threatening and grading the students. In the modern format evaluative or assessment activities commonly are provided for each behavioral objective so that both teachers and learners can receive day-to-day feedback on the effectiveness of their efforts. These evaluative procedures often become learning activities in themselves as learners are encouraged to discuss, apply, or in some cases dramatize through role playing the things they have learned in the classroom. The visible results of learning, such as increased knowledge or perhaps obvious attitudinal changes that can be observed in the classroom, are the focal points for this type of evaluation. The larger task of overall program evaluation, which often includes efforts to identify improvements in real life behavior that typically take place outside the classroom, usually requires more elaborate procedures as described in Chapter 20.

Planning documents. The curriculum-planning process basically consists of a series of decisions as to what educational experiences should be presented to particular groups of students at particular maturity levels. As noted, teachers play a crucial role in this general task; however, there are limitations to their planning effectiveness resulting from both their training, which typically included heavy emphasis on methodology rather than content selection, and the situation within which they typically operate. The heavy demands of the daily details of classroom teaching make it difficult for them to retain the perspective needed to select content that articulates effectively with that presented at other grade levels (the vertical organization of the curriculum). Also, at the secondary level the problem of coordinating health content with that of such related subjects as science and social studies (horizontal organization) becomes more than any one teacher can manage. These and other reasons make it necessary for planning groups to make many important curriculum decisions on the basis of a broader perspective. However, these decisions, suggestions, directions, or whatever are of little value unless they are communicated in some effective manner. This function is provided by various curriculum documents.

SHES model. During the late 1950's and throughout the 1960's many national study groups were formed for the purpose of bringing together the human and material resources necessary to produce model curricula related to specific teaching fields. The School Health Education Study (SHES) represents such an effort as applied to the specific field of health education. This project is outstanding both in terms of its ultimate result, that is, its curriculum recommendations, and in the very thorough procedures that were used to achieve this result. The work began with a thorough review of recent research pertinent to health instruction as a means of taking full advantage of what was already known about this complex endeavor; the results of this effort were published in the form of a useful monograph.* Program improvement logically begins and builds upon the programs currently in place. Therefore, a national survey was conducted to determine the status of such programs both in terms of such external conditions as class size, time allotments, and the training level of the teachers and on the basis of the health knowledge and practices of the young people whom these programs were designed to help; the results of this phase also were published as a special report.†

With the data base thus established, a writing team was assembled consisting of persons whose backgrounds included training and experience in health content, curriculum design, and program implementation. They devised a somewhat complex but very sound and logical curriculum structure that included among other components ten topical areas, which were designated by conceptual statements rather than by simple labels, as is the traditional practice. Authoritative reviews were obtained for all por-

tions of the first draft of this new curriculum, and the curriculum recommendations for two of the ten major content areas received extensive field trials in the schools of four major systems, which were widely separated geographically. On the basis of the information gained from these reviews and field tests, a final draft of the curriculum was prepared. The rationale and basic structure of this model health curriculum is described in the study's basic document entitled *Health Education: A Conceptual Approach to Curriculum Design.**

SHES in all its phases and operations had a strong positive effect upon the general effort to initiate and improve school programs of classroom health education. Some school districts chose to adopt the program in its entirety; some adopted certain portions and/or adapted the material in accordance with their best judgment of their situation. A great many other school systems who chose to develop their own health curricula from the ground up modeled their procedures and the structural framework of their curricula along SHES lines even though the actual content may have taken a different form.

State guides. In order to provide a helpful resource for individual teachers and planning groups at the local level, many state departments of health or education publish state guides. Although their purposes are similar, they vary greatly in their format and their recommendations. The *Maryland State Guide* is one of the more elaborate of these documents. Based on a comprehensive conceptual structure, it provides behavioral objectives for each of four school levels together with specific content, learning activities, and assessment tasks (evaluation). Within the supporting components for each behavioral objective, more suggestions are provided than any one teacher can use, thus allowing for selection according to local needs. It should be noted that the health edu-

---

*Veenker, C. H., editor: *Synthesis of research in selected areas of health instruction,* Washington, D.C., 1963, School Health Education Study.
†Sliepcevich, E. M.: *School health education study: a summary report,* Washington, D.C., 1964, School Health Education Study.

---

*School Health Education Study: *Health education: a conceptual approach to curriculum design,* St. Paul, Minn., 1967, 3M Education Press.

cation content mandated by the various state legislatures is generally quite broadly defined with considerable overlap from state to state. Therefore, well-developed state guides as can be found in the curriculum materials centers of colleges and universities or ordered directly from their source can be helpful to curriculum planners throughout the nation.

District guides or courses of study. Although state legislatures have the legal authority to control the content of school curricula, in actual practice most important curriculum decisions are left to the individual school districts. Therefore, one distinctive characteristic of a district guide is that teachers are generally expected to follow them reasonably closely. They tend to be prescriptive rather than suggestive; however, this prescriptive nature is seldom absolute. In a well-administered health program, for example, the teachers may be required to teach the basic concepts and behavioral objectives but are given a free hand in the selection of methods, materials, and means of evaluation. Also, there are often oppor-

---

Goal: The learners feel at ease in the presence of other persons and are effective in their interpersonal relations.
Content area: Mental health
Concept: Emotions and feelings are expressed in a wide variety of ways, which makes their observance in others sometimes relatively easy and on other occasions very difficult.

Unit of study: Understanding others: social communication—Grade 6

Behavioral objective: Given a description or a dramatization of a social situation in which a person attempts to hide his true feelings, the learner will identify the underlying emotion and present a logical motive for its concealment.

Content	Methods and resources	Evaluation
I. Motives for suppression A. Embarrassment B. Fear of retaliation C. Social customs D. Concern for others	1. Find situations in which feelings are concealed in appropriate children's fiction; read these to the class and discuss them.	1. Present in a multiple choice format short narrations that require identification of feelings.

II. Methods of suppression
A. Conscious self-control
B. Displaying opposite emotion (love-hate)
C. Fooling one's self
  1. Sour grapes
  2. Blaming others
	2. Ask each learner to write a short story in which a feeling is concealed; allow children to read their stories to the class if they wish. Discuss.
	
	3. Ask for volunteers to dramatize appropriate situations in which feelings are concealed.
		2. Observe class responses to the situations; be alert for emotions that were commonly misconstrued.

Fig. 5-3. Page of a hypothetical teaching-learning guide. More than the usual number of components is displayed here in an effort to show their relationship to one another. The goal was deemed valuable in itself; the concept is one of several deemed necessary to the realization of the goal; the behavioral objective represented one of several learning tasks deemed necessary to the formation of the concept; this task was grouped with a number of similar tasks to form a meaningful unit on social communication for sixth grade classes.

tunities for supplementary topics to be added at the classroom level to meet special interests, particularly for topics related to current events in the health field that the district committee could not have foreseen. This balance of freedom and control can provide for a well-articulated series of learning experiences as students progress from grade level to grade level throughout their school careers without stifling the creative ingenuity of individual teachers. This built-in flexibility is reflected in the recent tendency to use the term "guide" rather than "course of study" with its more restrictive connotations (Fig. 5-3).

Within many districts the essential control of the health curriculum may revert to the individual school or building; this allows good coordination within school levels, such as between grades 10, 11, and 12 of a senior high, but makes the articulation of the curriculum between school levels difficult to manage.

Unit plans. Thus far the curriculum documents discussed have tended to focus upon what students "ought" to learn and what they are capable of learning at various maturity levels. The concept of unit planning takes into account the very necessary ingredient of student interest, that is, what they "want" to learn. The *teaching units* are typically prepared by individual teachers who have the opportunity to incorporate a knowledge of the particular characteristics of their students and their own personal strengths, limitations, and preferences into the planning process. A key feature of any unit is a central theme that serves to define a manageable portion of content in an interesting way. The study of community health can be very unattractive if the students are merely led through a role call of agencies extending through various government levels; however, a unit based on the theme "society versus disease" can shift the students' focus from the agencies and organizations themselves to the disease entities they seek to combat. Rather than reporting on the Department of Health, Education, and Welfare, for example, students can report on "the war against cancer" following an investigation of federal, state, and local efforts against this intrinsically interesting problem. Other individual students or groups can trace community activities as applied to heart disease, communicable disease, and so forth as the unit develops.

Another important feature of most teaching units is the division of the learning activities into those designed as (1) initiating activities to build up interest at the beginning of the unit, (2) developmental activities to utilize this interst in the investigation of the subject matter, and (3) culminating activities to pull together the various concepts studied and allow for the formation of conclusions and implications.

Resource units are similar in their general scope and format to teaching units except that they include more recommendations for activities and materials than could be used in any one teaching unit. They thus constitute a "resource" from which individual teachers may construct teaching units.

Lesson plans. The specific activities planned by an individual teacher for a particular day are written into a lesson plan. As with other planning documents the degree of detail commonly found in lesson plans varies greatly according to a number of conditions. Some schools require that detailed lesson plans be prepared a week or more in advance so that a substitute teacher can carry on effectively should the regular teacher be absent. Also, beginning teachers and veteran teachers working with a new topic or in a new school situation are generally advised to prepare written plans in some detail. On the other hand, teachers who are thoroughly familiar with both the topic and the general school situation can often function effectively with only a brief outline to ensure a proper sequence and to avoid serious omissions. Regardless of how brief or how detailed they may be, however, effective lesson plans generally include such key elements as:

1. A clear idea of what they [the teachers] wish to accomplish by the end of the lesson (i.e. a clear purpose or objective). . . .

2. A clear idea of the procedures and activities they will use to help students attain the objectives they have in mind. . . .
3. Ensuring that the materials (books, newspapers, magazines, records, tapes, etc.) that students will need to obtain information are available.
4. A clear idea of the order in which they will proceed to use the material and activities. . . .
5. Provision for some means to evaluate whether or not the lesson was achieved. . . .*

For example, if these five points were applied to a unit on beverage alcohol at the senior high school level, a fairly thorough lesson plan might look like the one below.

In actual practice most lesson plans are not as thorough as the example presented here. It was selected as a means of showing how a variety of procedures might be described. Also, the various entries are more complete than most veteran teachers would need for their own purposes; however, they are none too complete if they were to be used by a substitute teacher.

---

*Fraenkel, J. R.: *Helping students think and value: strategies for teaching the social studies,* Englewood Cliffs, N.J., © 1973, Prentice-Hall, Inc., pp. 380-381. By permission of Prentice-Hall, Inc., Englewood Cliffs, N.J.

PLANNING PROCESS

The responsibility for planning the total school curriculum of any single portion of it, such as health, education, is seldom delegated to any one person. For a variety of reasons curriculum planning generally involves the concerted efforts of several persons, and therein lies one of its principal strengths as well as one of its most frustrating weaknesses.

Selection of personnel. There are at least three purposes that must be served by the makeup or the selection of a typical curriculum development committee: representation, expertise, and generation of support. Both wise selection and good organization are needed if these diverse objectives are not to conflict.

Representation. From a purely legal standpoint the only irrevocable right individual citizens have to particpate in curriculum decisions is by the extremely indirect route of their representation in their state legislatures. However, as noted previously, state legislatures largely delegate responsibility for the curriculum to the various

---

Sample lesson plan

Friday 4/15   Health—Beverage Alcohol

Objective

Given the information commonly provided on the labels, the learner can compute the amount of absolute alcohol various bottles of common alcoholic beverages contain.

	Activities	Materials
10 min.	1. Show overhead transparencies on content of alc. beverages. Discuss basic points.	OH transparencies (teacher prepared)
5 min.	2. Demonstrate typical levels of absolute alcohol by adding colored water to appropriate glassware.	Water, food coloring, beer bottles, wine glass, highball glass, whiskey glass
15 min.	3. Organize class into groups of three to five students. Distribute paper bags containing three empty bottles to each group. Ask them to compute the amount of alcohol that each bottle originally contained.	6 bags each with variety of empty wine, whiskey, cordial bottles, etc.

Evaluation

10 min.	Ask one student from each group to show on the blackboard the computation for their most interesting bottle.

school districts, and these, in turn, usually feel a responsibility to provide interested groups with an effective voice in important curriculum decisions. Partly for this reason district health curriculum committees properly include representatives from the teaching staff, the school administration, health services, students, parents, and community health departments and organizations.

Expertise. Fortunately, most persons appointed to a curriculum committee for purposes of representation can also bring special knowledge and skills to the curriculum development process. Health teachers commonly possess both a knowledge of subject matter and a knowledge of their students' needs and learning characteristics. Administrative representatives often provide ready answers when questions of budget, resources, regrouping of students, and other such matters are raised. The school nurse and school physician can provide input relative to the common health problems of the students as well as subject-matter expertise in many areas of the health curriculum. Student representatives can provide valuable insights as to topics of high interest among their classmates and attractive teaching approaches. Parents can acquaint the committee with certain health-related problems that young people may not display at school. Community health leaders can provide information concerning the availability of the resources of their organizations as learning opportunities as well as a special knowledge of certain community health problems.

A specialist in curriculum structure and development obtained as a hired consultant from an area college or university is generally essential to the committee's work unless the school district can provide such expertise from among its own personnel. Also, subject-matter specialists in the form of psychologists, ecologists, and so forth are sometimes needed as consultants to augment the competencies of the committee members.

Generation of support. Even the best curriculum plans are of little value until they are put into action in the classroom. This step requires the firm support of the teach-

ing staff, as a new or revised curriculum generally means that old, comfortable ways of teaching must be disrupted. The district administration must do its share if the necessary materials, facilities, time allotments, and so forth are to be available. Parents must often accept innovations in sensitive areas such as human sexuality and drug abuse if a new curriculum is to succeed. Health service personnel must lend their support; and most important is the response of the students themselves.

Ideally this necessary support will be based solidly on the intrinsic merits of the health curriculum itself rather than on local politics or public relations. However, a preliminary attitude of acceptance is needed if the curriculum is ever to have a chance to demonstrate its worth. Those who participate directly in the development of a curriculum generally become its most enthusiastic advocates and serve as communication links with their respective groups. This is another important reason for the selection of a broadly representative committee for any major curriculum development project.

Organization of personnel. The task of organizing and leading a curriculum development effort in health education or in any other subject matter area is complex and requires special skills. Personnel must be selected who possess enthusiasm for the task and the ability to work in groups in addition to their other assets. Support for the operation itself must be obtained in the form of release time or direct compensation if this enthusiasm is to be maintained. The committee members must be organized into working groups on the basis of their individual competencies. The proper information and data must be gathered and new people must often be brought into the organization to handle detailed assignments. A uniform format must be established for the various components, and considerable editing will be required as different individuals and groups contribute copy. The total task is a demanding but highly important one; once a health curriculum is established, it often has a major effect on the activities of teachers and students for years to come as they seek to implement its provisions.

QUESTIONS FOR STUDY AND DISCUSSION

1. Compare the relative importance of good curriculum planning versus good implementation by discussing the consequences associated with the lack of either one of these factors.
2. Explain how the same behavioral objective may sometimes be attained even though the content presented to various groups of students may differ considerably.
3. Compare the roles, as they apply to the health curriculum of (a) the state department of education, (b) the school district, (c) the building committee, (d) the individual teacher, and (e) the learner.
4. Present and discuss at least three reasons why it might be necessary or desirable for teachers to deviate from their planned lesson after class begins.
5. Present and discuss at least three factors that could affect the way a particular learner receives and interprets a particular item of health information.
6. Explain one essentially positive and one essentially negative way teachers often gain some flexibility in their selection of the content to be presented.
7. Discuss the relative strengths and weaknesses of curriculum committees versus individual teachers as selectors of curriculum content.
8. What purpose should a statement of philosophy serve? What factors limit the effectiveness of most statements of philosophy?
9. Distinguish between goals and behavioral objectives in terms of both their function and their general form.
10. Describe two essential features of a content area (organizing element) as a curriculum component.
11. Discuss the implications of Woodruff's definition of a concept.
12. Explain the relationship between content outlines and behavioral objectives within the structure of modern curricula.
13. Distinguish between classroom evaluation and program evaluation.
14. Discuss the basic sequence of procedures followed in the development of the SHES model curriculum.
15. Discuss the various ways individual school districts have benefited from the work of the SHES.
16. Identify the distinguishing features of a teaching unit as compared with other related curriculum documents.
17. List and discuss five components found in well-prepared lesson plans.
18. What factors should affect the degree of thoroughness incorporated into a given lesson plan?
19. List and explain three reasons why a particular individual might be appointed to a health curriculum committee.
20. Identify at least four specific tasks involved in the leadership of a curriculum development committee.

REFERENCES

Fodor, J. T., and Dalis, G. T.: *Health instruction: theory and application,* ed. 2, Philadelphia, 1974, Lea & Febiger.

Fraenkel, J. R.: *Helping students think and value: strategies for teaching the social studies,* Englewood Cliffs, N.J., 1973, Prentice-Hall, Inc.

Goodlad, J. I., Von Stoephasius, R., and Klein, F. M.: *The changing school curriculum,* New York, 1966, Fund for the Advancement of Education.

Health concepts: guides for health instruction, Washington, D.C., 1967, American Association for Health, Physical Education, and Recreation.

Health education: a curricular approach to optimal health, Baltimore, Md., 1973, Maryland State Department of Education.

Mager, R. F.: *Preparing instructional objectives,* Palo Alto, Calif., 1962, Fearon Publishers.

Saylor, J. G.: *The school of the future now,* Washington, D.C., 1972, Association for Supervision and Curriculum Development.

School Health Education Study: *Health education: a conceptual approach to curriculum design,* St. Paul, Minn., 1967, 3M Education Press.

Short, E. C., and Marconnit, G. D., editors: *Contemporary thought on public school curriculum,* Dubuque, Ia., 1968, William C. Brown Co., Publishers.

Sliepcevich, E. M.: *School health education study: a summary report,* Washington, D.C., 1964, School Health Education Study.

Taba, H.: *Curriculum development: theory and practice,* New York, 1962, Harcourt Brace Jovanovich, Inc.

Tanner, D.: *Using behavioral objectives in the classroom,* New York, 1972, Macmillan, Inc.

Tyler, R. W.: *Basic principles of curriculum and instruction,* Chicago, 1949, The University of Chicago Press.

Woodruff, A. D.: *Basic concepts of teaching,* San Francisco, 1961, Chandler Publishing Co.

CHAPTER 6 ❧ Health curriculum
in action

It is considerably easier to discuss the health curriculum planning process and the various components of the curriculum in general terms than it is to apply them to specific school situations. There is relatively little disagreement among health educators as to basic planning procedures and the general shape of the health curriculum; however, a review of curriculum guides as developed by various state and district level planning groups will reveal many differing concepts as to what should be emphasized at various grade levels that cannot be accounted for by variations in local needs. In other words, it seems clear that there are more differences among health curricula than there are among the children for whom these curricula are planned.

Philosophical differences among planning groups obviously account for some of the differences in curriculum guides, but the larger portion probably results from the complexities inherent within the general task of selecting educational experiences for specific situations. The farther one moves from the "clean," logical world of curriculum theory toward the increasingly "cluttered," emotional world of the real classroom, the more one encounters the necessity to make decisions based on value judgments, estimates, and compromises necessitated by limitations of time and resources. An attempt is made in this chapter to provide some help in making these difficult decisions by first discussing some basic criteria for the selection of content and then by providing specific examples of content appropriate at various school levels expressed in the form of behavioral objectives. Also, in the latter portion of this chapter such practical features as time allotments, class size, and equipment and facilities are

described. These sections as a group are designed to provide the reader with a clearer impression of the real nature of the health curriculum as it moves from theory to action.

SELECTION OF CONTENT

Curriculum committees typically divide the study of health into major content areas, an thus define generally what is to be taught on the basis of a consideration of such foundational factors as the health problems of society and the committee's philosophical concept of the scope of health education. These "global decisions" are soon followed by the more detailed task of selecting specific facts, topics, issues, and other items of content for presentation at particular grade levels. A great many factors can be helpful in this selection process; however, three basic criteria are commonly used.

1. *The immediate health needs of the children involved.* Perhaps more so than those in any other teaching field, health educators have endorsed the traditional educational dictum to base instruction on the "interests and needs" of the learner. Consequently, we find pedestrian safety stressed in the primary grades where young children are often making their longest "solo" journey on neighborhood sidewalks as they walk to school; in the seventh grade we may find a strong emphasis on mental health as these preadolescents and early adolescents display the typical emotional instability of their period of development; in the ninth grade we may find considerable stress placed on venereal disease problems in response to the acceleration in the incidence of VD, which often begins somewhere near this grade level.

The logic of presenting learning experiences designed to help young people with the problems typical of their age group is obvious, and thus the criterion of immediate needs should always receive proper consideration; however, when it is followed to the neglect of other equally important factors much precious time and energy can be wasted. During the height of the drug hysteria of the late 1960's and early 1970's many school systems found that drug abuse problems began to occur in significant numbers in their high schools and promptly directed a heavy drug education effort at that school level. Many of these programs failed because they were poorly planned and presented. Even good programs, however, made little visible impact on the drug use patterns of these high school students. Although it is always dangerous to generalize about human behavior, it seems clear that the personal concepts and values that lead many high school students into drug abuse had been forming for years prior to their actual encounter with drugs. This situation typifies the need for a second criterion.

2. *Preparation for life situations in the future.* The School Health Education Study group* and others have presented persuasive arguments for concepts as the principal determinants of health behavior. More recently others have cast values in this role, but regardless of differing theoretical viewpoints, there is general agreement that important changes in behavior, whether for better or for worse, take time. Too often health educators wait for the problem to appear before they attempt to deal with it and thus find themselves always playing fruitless games of "catch up ball."

3. *Preparation for future learning experiences.* With mathematics and science curricula the learning experiences at one grade level typically build upon those the children have experienced at lower levels. Pupils in the fifth grade may learn the concepts related to common fractions so that they will be prepared to learn about decimal fractions in the sixth grade. The learning experiences regarding common fractions were prerequisite to the learning experiences related

*School Health Education Study: *Health education: a conceptual approach to curriculum design,* St. Paul, Minn., 1967, 3M Education Press.

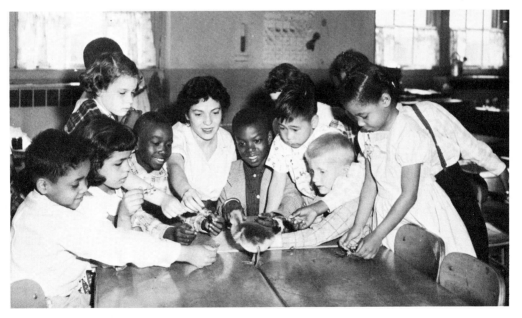

Fig. 6-1. The health curriculum typically includes informal as well as highly structured learning experiences. (Courtesy A. Devaney, Inc.)

to decimal fractions; and the need for prerequisite learning becomes a third criterion for the selection of content at a particular level. Although the need to provide children with subject matter of immediate practical usefulness should perhaps always predominate as health content is selected, the process of pyramiding learning experiences upon one another into an ever more mature understanding of the factors that affect one's health both now and in the future represents a consideration of almost equal importance.

K-12 CURRICULUM

Traditionally well-established subjects such as English, mathematics, and social studies are planned on a kindergarten through grade twelve (K-12) basis to allow for proper progression and to avoid undue overlapping of content from grade to grade. The advantages of such a planning approach are almost universally accepted among educational authorities; however, within many school districts K-12 planning in health education remains an ideal rather than a reality. Too often the initiative to develop adequate programs of health education must come from the school nurse or a combined health and physical education teacher within one building rather than from a districtwide effort sponsored by the administration and led by fully trained health educators. Under such circumstances the school personnel pressing for a good program must do heroic work simply to get something started in their own building; they have little immediate opportunity to involve teachers at the other school levels in their planning. Thus, many health education programs begin in a single junior high school, for example, and then over a period of years spread horizontally to other junior high schools in the same district and vertically to the elementary and high school levels.

With the advent of new state legislation in many states that mandate comprehensive health education, the building by building, level by level, piecemeal approach to planning is becoming less frequent. But

when the circumstances necessitate this pattern, those persons planning for a particular grade would do well to lengthen their perspective and give attention to the long-term needs of the students as well as to the problems that are already upon them.

ELEMENTARY SCHOOL LEVEL

A number of factors combine to make the years children spend in elementary school an ideal time for educating them about health. Each child normally enters kindergarten or first grade as a person whose day-to-day actions are in large part decided by other persons; teachers, parents, and older siblings often tell them what to eat, when to cross the street, what games to play, and with whom to play. Some years later the child leaves for the next school level as a person who has developed considerable personal autonomy. The guidance of other persons is still relied upon, but the child now typically has some very definite ideas about what to eat, what to wear, what time to go to bed, how to act toward friends and antagonists, and perhaps of prime importance, how to influence and pressure parents and teachers so that he or she can do more things "my way." In other words, the elementary school years are times during which many important lifelong habits are formed.

Developmental characteristics. These years of habit formation are also years during which children tend to be quite responsive to adult leadership. Things that "the teacher said" tend to be accepted as true and binding particularly among children of the primary grades; therefore, when good health procedures are clearly presented with consistent reminders, much can be accomplished without the necessity for dealing with the dynamics of the peer group as secondary teachers must do. A closely related factor is the general child-centered philosophical environment that tends to exist within elementary schools as opposed to the colder academic or vocational orientation that one often finds at the secondary level. In such circumstances teachers of health education are likely to receive both a better response from the children and more support for their efforts from parents and administrators than is often the case at the secondary level, where a "pecking order" of major versus minor subjects often prevails.

Curriculum emphasis. In terms of major health topics or content areas, there is little need for a different pattern or emphasis at the elementary as compared with the secondary levels. Most K-12 health curricula are organized so that the same areas (organizing elements) such as nutrition, disease, sexuality, and consumer health extend throughout all grade levels. The main difference, of course, is the level of complexity and the specific nature of the subtopics and examples used within these broad areas. The traditional but very worthwhile admonitions to choose learning experiences at the elementary level that actively involve the child and that are focused within the realm of his immediate experiences are very compatible with the teaching of health. These features have been incorporated in a number of comprehensive health education teaching-learning guides, which provide detailed suggestions for each school level. In this section samples of the general type of material found in such guides are presented and discussed as they apply to typical health content areas.

Disease prevention. Although there has been some tendency in recent years to reduce the traditionally heavy emphasis on personal hygiene and disease control in health curricula, this area still retains an important place in virtually all health education programs. At the kindergarten-primary level (K-3) both the immediate needs of the children and their long-term educational goals can be met by learning activities designed to improve their day-to-day living habits related to disease prevention. Typical behavioral objectives for this area and level are:

Pupils will be able to describe four ways by which they can help prevent the spread of disease germs.

Given a narrative description of a young child's behavior during a typical day, the pupil will be able to identify those actions clearly related to disease prevention.

For the first of these objectives it is easy to visualize first-grade pupils drawing posters that depict children covering their nose and mouth when they sneeze, washing their hands before eating, and staying home when they have colds. For the second, one can easily imagine a third-grade class listening to a story read by the teacher and checking off items on their "health score sheets," such as "had fruit juice at breakfast," "brushed his teeth after breakfast," and "went to bed by 8 o'clock."

Many of these same types of practical objectives are appropriate at the upper elementary level (4-6), but the broad interest patterns typical of this older age group provide the health teacher with the opportunity to begin dealing in a modest fashion with some basic principles of disease and its prevention. Typical objectives of this type include:

Pupils will be able to list the basic conditions that favor the growth of bacteria.

Given a list of various body structures, pupils will be able to describe the role of each in disease control.

The first of these objectives would lead to learning activities in which the children would discover that bacteria need starchy or sugary food such as candy, which nourishes the organisms that produce tooth decay, and warm temperatures such as those that often encourage spoilage in cream-filled pastries that sit out too long on a warm day, as well as moisture and darkness as provided by a musty sleeping bag that was not properly aired out after a camping trip. The second objective dictates learning experiences leading to an understanding of the importance of healthy skin and mucous membranes, the acid secretions in the stomach, the cilia of the respiratory passages (which cigarette smoke tends to paralyze), and the white blood cells and antibodies of the bloodstream.

Nutrition. Older children often reach a point where they have "heard too much about what I should eat," but foods and eating practices retain a constant appeal for the primary child as a topic of study. Health curricula for this level frequently include such behavioral objectives as:

Pupils will be able to tell three benefits resulting from a well-balanced diet.

Given a selection of common in-between-meal snacks, pupils will be able to identify those with definite health value.

Many teachers have had considerable success with a "snack tray" learning activity for the second of these objectives wherein the children have an actual chance to make selections and demonstrate both their knowledge of nutritious food and their ability to resist temptation. The first of these would lend itself to role playing with a second-grade "father" telling his "children" that their dinner would help them grow, stay well, and become stronger.

Children of grades 4-6 show a particular interest in animals, and when available, classroom pets in the form of rats, mice, hamsters, or guinea pigs can serve as media for teaching many nutritional concepts. These experiences may take the form of nutritional experiments or simply occur as children learn to care and feed these interesting classroom companions. In this manner the following objectives could be completed:

Pupils will be able to describe at least three important functions of nonenergy foods (such as vitamins, minerals, and water).

Pupils will be able to discuss the term "empty calorie" in terms of its significance to good nutrition.

Consumer health. Access to quality health care and essential health products is coming to be recognized as a right rather than a privilege restricted to those who can pay the price. But under any circumstances the quality one receives in this realm is highly related to the wisdom of one's choices; therefore, it is none too early to begin educating elementary school children as to the differences between various health practitioners, the protocol for prescribing and dispensing drugs, the interpretations of advertising material, the characteristics of health quacks, and similar topics. These behavioral objectives illustrate ways to get started at the kindergarten-primary level.

Pupils will be able to describe the basic function of television advertising.

Given a narrative description of a child's trip to the hospital for an operation, pupils will be able to describe the purpose of each major procedure, (for example, identification bracelet, medical exam, and anesthesia).

Teachers pursuing the first of these objectives, for example, might ask their second graders to describe a few of the TV ads that they have recently viewed before asking for ideas on why these ads are shown; the conclusion will probably be that "they want to get your money." The second objective is appropriate for any grade level, depending of course on the detail of the required descriptions. Occasionally hospitals will make special provisions to allow class field trips to their facilities.

Psychoactive substances. Many school systems have shown an unfortunate tendency to delay the study of drugs and alcohol until a significant number of these problems appear, which in most cases is at the secondary level. It is not surprising that such an approach generally fails to yield any solid evidence that any favorable changes were effected in the drug use behavior of the children involved. Elementary school children are interested in alcohol, tobacco, and drug problems but in most cases have not yet formed the habitual use patterns that lead to a firming up of attitudes. Drug use of all types remains an open question in their minds, and thus the conditions are good for the formation of valid concepts and constructive attitudes. At the K-3 level this general learning task can be based on such behavioral objectives as:

Pupils will be able to describe several examples of adult use or nonuse of psychoactive substances.

Pupils will be able to tell three reasons why the use of certain substances is restricted to adults.

These two objectives basically call for the development of a simple awareness on the part of young children as to the existence of psychoactive substances without implying any "heavy" interpretations or ethical judgments that would be inappropriate for this level. Children in grades 4-6 are ready to develop a more sophisticated understanding of this topic, as suggested by such objectives as:

Pupils will be able to suggest and discuss factors that may logically account for different use patterns regarding psychoactive substances.

Given a list of commonly used psychoactive substances, pupils will be able to describe their basic effects on body functions.

Probably the large majority of the films, filmstrips, and other media dealing with psychoactive substances is directed toward teaching the effects of these substances. Consequently, the second of these objectives can be accomplished via the media route, provided a careful selection is made. The behavioral aspects typified by the first objective are a bit more difficult to teach and call for more innovative approaches, such as polling parents and relatives on the reasons for their use or nonuse of tobacco and alcohol, or perhaps role playing to illustrate the influence of peer pressure on drug use.

Mental health. The study of mental health can be roughly divided into two broad categories: (1) understanding one's self (self-concept) and (2) getting along with others (interpersonal relationships). In one sense the entire elementary school serves as one vast learning laboratory for the mastery of these two important tasks. Obviously the children's school experiences, which provide them with insights into themselves and strategies for dealing effectively with others, occur in a variety of situations, and a large majority of these have little to do with formal health instruction. But regardless of its minority role, direct instruction in mental

health can correct misconceptions and provide a forum in which children can discuss typical emotional problems or situations and thus contribute to the development of healthy personality structures. For example, it is helpful for children to begin looking for the causes of both their own behavior and that of others, as suggested by the following behavioral objectives:

Given a basic narrative description of behavior typical of a specific mood (such as happiness, sadness, or anger), pupils will be able to identify the mood and suggest its possible causes.

Children will be able to describe two situations that commonly make them feel fearful or depressed and will suggest possible reasons for these reactions.

Both of these objectives could be approached by use of suitable discussion techniques, and both could help children understand that there are many factors outside themselves that account for the emotional reactions they see or experience. Children often tend to blame themselves unduly for temporary bouts of hostility or moroseness on the part of their parents and to likewise feel that something must be drastically wrong when they find themselves fearful of trips to the physician or dentist. At the upper elementary level, children can become slightly more analytical as they deal with the emotional dynamics of various situations. Typical behavioral objectives for this level include:

Pupils will be able to suggest methods for the effective resolution of arguments or conflict situations.

Pupils will be able to list characteristics that serve to identify personal problems requiring outside help.

The first of these situations would lend itself to role playing in which disputes were resolved through good communication, compromise, or perhaps appeals to the judgment of a trusted third party, such as a parent, counselor, or friend. The second of these could be accomplished through use of case studies presented either in written form or, if available, on film. Ideally, situations involving prolonged depression or anxiety, interference with school work or normal social relationships, or inability to control anger and hostility would be presented and discussed.

Human sexuality. Teachers at the secondary level often spend considerable time in efforts designed to help their students become accustomed to discussing sexual matters in the classroom. This task is greatly minimized in well-organized health education programs wherein children have the opportunity to grow up in classrooms in which the study of sexuality represents a regular topic of study. The basic curricular task in this area at the K-3 level thus becomes to provide basic information and, perhaps more important, to "normalize" its study. Typical objectives include:

Pupils will be able to describe both the male and female roles in the reproductive process.

Pupils will be able to describe examples of the ways adults typically treat girls and boys differently.

Classroom pets such as guinea pigs or hamsters provide a very natural way to acquaint children with the male's basic role in reproduction; they soon discover that both sexes are necessary if there are to be any babies. The many good films and filmstrips on the market can substitute for or supplement the experiences with pets. The second objective illustrates another vital aspect of sex education, namely, an understanding of sex roles and how they develop. This is useful regardless of one's personal views as to their validity in their modern form.

At the upper elementary level typical behavioral objectives for this area of study include:

Pupils will be able to trace the pathways of the sperm and the ovum in human conception.

Pupils will be able to compare the strength of the sex drive with other examples of human motivation.

The objective related to the pathway of the sperm and ovum is relatively conventional in the sense that it deals with traditional biological content. The second example related to the strength of the sex drive is often overlooked at this grade level; however, this is a good time for children to develop a concept of this human force as strong but manageable, as being channeled, redirected, and inhibited by social mores and customs, and as being affected by various forms of stimulation. In a thorough program, which many districts still would not permit despite the trend toward increasing acceptance of sex education, learning activities based on films and narratives involving examples of both constructive use of the sex drive as in a good marriage and destructive as with an unwanted pregnancy could lead to good class discussions. In this manner children could gain some understanding of the task of managing the sex drive.

MIDDLE SCHOOL LEVEL

As with any activity dealing with human behavior, the field of education is characterized by persistent problems and equally persistent efforts to find better ways of coping with these problems. This is nowhere more apparent than in the recent attempts to better provide for the "transescent" student, that is, for the 10-14 age group in transition between the relatively more stable and well-defined periods of childhood and the traditionally unstable and less understood adolescent stage.* A significant number of school systems have been deserting the traditional 6-3-3 and 8-4 patterns in favor of 4-4-4, 5-3-4, and similar configurations. The inherently complex educational and developmental considerations that have produced these changes have been further complicated by those situations wherein various grade levels are shifted from building to building simply to use space more efficiently as changing birth rates or shifts in population affect school enrollments.

---

*Eichhorn, D. H.: *The middle school,* New York, 1966, Center for Applied Research in Education.

What all this means is that teachers responsible for teaching health education in any of the 5-9 grade levels may (depending on the grade level, the organizational pattern, or the philosophy that prevails) find themselves working in a typical elementary school type of environment or a relatively new situation wherein a rigorous effort is made to truly design a school to accommodate the needs of this challenging age group. Where the elementary school point of view prevails, for example, one teacher may teach all the major subjects with the help and support of coordinators, supervisors, or resource teachers in the self-contained classroom; here the health education specialist would more likely take the form of "helper" or coordinator. At the secondary level where classes are often organized along the lines of subject fields or disciplines, the full-time health teacher is most appropriate. In the middle school, however, either of these roles might prevail according to the manner in which the particular school is organized.

The continual effort to restructure schools and school systems in search of better patterns is no doubt worthwhile and should continue, but it is well to note that an eighth grader remains an eighth grader regardless of whether his or her school building is called an elementary school, a middle school, or a junior high school. Therefore, those who are involved with the "transescent" grade levels should find the material presented in upper elementary and/or junior high school sections of this text helpful to them depending on the grade level or levels for which they are responsible.

SECONDARY SCHOOL LEVEL

In comparison with elementary school children, secondary students present the teacher with an interesting pattern of advantages and disadvantages. On the positive side this older group's larger repertoire of experience and skills makes it possible to use a greater variety of teaching techniques. The whole realm of mass media, including newspapers, magazines, and television documentaries, becomes available as teaching tools; assignments involving writing and library reference skills are generally appropriate throughout all secondary grade levels. A larger proportion of the available resource speakers are able to communicate with secondary students than is the case with elementary school pupils, where more specialized approaches and materials are normally required. Unlike younger children who typically require constant supervision and stimulation in the completion of their assignments, secondary school students can carry out relatively complex projects, experiments, and other assignments on their own once they have developed an interest in the task.

Developmental characteristics. The phrase "once they have developed an interest" exemplifies what is perhaps the health educator's greatest challenge at the secondary level, since preadolescent and adolescent youths typically have more of their own individual ideas about what is "relevant" or otherwise worthy of their time than do younger children. This is particularly the result of the older child's increased degree of individuality, which is the normal outcome of his or her more advanced state of personality development. As the years pass various maturational factors produce differences in physical size, appearance, perception, and reasoning ability. These interact with environmental factors, such as a particular pattern of values and traditions within the home, and with chance factors, such as distinctly good or poor first experiences with some new endeavors such as sports, music lessons, and even perhaps long division. These characteristics and experiences tend to channel each child into patterns of likes and dislikes that tend to become permanent with time and thus form a personal structure that may become more elaborate in some areas or erode and wither away in others but will essentially retain its basic shape.

One of the major environmental factors contributing to this process is the influence of the peer group. In their natural effort to become fully competent and independent human beings, children at the secondary level set up their own subculture to serve as a source of emotional support and guidance for problems and concerns that they feel they can no longer take to their parents. To many adults the peer group looks like one cohesive and highly integrated entity that enjoys the freely offered allegiance and loyalty of each and every member. This is true, but only to a certain point, for the peer group also represents another outside force that each child must accommodate in his or her individual way. Secondary school youths also soon find that the group can be even more unreasonable and tyrannical than the parents whose dominance they are seeking to avoid. Thus, young people often find themselves in conflict with various combinations of parents, peers, and their own emerging value structures.

Health educators at the secondary level can learn to function effectively within this maelstrom of emotional forces, if they will, to borrow a concept from the advocates of transactional analysis, avoid becoming another parent calling for compliance for the sake of compliance, or another peer (child) calling for rebellion for the sake of rebellion, and appeal to the emerging adult within the student who is seeking to become effective in making decisions that serve his or her own self-interests.* Self-interest is intended here in a humanistic sense and is related to actions that are inner directed and based on one's own value system. The resultant behavior is often directed toward helping friends and loved ones and serving society as well as one's self in a narrow sense. Truly selfish individuals, of course, eventually damage their own personality and thus systematically act against their own self-interest.

Curriculum emphasis. Young people at both the junior high and high school levels have educational needs within all the typical content areas of the health curriculum. At the junior high level, however, a systematic

---

*Berne, E.: *Games people play,* New York, 1964, Grove Press, Inc.

shift is needed within each area from any heavy concern with the external environment and community affairs toward more consideration with personal problems in sexuality, relations with peers and parents, attitudes toward one's self, one's growth and development, one's figure or physique, and drug and alcohol concerns. At the senior high level, students once again are ready to turn outward and begin to take an adult interest in the problems of society. Here such topics as pollution control, overpopulation, and the delivery of medical care become possibilities as topics with high interest value.

Disease prevention. During the junior high school years the threat of VD begins to make its presence felt. Although the incidence typically is not high within this age group, these years constitute the ideal time to educate young people against the VD risks that many of them will incur at later age levels. Also, the emotional stress and instability associated with pubescence and prepubescent development make junior high school children particularly susceptible to various psychosomatic complaints. The headaches, stomach upsets, sleeplessness, and other such problems typical of this level can be reduced or, at the very least, more easily endured as children gain a better understanding of the underlying dynamics of such problems. For this area and level the following behavioral objectives are appropriate:

Students will be able to describe the role of prompt treatment in the control of venereal disease.

Given a description of a disease condition, students can suggest the probable contributing causes.

Although such immediate threats as respiratory tract infections, skin disorders, and VD still merit attention at the senior high level, these older students are ready to progress beyond these more personal concerns. The more advanced students can benefit from educational experiences leading to a more sophisticated understanding of the natural disease-resistive mechanisms of the body. The antigen-antibody reaction merits study because of its important relationship to a wide variety of topics such as resistance and immunization, allergies, autoimmune diseases, organ transplants, and because of its probable role in cancer prevention. Also, in other realms of disease study, high school students can be taken beyond their immediate problems; they are ready, for example, to consider matters of public policy such as pollution control, public supported research efforts, and the improvement of public health services. Typical behavioral objectives for this level are:

Students can list the typical series of events in the development of an allergy in their proper sequence.

Given a values continuum on the importance of heart disease, ranging from "most important problem in the world" to "not really a problem," students will be able to locate their personal positions and discuss the probable reasons for these positions.

Nutrition. The emphasis within the study of nutrition at the secondary level should normally follow the general pattern described above for disease in which there is somewhat more concentration on immediate, personalized concerns in grades 7-9 and some effort to reach out toward the more challenging areas related to scientific bases and public policy at the senior high level. In the lower grades, for example, there is a particular need to correct and prevent popular misconceptions related to dietary practices and such factors as growth, energy level, and weight control. Children at this level are particularly susceptible to fads, quackery, and the distortions of hard-sell advertisements. Behavioral objectives for the junior high grades include:

Students can describe the effects of specific dynamic action as applied to various dietary approaches to weight reduction.

Students can plan daily menus including a well-balanced selection of essential nutrients and traditional foods for three different cultural groups.

Consumer health. The study of health products and services at the junior high level normally focuses on the general area of the choice behavior of the consumer. On one hand this involves learning ways to avoid quackery, price gouging, and so forth, and on the other the students need to increase their knowledge of the legitimate members of the health profession in terms of their particular roles and special areas of expertise. Children at this school level are learning to manage their own money in the forms of allowances and wages received for odd jobs, and they are particularly sensitive to what is known, at this writing, as a "rip off." Also, they tend to be fascinated by competent, independent adults other than their parents, and they are ready to distinguish between dentists, dental hygienists, medical technicians, and the various medical specialties. Typical behavioral objectives for this area include:

Students can list four characteristics that can be effectively used to distinguish quacks from legitimate practitioners.

Students can describe the general types of services provided by each of the major specialties within the medical and dental fields.

At the senior high level a further study of the various occupational specialties within the health field, particularly in terms of the nature and duration of the training required, serves both to prepare students as present and future consumers of these services and to acquaint them with the vocational and professional opportunities that exist in the health fields as possible career choices. Also the youthful idealism typical of late adolescence and early adulthood can be used to lead senior high school students into a productive study of the ever present problems in the health delivery system, or nonsystem as many currently prefer to term it. Although students of all age groups have a limited tolerance for the details involved in comprehensive regional health planning and the relative efficiency of private insurance carriers versus government-sponsored coverage, senior high students do respond quite well to such basic issues as "medical care as a right rather than a privilege" and "the role of the nurse practitioner or medical assistant" as a practical solution to health manpower problems. Behavioral objectives in this area include:

Students will be able to provide three criteria that distinguish the roles of fully trained professionals from those of the various health technicians.

Students can compare the major features of the health delivery systems of two other countries with the health care situation in our nation in terms of relative advantages and disadvantages.

Psychoactive substances. Except for cigarette smoking and scattered cases of schools with heavy abuse problems, drug use among junior high school students tends to be relatively light in comparison with use in high school populations; however, there is enough use to make these students generally aware of and interested in a wide variety of psychoactive substances. As noted earlier, it is well to warn children about the hazards of drug abuse at the upper elementary level when adult opinions tend to carry more influence. At the junior high level anything resembling a hard-sell effort at dictating behavior will most likely be ineffective or perhaps even encourage rebellious experimentation. Junior high students will respond quite favorably, however, to a more objective approach and allow themselves to be drawn into a quite detailed study of the nature and effects of various drugs and the various drug-related problems of intoxication, dependency, and increased accident risks. Appropriate behavioral objectives for this level include:

Students will be able to trace the pathway of a commonly used drug through the body and describe its interaction with major organs.

Students will be able to distinguish between various types of drug dependency in terms of typical stages and symptoms.

At the senior high level students are ready to develop a more mature understanding of the psychosocial aspects of drug use including factors that motivate various use patterns, such as moderate versus abusive use of alcohol, and the behavioral benefits or consequences of such patterns. They are capable of developing a useful degree of tolerance toward persons whose habits and attitudes differ from their own, and they are also capable of becoming effective referral persons who can identify classmates with drug problems and encourage them to seek help from a counselor, family physician, or some appropriate agency. The general realm of needed legislation or government support for drug abuse prevention or treatment is another topic that merits emphasis at the senior high level. Examples of behavioral objectives for this level are:

Given a series of case studies involving a variety of drug use patterns, students will be able to suggest the probable effects of each pattern on general living effectiveness.

Students will be able to compare two different approaches to drug control on the basis of logically determined criteria.

Mental health. In terms of personality development children typically make the stormy transition from childhood to adolescence during their junior high school years. In many respects this is the most trying period of their development. As seventh graders most children come to realize either consciously or more often subconsciously that adults can no longer serve as sole providers for their important emotional needs for support and companionship. Later as senior high students, they will "rediscover" their parents and teachers as helpful, if no longer omniscient, sources of strength in times of difficulty. But now, in the early stages of their emotional emancipation, their natural tendency is to turn their back on these benevolent tyrants and seek support from the peer group. However, they soon find that the "group," although promising much, often do not deliver as the interests, activities, and friendship patterns vary from one week to the next; a child securely established in the mainstream of things one weekend may find himself stranded with nothing to do the following Saturday morning.

No educational program can or should take all the stress out of this process or drastically change the often moody and introspective qualities of the normal junior high school child; however, the wholesome aspects of this growth period can be augmented by providing opportunities for them to get outside themselves and gain insight into their emotional experiences. They need, perhaps most of all, to accept and understand the inevitability of change and to realize that strong feelings, whether they involve elation or despondency, do not last forever. They must also begin to accept an appropriate amount of responsibility for their own development as unique human beings. Individual personalities are, for the most part, formed slowly but relentlessly by day-to-day experiences. Much of the content of these experiences is determined by individual children as they decide how to "spend their time." Learning activities that can help meet these needs are suggested by the following behavioral objectives:

Given an example via role playing, sound film, or written narrative of a person experiencing some strong emotion, students will be able to suggest whether the emotion represents a healthy or pathological response to the circumstances involved.

Given a description of the circumstances surrounding a person who experiences personality growth or change, students will be able to identify the probable causes of this change.

In comparison with junior high school children, youth of high school age have typically achieved a considerable degree of stability, or at least dynamic stability in their behavior and in their feelings about themselves. Their preliminary struggles toward adulthood usually lead to a measure of grudging respect for and some accommodation with their parents or parent substitutes, and they often find a relatively secure and comfortable place within a now more stable group of those their own age. Simply stated, high school students are full-blown adolescents; their struggles with themselves and with others are slightly less stressful than

their preadolescent counterparts, but they are embroiled in the same basic emotional problems. They have simply become a bit better adjusted to the problems involved in personality growth, and they now can take a more mature, empathetic interest in other people and in the larger problems of society. Typical behavioral objectives in mental health for this level include:

Given the information provided by discussions with others and their own self-analysis, students will be able to identify their distinguishing personality traits and suggest the advantages and disadvantages related to these traits.

Given an opportunity to study the nature and extent of mental illness in the present society, students will be able to devise a hypothetical program designed to reduce this general problem.

Human sexuality. Elementary school–age children seem to enjoy speculating about what they are going to be and do when they grow up, and in these fantasies it is easy for them to see themselves as powerful and capable adults. To junior high school children, however, manhood or womanhood is not some distant possibility but is something that seems to be almost already upon them. The girls with monthly menstruation and developing breasts and the boys with nocturnal emissions and changing voices find that physiological maturity is arriving on schedule, but as functional persons they find that they are still bumbling, insecure children who are still "bossed around" by adults and who have little idea of how to handle their new-found potential. Although this characterization is admittedly somewhat extreme, it serves to illustrate the role of sexual maturity with its physiological changes and its erotic strivings as one of the major adjustment tasks of this age group. The role of the health educator in this adjustment process is to provide experiences leading to better insights into the significance of these normal changes. The following objectives suggest these needed experiences:

Students will be able to describe in general terms the role of hormones in the development of primary and secondary sexual characteristics.

Students will be able to describe commonly observed differences in the way the sex drive is experienced by males and females.

As psychologists and many novelists accurately describe, human sexuality can be used as a means to greatly enhance human relationships or as a vehicle for unwittingly or intentionally harming a person or relationship. Although sexual intercourse is, of course, a prominent manifestation of one's sexuality, it is only one aspect of this complex entity. It would be presumptuous to assume that any school program could make more than a small inroad into the present or future sex-related problems of its students; however, during the past 2 or 3 decades there has been a dramatic increase in the degree of openness by which sexual matters may be discussed. These investigations and discussions are beginning to yield knowledge and insight from which all persons, including high school students, may benefit. Simply stated, this means that some of the basic features of constructive as opposed to destructive uses of sexuality are beginning to emerge. The degree to which individual school districts will permit this material to be presented in the high school classroom varies, but here are some sample behavioral objectives related to this content:

Given a case history of the relationship between two persons that involves sexual aspects, students will be able to suggest the probable effects on the well-being of each person involved.

Students will be able to describe their personal views concerning the privileges and responsibilities of each member involved in an ideal marriage and defend these views on the basis of logical criteria.

IMPLEMENTING THE HEALTH CURRICULUM

The most carefully planned curriculum will fail to achieve its goal if practical circumstances within the school hamper its proper implementation. Although highly complex, the factors related to the support of any aspect of a school's program, including health education, may be eventually reduced to considerations of time and money. Both of these are limited commodities; thus, the competition for both the school child's time and the budget dollar is exceedingly vicious in most school districts. Since health educators will seldom get everything they request, it is necessary to review these practical factors to determine essential minimums and to establish priorities for program development.

Personnel. The starting point for any program is the obtaining of competent personnel. Once this step is accomplished, the energy and the expertise that the term "competent" implies become available for the remaining steps of program development.

Elementary level. Although opinions vary, the regular classroom teacher is commonly considered to be the best person for the teaching of health in the elementary school. This seems particularly true at the primary level. Effective health teaching requires good rapport between teacher and child. The child must feel comfortable with the teacher, and the teacher must know the child well. Such a relationship generally requires day-to-day contact. Another advantage that the classroom teacher offers over a floating specialist is a high degree of knowledge of health-related learning experiences that the child has received and will receive in other school subjects. As the teacher of science, social studies, and language arts, he or she knows not only what the curriculum guide prescribes for these topics but what was actually taught; therefore, unnecessary duplications and important omissions can be avoided.

If elementary schoolteachers are to do an effective job, they must possess (1) the necessary competencies and (2) a willingness to treat the study of health as a serious responsibility on a par with the other subjects within the elementary school curriculum; in other words, proper motivation.

These are somewhat demanding require-ments; however, they are well within the reach of any school district that is willing to place proper emphasis on the long-term health needs of its children.

In terms of competencies, good health teachers at the elementary level must relate well to children, be skilled in general class-room methodology such as those used in science and social studies, and have a good general education that enables them to interpret the elementary scientific and be-havioral aspects of the issues and topics covered in the typically broad elementary school curriculum. These qualities are highly desirable in any teacher at this school level. To this foundation the addition of one three-semester-hour health course will equip such teachers to do an adequate job of health teaching. More training would of course be highly desirable; however, health educators have a tendency to characterize their subject as something so unique and exotic that it often gets pushed out of the regular curriculum, confused with health services, and generally neglected. More often lack of concern rather than lack of ability constitutes the more serious obstacle.

If teachers are to develop this proper de-gree of concern about the health education of their pupils, they must (1) see such in-struction as one of their responsibilities and (2) feel that someone cares about how well they meet this particular responsibility. The first step in developing this perception of health is the requiring or encouraging of all prospective elementary school teachers to take the aforementioned health course as part of their professional training. It is diffi-cult to view something as an important part of one's job if it is never mentioned during one's training program. Next, those re-sponsible for the curriculum must see that health appears as a regular subject with a regular weekly time allotment. Finally, there must be a health education supervisor, coordinator, or resource teacher to circulate among the various classroom teachers as visible representatives of the school sys-tem's concern for health instruction. Such

a resource person can offer much tangible support in the form of suggestions about methods and material for specific topics and perhaps some demonstration teaching of model lessons; however, the motivation value is equally if not more important.

Secondary level. Somewhere between the fourth and eighth grades, depending on the particular form of vertical organization, most school districts begin to reorganize their teaching staffs along the lines of subject matter. This is commonly prompted by the increased demands for subject-matter profi-ciency at the higher grade levels. The rela-tive value and exact nature of this type of "compartmentalization" at particular grades remains an area of educational controversy, as shown by the great variety of organiza-tional plans whose diversity far exceeds that of the underlying needs of the various school systems involved. But regardless of the theoretical aspects of this matter, health education typically fares best when it is treated on the same basis as other subjects. When teachers in a junior high school, for example, are hired as science teachers or English teachers, their interests and con-cerns are usually channeled along the line of their discipline. Efforts to involve them in "correlated health programs," wherein each specialist is to give appropriate attention to health, generally look good on paper but fail in practice as each teacher's real en-thusiasm goes into the teaching of the basic concepts of his or her own subject.

In view of these considerations most health education authorities feel that health education at the secondary level should be taught by specialists in health education.* Such persons are commonly defined as those who have the equivalent of a bachelor's de-gree and state teaching certification in the specific field of health education. Although health specialists are still in the minority at this writing, an increasing number of states

*For example see National Committee on School Health Policies of the National Education Associ-ation and the American Medical Association: *Suggested school health policies,* Washington, D.C. and Chicago, 1966, NEA and AMA, p. 2.

have mandated the health specialist as a certification specialty in recent years; thus, this long-recommended but commonly ignored policy is becoming a reality in many school districts. Where such specialists are not available, the common pattern is to hire the combined health and physical education major to teach health in secondary schools. Where such is the case a definite effort should be made to shift the major burden for health teaching to those particular dual majors who have higher levels of interest and aptitude in health rather than arbitrarily assigning an even balance of health and physical education teaching to all. Once this organization is accomplished, these designated specialists can be encouraged to seek inservice and graduate training designed to bring their health education competencies up to the level of the specialist.

Time allotments. Next to good personnel, time is probably the most precious commodity needed to nourish a good health education program. An inspirational speaker can make a big splash in a 1-hour school assembly program, but one will be hard pressed to find any effects on student behavior that last more than a week or two. Any hope for favorable changes in health practices and/or a workable understanding of basic health concepts is dependent on meaningful involvement with subject matter and requires a well-planned progression of experiences over an extended period of time.

Elementary level. The common recommendation for the elementary level is that health receive the same time allotment as other instructional areas. With the shorter attention spans and less complex subject matter that prevail at the kindergarten-primary level, a daily health lesson of 20 or 30 minutes seems close to the optimal pattern. In the upper elementary grades the equivalent amount of time can be concentrated into two or three sessions per week to provide the opportunities for more involved learning activities. However, with only one teacher involved in the self-contained classroom, a great variety of time patterns are appropriate since health may be emphasized heavily one week to accommodate some large project, such as producing an assembly program for the total school or putting on a health fair, and then given proportionately less time the following week.

Secondary level. Ideally, students should receive the equivalent of a full year of health on a 5 day per week basis at the junior high level and another year at the senior high level. Opinions vary about whether to concentrate this allotment in a single year, divide it into separate semesters in alternate years, or perhaps offer a block of 12 weeks every year; however, 5 days per week are definitely favored over alternate day patterns that make it difficult to maintain interest and continuity of instruction. Also, holding to the full semester rather than to a fractional block of weeks in many school districts makes it more likely that health education will receive the status and support accorded to a major subject. Although a growing number of schools are meeting this standard, most are considered fortunate if they receive half this time allotment. Those health educators who find themselves struggling with the practical realities of limited support are well advised to first establish the policy of the 5 day per week pattern, then pressure to extend this block to 6 weeks, 9 weeks, 12 weeks, and so forth until the full semester has been allotted.

Class size. Instructional health objectives involve both complex cognitive behavior in the form of analysis, synthesis, and so forth and effective changes in the realm of values and attitudes. Both categories require the personal interaction between teacher and student that can occur only when class size is held to reasonable maximums. In our experience the person-to-person atmosphere of a class tends to deteriorate rapidly as the number of students moves above 28 or 30. About 10 to 15 would probably be ideal in the sense of allowing for both individual instruction and diversity in group discussion, but this low number is seldom possible. Large group activities to hear

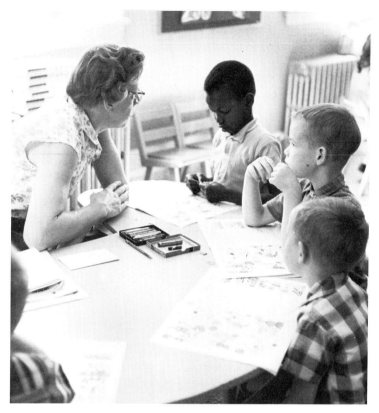

Fig. 6-2. Individualized instruction becomes possible when class size is held to a reasonable number.

speakers, view films, or participate in similar activities can be useful if they are followed by small group meetings wherein the material can be discussed.

Sex grouping. Unfortunately, sex grouping of boys and girls for health instruction often begins in the fifth grade when the school nurse comes to talk to the girls about menstrual hygiene while the boys are excused to play basketball in the gymnasium and continues at the secondary level when health education is taught as part of physical education. Menstrual hygiene is most properly taught within the contex of a comprehensive unit or human sexuality and reproduction, which both boys and girls obviously need. Also, one of the main goals of each unit is to demystify and normalize its study, and this is hardly accomplished by separating the sexes. In health as with most other subjects there are few educa-

tional needs that are exclusively female or exclusively male. Where sex differences in viewpoints with respect to specific topics commonly exist, both sexes usually benefit from a sharing of these viewpoints.

Facilities and equipment. The teaching activities in health education in their simplest analysis represent a combination of techniques commonly used for science and social studies; therefore, any elementary school classroom equipped for the effective teaching of these subjects will also be found adequate for health instruction. With both elementary and secondary schools the needs will naturally vary somewhat according to the emphasis of particular programs. However, the following items or features have been found very useful at both these levels:

1. Movable seats to facilitate a variety of seating arrangements for discussion and small group meetings.

2. Two or three tables of various sizes to accommodate panel discussions, displays and exhibits, and similar uses.
3. Adequate bulletin board and chalkboard space.
4. Ready access to audiovisual equipment with darkening drapes and preferably a permanently installed screen and permanently assigned items of AV equipment that receive heavy use, such as an overhead projector, tape recorder and/or classroom television receivers.
5. Adequate storage space for mimeographed handout sheets, filmstrips, overhead transparencies, and similar items.
6. A laboratory demonstration table as a preferred optional item. This is particularly useful at the secondary level as are "wet carrel"-type facilities for the students. The priority that such items receive should vary according to the emphasis of individual programs.
7. A small committee room separated from the regular classroom by a regular or glass-windowed partition. This is another nonessential but highly useful item at the secondary level.

Within almost any school a gap exists between what teachers of health would like to have and what is realistically possible in the way of equipment and facilities. Within the self-contained classroom of the elementary school the interests of health education merge with those of the other subjects and tend to share their fate. In those situations where health is taught on a compartmentalized basis, which include most junior and senior high schools and some middle and elementary schools, it is placed on a competitive basis with other subjects. In these situations the first priority is to secure a permanent "health room or rooms" so that bulletin boards, magazine tables, exhibits, and other items that create a warm, inviting classroom environment become possible. The next priority is generally assigned to attractive, movable furniture, then perhaps shelves and storage space according to program needs and economic realities.

QUESTIONS FOR STUDY AND DISCUSSION

1. Name three basic criteria commonly used for the selection and grade placement of health content.
2. How are the specific characteristics of these criteria determined?
3. In what ways may these criteria conflict with one another in specific situations?
4. Compare the real with the ideal in regard to K-12 planning in health education.
5. Describe some of the common developmental characteristics of elementary school children that provide important implications for health instruction.
6. Compare the specific emphasis appropriate for the elementary and secondary levels in regard to the major topical areas of the health curriculum.
7. What are the major advantages and disadvantages of assigning health-teaching responsibilities to the regular elementary school teacher as opposed to a "floating specialist"?
8. What important functions can a health coordinator perform within an elementary health education program?
9. What are the basic considerations at the elementary and the secondary levels with regard to time allotments, time patterns, class sizes, and sex grouping of students?
10. Describe the basic needs of a health education program in terms of classroom facilities.

REFERENCES

Byler, R. V., Lewis, G. M., and Totman, R. J.: *Teach us what we want to know,* New York, 1969, Mental Health Materials Center, Inc.

Maryland State Department of Education: *Health education: a curricular approach to optimal health,* Baltimore, Md., 1972, The Department.

Mayshark, C., and Foster, R. A.: *Health education in secondary schools,* St. Louis, 1972, The C. V. Mosby Co.

National Committee on School Health Policies of the National Education Association and American Medical Association: *Suggested school health policies,* Washington, D.C. and Chicago, 1966, NEA and AMA.

Pennsylvania Department of Education: *Conceptual guidelines for school health programs in Pennsylvania,* Harrisburg, Pa., 1970, The Department.

Read, D. A., and Greene, W. H.: *Creative teaching in health,* ed. 2 New York, 1975, Macmillan, Inc.

School Health Education Study: *Health education: a conceptual approach to curriculum design,* St. Paul, Minn., 1967, 3M Education Press.

Stone, L. J., and Church, J.: *Childhood and adolescence,* ed. 2, New York, 1968, Random House, Inc.

CHAPTER 7 🌿 Teaching techniques

Perhaps the most challenging aspect of the total process of health education is the task of selecting and applying teaching techniques that will effectively "deliver" content to young people in the classroom. "Delivering" in this case does not imply presenting content to passive students but actively involving them in learning experiences in such a way that their health knowledge, understanding, attitudes, and practices will develop along constructive lines. Actually, the nation's schools are full of health education programs that look good on paper, that favorably impress school boards and parents with their worthy goals and relevant subject matter, but that do little for the students except to produce negative attitudes toward the study of health because of the boring and ineffective classroom techniques used in their implementation. There are a number of reasons for these unfortunate situations, many of which are beyond the individual teacher's control, such as inadequate resources, excessive class size, and insufficient time allotments; however, even under the best of conditions the actual teaching process is a highly complex and demanding activity.

SELECTION OF TECHNIQUES

The selection of specific techniques to meet the needs of and comply with the limitations of particular teaching situations requires the consideration of a number of pertinent factors, many of which apply to the relationship between teaching techniques and other major components of the total teaching-learning process. A second broad category relates to the internal qualities or dimensions that give each technique its particular qualities.

Some important distinctions. The relationship between such factors as content, technique, and resources is often so close as to make it impossible to distinguish between

them. The use of a sound film is an example of a teaching *technique;* the film itself represents a teaching *resource;* and the information the film conveys represents part of the *content* of the course. Similarly, in many values clarification techniques the content to be acquired by the learners is an ability to use the technique to identify and clarify their own values; here again, medium and message overlap. These blurred distinctions cause few problems to individual teachers, who are understandably more concerned with assembling the components of a good classroom experience than with labeling each one; however; they do cause some communication problems as one discusses the teaching process with others.

Many educators also distinguish between specific teaching techniques or devices and the general *method* or *approach* that individual teachers or schools might use. The term approach (and to a slightly lesser extent, method) refers to a broad and consistent manner of teaching that is guided by certain basic assumptions and beliefs. It is characterized by the way content is commonly organized, by the teaching techniques commonly used, by the degree of learner involvement in the planning process, and so forth. The problem-solving approach is a typical example. Teachers consistently lead their classes toward the investigation of one central problem that lies at the heart of the subject matter to be studied; often they will use a student committee structure as the usual vehicle for organizing the learning experiences.* Other teachers with a more biomedical view of health education might adopt a lab-centered discovery approach, with consistent use of classroom experiments and dissections. Although many stereo-

---

*Eberle, R.: Problem-solving modes of classroom instruction, Educational Leadership **30:**726-728, May 1973.

typed approaches exist, perhaps the majority of teachers develop their own personal pattern over a period of years as they gain classroom experience.

Some important dimensions. With respect to the use of a particular technique, perhaps the first aspect to consider is the degree to which the technique provides the learner with a *direct, concrete learning experience* as opposed to one that is more abstract. If a unit of study, for example, calls for acquainting high school students with the problems and complexities of modern hospital care, a teacher in some situations might be able to arrange for the students to actually work in the hospital as part-time volunteers and thus provide close to the ultimate in a direct learning experience. At the other extreme, the teacher in another situation might seek to attain the same objective by asking the students to read a chapter on hospital care in their textbooks, thus leading them into a relatively abstract experience. Still another teacher might show a film on hospital care, thereby providing an experience ranking between the two extremes of the abstract-to-concrete continuum. Edgar Dale has categorized common learning activities in terms of this dimension, as shown in Fig. 7-1.

Concrete versus abstract. Although it seems obvious that the more direct a learning experience is the more effective it will be, it is also true that the more direct a learning experience is the more costly it is likely to be both in time and resources. A good film is usually more meaningful to students than a well-written chapter; however, it is more expensive and takes longer to present the same number of facts and concepts. A field trip can be even more meaningful, but unfortunately even more costly, particularly in terms of the time consumed. Therefore, a balanced mixture of teaching devices is both more feasible and more efficient in most school situations. The use of a field trip, resource speakers, or projects and experiments can add depth to learning within a particular unit, whereas the use of textbooks and library resources

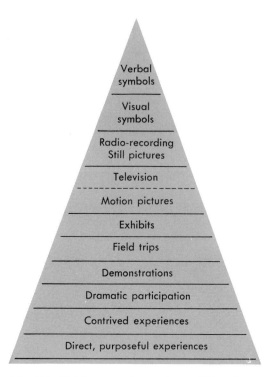

Fig. 7-1. Dale's cone of experience. This scheme provides a means of categorizing learning experiences according to their relative degree of abstractness or concreteness. (From *Audio-visual methods in teaching,* revised edition, by Edgar Dale. Copyright © 1946, 1954 by Holt, Rinehart and Winston, Inc. Reprinted by permission of the Dryden Press.)

can add breadth and scope to the same area of study.

Cognitive versus affective. Teaching techniques also vary along a cognitive-affective continuum. Some techniques are particularly useful for increasing the learner's knowledge and understanding about a health topic, and others are more valuable as a means to deal with the learner's feelings or attitudes toward it. For example, charts, graphs, and laboratory demonstrations might be used to provide students with the opportunity to learn about the physiological aspects of weight control, whereas the emotional aspects of efforts to restrict one's eating when confronted with social pressure to join in a festive meal might better be experienced through role playing or similar classroom dramatizations. In a similar fashion a visit to a nursing home might give

Table 7-1. Cognitive-affective classification of teaching techniques

Cognitive	Affective	Composite
Reading assignments	Role playing	Films
Lecture-discussion	Playlets	Slide-tapes
Oral reports	Affective discussions	Field trips
Resource speakers	Values clarification techniques	Demonstrations
Overhead projector		
Charts and graphs		
Programmed instruction		

students some appreciation of the loneliness and despair that many older persons must endure; however, any detailed understanding of the economics of medicare and social security could well require the cooler, more detailed medium of the chart, graph, and written explanation. The Table 7-1 organizes common techniques on the basis of their relative usefulness in dealing with cognitive versus affective objectives.

Although it is useful to classify techniques in this manner, it is important to bear in mind that all learning experiences contain both cognitive and affective elements; it is virtually impossible to separate what students "know" about a given topic from how they "feel" about it. Almost all "feelings" are attached to "objects," and almost all "objects" evoke some "feeling" even if it is limited to simple apathy. Likewise all teaching techniques have some impact, however minimal, on both knowledge and feelings. The relative balance of these impacts produced by any technique in a given instance of use varies greatly in accordance with the content of the lesson and the specific way the learning experience is handled. Small group discussions may be used to discuss and digest scientific facts and principles (cognitive) or to share personal problems and experiences (affective); the printed word is commonly regarded as a "cool" medium, but a talented writer can on occasion evoke anger or tears. Therefore, no techniques are purely cognitive or affective, but some generally tend to be more useful when the objective to be attained deals mainly with one or the other of these two types of behavior.

Teacher-centered or student-centered. Another consideration in the selection of teaching techniques is the degree to which a given device centers on teacher behavior or student behavior in its operation. When teachers lecture to the students or dominate classroom discussions, they are obviously using teacher-centered techniques. When students are stimulated to select and carry out their own individual projects, the focus is obviously on student behavior. Within this general teacher-student dimension it is also useful to make a distinction between activities per se and decision making; these aspects are closely related but not synonymous. For example, students might be busily involved carrying out nutritional experiments in which they observe the effect of different diets on the general health of rats according to specific procedures prescribed by the teacher; in this case the students are active but are minimally involved in decision making. In another situation we might see students passively listening to a resource speaker who they, as a group, had selected and invited. Here the activity level of the students is low, but they obviously had a large role in classroom decision making.

It is generally believed that techniques that both produce active student involvement and allow them a strong voice in decision making are the most effective in generating meaningful learning experiences. However, as with most other aspects of education, there are a number of exceptions to this generalization. The use of student-centered methods must often be limited somewhat to conform to the curriculum; even under the most ideal of circumstances, the

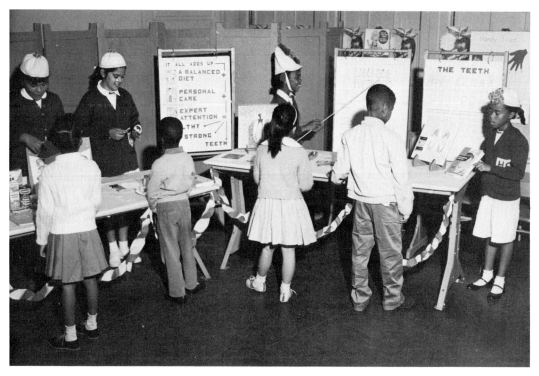

Fig. 7-2. Student-centered teaching techniques often stimulate enthusiasm and creativity.

experience and knowledge of teachers should not be underutilized by their adoption of excessively passive roles in the teaching-learning process. Thus, there are both practical and theoretical limits to the desirable level of student involvement in classroom learning activities; however, in actual practice these are seldom exceeded. The general tendency is to underplay student activity and decision making; therefore, teachers should seldom neglect any opportunities to bring some balance to this situation.*

OVERVIEW OF BASIC TECHNIQUES

Because of the many different teaching techniques that exist, only a limited sample was selected for discussion in this chapter. However, an attempt was made to include examples within all major categories and to describe each one in sufficient detail to

*Kelly, B. J.: A place for both student-centered and teacher-centered instruction, School Health Review **3:**34-37, Jan.-Feb. 1972.

provide a practical understanding of how each can be used. Once teachers have gained experience in the use of standard techniques, they often begin to develop variations or innovations that are well suited to their individual style and to the demands of their situation.

Large group discussion. The large group discussion with genuine student involvement and broad participation is one of the most convenient and versatile classroom tools that a teacher can use. As the students respond, they must think about the topic and often manipulate or apply supporting facts to make their point; they gain insights not only into the topic itself but into the views of their classmates. As differences of opinion are expressed, the antagonists are stimulated even further in their thinking as they lobby for their personal position. Although disagreements provide potent fuel to move a discussion, it can be equally as stimulating to students to receive support for their ideas—to find out that others feel the same way and to experience the genuine satisfaction of reaching someone else with a relatively complex idea.

The skill and planning necessary to good discussion leadership often go unappreciated by casual observers, such as parents and others untrained in discussion leadership and often by the student participants themselves. A good discussion looks like something that occurred merely because the students happened to be interested in the topic and happened to feel like talking that day. Although chance factors do appear to affect the quality of any given discussion, teachers can do much to increase the odds in their favor by (1) establishing a good general classroom environment for discussion, (2) devising good discussion questions, (3) applying specific discussion management techniques, and (4) learning to recognize spontaneous discussion opportunities.

The classroom environment. The only suitable foundation for a good classroom discussion is the same healthy emotional environment that is essential to any classroom; this can be described very briefly as an environment in which each person feels respected. However, this is simply a starting point; beyond this basic respect for people the teacher must cultivate a respect for ideas and place value on the process of drawing them out, clarifying them, and examining their implications. Many otherwise pleasant and constructive teachers are too busy "covering the material" to devote significant class time to exploring and digesting it through class discussion. Students never get a chance to work through their own misconceptions and immature observations; these are nipped in the bud by the impatient teacher to save time and to move the class along to the next topic.

Discussion questions. A discussion implies an exchange of ideas; therefore, a good discussion question must be (1) broad enough to serve as a focal point for many related facts and ideas and (2) controversial enough to elicit differing points of view. Questions such as "How many traffic deaths were reported for the U.S. last year?" or "Who is the Surgeon General of the U.S. Public Health Service?" are obviously too narrow to support a discussion. Others such "What is the nature of the antigen-antibody reaction?" or "What are the functions of a local health department?" are broad enough but generally do not lend themselves to different points of view as they are normally presented at the public school level. Examples of questions with more discussion potential are:

Should the United States do more to help nations experiencing famine or chronic food shortages?

Should the legal penalties for marijuana possession be reduced or eliminated?

Should a system of trial marriage be established wherein procreation is discouraged until the relationship is finalized?

These questions would work well with many groups of students at the secondary level who had completed some preliminary study within the general areas they are covering. The potential of elementary school pupils to express ideas often goes untapped by teachers who underestimate their capacity for original thought. Questions such as these can often produce good results with this age group:

Of all the safety rules you know, which one do you think is most important?

How would you try to help a friend who was sad and unhappy about something?

If you could discover a cure for one disease, which one would you choose, and why?

Discussion leadership. Good discussion leadership is more an art than a science and requires considerable experience for the development of real effectiveness; however, a few simple hints can serve to get one started in the proper direction.

1. *Avoid introducing too many of your own ideas.* There are proper places for teachers to present information and opinions, but the early stages of a discussion is not one of these. It is often useful to relate the contents of a pertinent newspaper item or

to display some related information by use of the overhead projector as a lead-in to the discussion question. Once the question is presented, however, give the class a chance to think for a few moments; learn to tolerate periods of silence. The first responses may not be of the highest quality, but when properly handled, they will serve to stimulate additional contributions. If the class must be prodded, one of the best techniques is to simply repeat the question.*

2. *Maintain an accepting and supporting attitude toward all replies.* As with generally unresponsive groups, the development of a good discussion in many situations is somewhat like starting a campfire under difficult conditions; the first spark must be nourished and tended properly if it is not to die out. The discussional fire can be quickly extinguished by such "killer statements" as "where did you get that idea?" or "Few people would agree with you." Even if the response is quite bizarre, it is better to say something like "That is an interesting view; I wonder if others agree with you." The general rule is to protect the contributor from embarrassment and use the response to draw new people into the discussion.

3. *Keep the discussion on the topic.* Although quite free wheeling, a good discussion still must be kept within the limits; this is probably the main characteristic that distinguishes it from a "bull session." At times the discussion may be permitted to wander from the original discussion to closely related topics, but when it begins to stray beyond acceptable limits, the teacher's best response in most cases is to ask a variation of the original discussion question that brings the class back to the last relevant topic before it got off the track. This can be smoothly accomplished by saying "Well that lets us know how you feel about . . . (the irrelevant point); now, can someone else tell us about . . . (the relevant point)?" or "Before we talk about . . . (irrelevant

topic), we should try to decide about . . . (relevant topic)."

4. *Turn questions back to the group.* Once the teacher starts answering questions on substantive points, the discussion may die or take on a "quiz the expert" quality as each query receives its authoritative reply; this may have value in some circumstances but not when a broad exchange of views is desired. A good way to handle a direct question is to say, "I have a few ideas on that point, but I'm more interested in what the rest of you have to say."

5. *Recognize irreconcilable views and move on to other aspects of the topic.* The discussion question was selected in part because it was one on which "good men might differ"; therefore, such differences should be expected (even welcomed) as a healthy sign of valid participation. As individual students or groups of students begin to get embroiled in controversy, a leader will occasionally ask clarifying questions designed to see if the opposing forces really disagree or are perhaps simply using terms differently. At that time utilize the controversy as a vehicle to stimulate the students to marshall facts and logic to support their point of view. Finally, as the intellectual resources of the participants have been exhausted and the exchanges degenerate into a simple restating of positions, it is well to move the group on to another topic.

Variations of the discussion format. One of the main virtues of classroom discussion as a technique is its general versatility. This intimate form of face-to-face communication has been with us since the early beginning of civilization and should never be underestimated as a teaching-learning device. However, like most forms of human interaction, its quality is significantly affected by a wide variety of situational factors. The need for a climate of trust and openness in the classroom merits continual reemphasis. Next in priority is the proper match between the assigned topic and the experiential background of the participants. Discussion is a relatively poor device

*Epstein, C.: *Affective subjects in the classroom: exploring race, sex, and drugs,* Scranton, Pa., 1972, Intext Educational Publishers.

for presenting new information; its strengths lie in the opportunities it provides to sort out, digest, compare relationships, and assign priorities to facts and ideas. Therefore, students must have had prior experiences with the topic in the form of films, assigned readings, and perhaps best of all, everyday living experiences. Once these two preconditions have been satisfied, the next aspect to consider is the most effective way to structure both the intellectual and the physical conditions of the discussion or, in simpler terms, to select the best format.

Small group discussion. One of the simplest ways to increase the opportunities for active participation in a discussion is to divide the class into small "buzz groups" of perhaps four to six students. In addition to the obvious reduction of competition, inhibitions are also reduced for those students who are reluctant to speak out in class; moreover, the removal of the teacher as a direct participant is a definite advantage in many situations. The question does arise, however, as to why class time should be allotted to an activity that the students do all the time outside of class in a spontaneous fashion. This objection, however logical it may seem, does not take into account the many tools teachers have for guiding these small group discussions by use of devices other than direct participation. These become apparent as one examines the specific procedures involved. Although the style of individual teachers varies, the following steps generally apply:

1. In most cases it is desirable to stimulate interest in the general topic to be discussed by a brief general presentation before placing the students in discussion groups. A brief report on a newspaper clipping or magazine article by the teacher is one good lead-in; others include one or two interesting overhead transparencies, a short film, or even a brief general discussion of a portion of the textbook.

2. The discussion task for the small groups should be clearly defined; often it is well to put the question or questions to be discussed on the chalkboard or in some cases on dittoed handout sheets. Next the student must be given a time frame in which to operate; this may vary from 10 to 30 minutes or more according to the situation.

3. Although well-motivated students with previous experience with small group discussions can often sort themselves out into groups of their own choosing, the teacher should usually take the lead in this task. This can be done on the spot by simply putting the nearest five or six students together, or it can be done more deliberately by arranging the group beforehand and then reading off the names, or better yet, displaying them on the overhead projector. This latter procedure enables the groups to be balanced for sex and leadership ability or to be changed periodically in membership when the technique is frequently repeated.

4. Either before the small groups assemble or immediately thereafter, leaders and/or recorders should be assigned; usually they are charged with the responsibility to report the conclusion or other main points arising from their group's discussion.

5. As the small group discussions begin, the teacher usually should first circulate and encourage slow-starting groups to begin the assigned task; thereafter the teacher can circulate among the groups, occasionally resolve conflicts, and in some cases sit in for awhile with individual groups.

6. The decision as to specifically when to terminate the small group discussion within the allotted 10 to 30 minutes and reassemble the class in most cases should be based on the teacher's estimate of the productivity of the various discussions. With experience most teachers can sense when the purpose of the discussion has been achieved.

7. Once the large group has been reassembled, the common practice is to

call for a brief report of the recorders and follow this with a general discussion of their more interesting points.

The fishbowl. Every type of discussion offers students the opportunity to gain insights into the mechanics of the discussion itself as a form of human interaction as well as into the actual content being discussed. Fishbowl discussions provide perhaps the best balance of these two advantages. In this technique a small group of perhaps six to eight students form a circle in the center of the classroom and carry on a discussion while the balance of the class observes them. The observers are usually asked to give attention to the dynamics of the discussion, such as who dominated the exchanges, who stayed with the issues, and who made irrelevant statements as well as give attention to the substances of their comments. One variation of this technique provides one or two vacant chairs in the inner circle, which outsiders may occupy temporarily when they wish to speak on a particular point. The same preconditions of a good classroom atmosphere and heightened interest in a particular topic are essential for good results.

The symposium. Teachers who prefer a more highly structured discussion format find the symposium quite useful. Here perhaps two to six students locate themselves at the front of the classroom and present brief prepared reports on a particular topic. Following their reports, the topic is opened up to general class discussion with the panelists serving as "experts" on their assigned aspect of the topic. The simplest way to organize a symposium is to simply assign oral report topics to all or a portion of the class and then form those with closely related topics into symposiums; however, better results will be obtained when the students are provided the opportunity to function as an investigating committee before presenting their reports. This also provides the teacher with an opportunity to assist in the planning of the information-gathering procedures and the organization of the presentation. It is also well to en-

courage students to support their reports with charts, posters, colored slides, or tape recordings. The overall benefits to the class are usually increased when the participants are selected from among volunteers or the better students insofar as speaking skills are concerned.

The lecture. Few practices in education have drawn as much justifiable criticism in recent years than has the excessive use of the lecture in the health education classes of junior and senior high schools. A good speaker with something interesting to say can hold the attention of a mature audience for an hour or more on a given occasion; however, few if any lecturers can hold an audience two, three, or even five times per week as some public school teachers try to do. In many cases the offending teachers are simply too lazy or too timid to use more student-centered techniques. Other very conscientious teachers, who find themselves with too much important material to cover under conditions of limited time and resources, tend to see the lecture simply as a no-nonsense way to get the job done. "When the health of our young people is at stake," they say, "we cannot afford to use time-consuming techniques—we must cover the material." The only problem with this point of view, however, is that it is not what the teacher *covers* that is so important; it is what the students *retain* and *apply* that really counts. Although it is true that well-organized lectures, coupled with a tight grading system, can motivate good students toward impressive performances in final examinations, many modern health educators feel that techniques that provide the opportunity for more student involvement hold much greater potential for producing long-term changes in real-life health behavior.

Applications. A common reaction to the recognition of overuse of any method is to abandon its use entirely even in those situations where it would be appropriate. Consequently, many teachers refuse to lecture under any circumstances. However, when judiciously applied, the lecture represents a very efficient way to transmit information. Visiting resource persons often combine a new face with new information and thus obtain good results with the lecture technique. The periodic large group instructional period in which two or more classes meet together often produces good student response in a lecture situation, particularly when supported by the use of overhead transparencies, colored slides, or other appropriate media applications. Within the more intimate setting of the individual classroom in which students often have day-to-day exposure to the same teacher, lecturing is generally less appropriate. However, even in this setting there are occasions when student interest is high in a given topic, which also happens to be reasonably complex, thus setting the stage for a short lecture. The concept of blood alcohol concentration, the hormonal control of ovulation, or the problems related to the Rh factor are possible examples. The lecture should seldom be used as the primary teaching technique, but if the conditions are appropriate, it should be used without any apologies.

Procedures. When the lecture is used, the traditional advice to (1) explain what you are going to say, (2) say it, and (3) explain what you have said should not be forgotten. Generally it is well to organize the presentation around a limited number of main points. As each point is introduced, it can be written on the chalkboard or perhaps displayed or represented on an overhead transparency. The point can then be developed with more detailed, supporting information. After the final point has been developed, all the main points should be reviewed.

Even the best preparation of the content of the lecture can be negated by poor mechanics of delivery. Within the classroom it is generally best for a teacher to develop an informal style, relying on spontaneous phraseology rather than on a written text. Both lecturing and discussion leadership are helped by the use of eye contact with first one and then another person as the room is scanned. Although voice volume must be high enough to reach all members of the group, one should try to retain a conversational style of inflection with suitable variations in pitch. Distracting mannerisms and the overuse of certain words or phrases should be avoided; the use of student forms for the evaluation of the instructor and classes are very effective in bringing these nuisance items to light.

Media-oriented techniques. The use of still pictures, slides, tape recordings, and other such media sometimes constitutes a technique in itself but more commonly provides support within the larger framework of class discussion, laboratory demonstrations, panel reports, and other comprehensive activities. The effective use of media is marked by a smooth transition to and from the media presentation and the ongoing activities of the class. The use of a sound film, for example, should augment rather than slow down the momentum a class has developed in its quest for information on a particular health topic, and this occurs when the teacher makes the effort required to tie in the content of the film to the objectives of the current unit of study by preparing the class properly for the film before it is shown and then discussing it effectively afterwards. This somewhat obvious need is too often neglected.

Motion picture. Literally hundreds of reasonably attractive films on health topics are available. Unfortunately, there are at least two main limitations to this availability. Although there are many attractive films available, only a relatively small proportion of these have real educational merit. For example, during the height of public concern over the problem of drug abuse an expert panel reviewed the drug education films that were then in most common use and pronounced over 90% of them essentially useless and judged a few of the worst to be more threatening to the health of young personalities than the drugs themselves.* This harsh judgment may do an

*DeLone, R. H.: The ups and downs of drug education, Saturday Review of Education, Sept. 11, 1972, p. 28.

injustice to the many really good films that are available; however, it underscores the need for careful and critical selection. Another barrier to effective film use is the frequent delay in the delivery of borrowed and rented films. Furthermore, those organizations that do hold to their promised delivery dates oftentimes require 2 months or more lead time in filling film requests, with the result that teachers must commit themselves to a rigid time schedule if they are to keep the current units of study in line with the arrival of the films. Because of this, a few carefully selected films that are purchased and kept readily accessible in the instructional materials center or film library of the school or school district are often more useful than are those that must be rented or loaned from distant sources.

When properly used, good films can meet a variety of educational objectives. A short film that incorporates color, music, and a lively narration can serve to build interest to a high pitch as a new unit is introduced. Time lapse, microphotography, and other techniques can often provide clear explanations of complex processes and principles; and as applied to one of the more difficult educational tasks, many films can communicate human feelings and emotions effectively. The achievement of these desired results requires both the wise selection of films (as discussed in Chapter 8) and their skillful use. Good teachers vary in their specific procedures; however, the more commonly accepted ones are provided below.

PREVIEWING. Even highly recommended films should be previewed so that the teacher can prepare to discuss points that may arise and to warn the class against unduly biased treatment of specific issues or aspects. More important, the preview can enable the teacher to relate the film content to the unit content derived from other sources.

MECHANICS OF PREPARATION. Although the new modern self-threading projectors are becoming increasingly reliable, one must still take considerable care in the mechanical details if time is not to be wasted. In a new situation, the teacher should check on the effectiveness of the darkening drapes well ahead of time, locate the wall socket to be used, see if it works and if an extension cord will be needed, and be sure the projector and screen are set up before the students arrive. If teachers are to operate the projector themselves, they should thoroughly familiarize themselves with the projector, including such skills as the use of the lever that corrects the frequent problem in sound synchronization and the replacement of bulbs that always seem to burn out at the most inconvenient time. When the film is completed, its rewinding should be delayed until the last few minutes of class or better yet during some natural break such as when pupils or students leave the room for lunch or for their next class.

INTRODUCING THE FILM. When other activities such as a lecture, discussion, or demonstration have preceded the film, a smooth transition can be effected by first pointing out any major points to be seen in the film related to these activities. If the class had been engrossed in values clarification activities (see pp. 104-105), it might be appropriate for the teacher to say, "We have just seen within our own class how people differ in their feelings regarding population control and the world food situation; see if you find similar differences among the people you are about to see in this film." Following this it is good to alert the class to one or two other main points to which they should give attention.

DEBRIEFING THE FILM. Once the film is complete, it is most appropriate for the teacher to lead the class into a discussion structured around the main points to which the class was alerted when the film was introduced. But in most cases, it is best to call first for general reactions; individual students will often pick up highly relevant points that the teacher overlooked. Occasionally these spontaneous reactions lead into facets of the topic more valuable than those preplanned by the teacher. Also, student criticism of the film itself is often valuable to air. Even the more useful films often contain undue biases or some aspects of commercial propaganda; although the teacher has a responsibility in this regard, another way to offset these negative aspects is to let the students themselves bring these points to light.

Filmstrips and slides. In recent years the sound filmstrip has become an increasingly popular medium for the presentation of health facts and concepts. The incorporation of vivid color photographs into a filmstrip is combined with background music and synchronized narration provided by an audiocassette; this combination can often approach the effectiveness of the conventional sound film for a fraction of the cost. In practical terms this often means that attractive, up-to-date sound filmstrips may be purchased and kept conveniently at hand within the school building or district media center. They would be used to cover topics that might have required less convenient rental or loan arrangements for regular sound films.

The mechanics of the actual classroom use of sound filmstrips are essentially the same for sound films; however, there are a few specific points to keep in mind.

When the audio portion is provided by a cassette rather than by a record, it is possible to interrupt the presentation by simply flipping the switch in order to discuss a particularly provocative point. Also, many teachers prefer filmstrips without the audio so that they can provide their own narrations, handle questions, and allow for ongoing discussion of the material with complete control and flexibility. The main barrier to this type of use is that the large majority of filmstrips produced these days come equipped with their own sound. Some more ambitious and creative teachers recapture this old-fashioned flexibility by making up their own 35-mm colored slide presentations on local health topics, thus achieving the added benefit of community relevance. Furthermore, the production of one's own slide-tape presentations with effective music and narrative is well within the capability of most energetic teachers with access to a modest amount of help from the school's media personnel.

The overhead projector. Few new teaching aids mesh so well with the habitual tendency of most teachers to stand up and talk before their students than has the overhead projector; herein lies both its most useful and attractive feature and its greatest potential for abuse. Simply taking the same lists of points, definitions, and so forth that one might otherwise write on the blackboard and displaying them on a lighted screen while retaining eye contact with the class can make an otherwise boring presentation tolerable, but this is hardly making the best use of this flexible tool. Although many teachers have been able to make a relatively smooth transition from use of the overhead projector as a vivid blackboard to its use as an exciting new teaching medium, all teachers can improve their effectiveness in proportion to the skill they develop in its use.

It is appropriate, particularly for many experienced teachers, to become acquainted with the overhead projector by first learning to handle it effectively at the "blackboard" level. It takes only a set of felt-tipped pens and a few pieces of clear acetate to get started. Even with this modest equipment certain advantages will soon become apparent. One can write the words to be displayed carefully and clearly well before going before the class (a feature that many appreciate), spelling can be straightened out ahead of time. Also, just the simple use of different colors for different points, labels, and so forth can serve to make a transparency better organized and more appealing. A few basic points to keep in mind at this beginning stage of overhead transparency use are:

The letters should be large and clear; one-quarter inch of letter height is the minimum needed for a standard classroom, and more height is preferable.

The wording should be sparse; lists and phrases are generally better than sentences. The temptation to fill up the transparency should be avoided. When it is necessary to present significant amounts of text, the dittoed or mimeographed handout is a more appropriate medium.

When the equipment is being set up, the projector and screen should be arranged so that neither the teacher nor the projector block the view of the screen; usually it is best to angle the screen across a corner of the room.

During the presentation it is often useful to cover with a piece of cardboard all but the first points of terms to be displayed; it then can be moved to successive stages as the discussion proceeds.

When it becomes necessary to point to any part of the material, the actual pointing should be to the transparency on the projector, while facing the class, rather than to the screen.

The overhead projector should be turned off any time the discussion or presentation moves to topics unrelated to the material on the transparency; otherwise class attention will be divided.

At the next level of use, the interested teachers can begin to experiment with simple drawings and diagrams; they will find that even relatively crude efforts will often be effective when projected in color. From here it is but a short step to the use of an infrared copying machine with heat-sensitive acetate to make transparencies from any appropriate pictures or diagrams. This process will make clear copies of any carbon-based material such as pencil drawings, newspaper graphs and illustrations, and mimeographed or typewritten copy. A large print (primary or bold-faced) typewriter must be used, however, for clear projection. Noncarbon-based illustrations or graphs of sufficient size that one might find in a book or magazine can be first copied in any common library duplicating machine and then fed into the infrared copier together with heat-sensitive acetate to produce an effective overhead transparency. This basic process can lead one into a whole system of transparency production that involves sophisticated materials but not an unreasonable amount of training or experience for the achievement of good results.

Although overhead transparencies represent one of the better media for the teacher preparation of visual materials, commercially prepared transparencies are appearing on the market in ever increasing quantities and varieties. These combine the advantages of vividly projected material with complete teacher control of the presentation. Also, simple black and white masters may often be purchased and reproduced on acetate to obtain the advantage of professionally prepared content at a greatly reduced cost.

The opaque projector. Occasionally it becomes important to project directly on a screen material from a book, magazine, or other original source. This can be done by use of the opaque projector. Although it is highly useful in special stiuations, there are several limitations to this method of projection. Unlike the overhead projector, the opaque projector must be operated from the rear of a darkened classroom. Also, unless the copy on the original material is exceptionally clear, the projected image will be of poor quality. Consequently, most teachers reserve the use of this technique for those situations wherein a limited amount of priority material must be displayed to a group on short notice. With material that will receive repeated use, it is better to make the added effort required to put it on overhead transparencies or some other medium. One creative use of the opaque projector, however, is the projecting of large images on paper or posterboard for the preparation of posters, bulletin boards, wall murals, and so forth. Finally, one unique feature of this device is that three-dimensional objects, if they are not too large, can be placed on its stage and displayed on the screen.

Television. As is so often the case with educational innovations, television was at first regarded by many educators as a revolutionary new tool that would solve many of the persistent problems associated with the teaching process. During the late 1960's, for instance, this belief was so strong that classroom teachers were often led to believe that they would be soon replaced by a centralized corps of master teachers operating from the television studio. This of course proved to be a gross exaggeration. However, as the myth was dispelled, television developed a more realistic role, not as a new system of teaching, but as a highly useful medium to be used as part of a balanced selection of teaching techniques.

Television in its various forms is so versatile a tool that it is easy to overlook many of its important applications. Some of these require considerable resources in the form of equipment and the support of media specialists, but others require nothing more extreme than the weekly TV guide found in most Sunday editions of the newspaper. A brief overview of television's uses includes:

1. *Use of major network television.* Many of the documentary programs produced by the major commercial networks have educational value that is often superior to that provided by commonly used educational films. Special educational guides are available that provide reliable descriptions of the program content; however, the regular commercial weekly TV guide often has the same information in a more available form. Well-motivated students will often be willing to view these programs when the teacher provides the necessary information and encouragement. Sometimes it is practical to offer students the alternative of viewing a program in lieu of a reading assignment. Also, students who have reports to complete can use television programs as a source of data. The incorporation of regular network television into the health education program not only meets immediate objectives but provides students with the opportunity to gain experience, under supervision, with a medium that will be the source of much of their health information in future years.

2. *Use of educational television.* After a number of false starts, educational television (ETV) as provided by the national public television network is beginning to realize its potential. Its frequently offered health-related programs can be used in much the same way as similar programs offered on the major commercial networks. Also, schools that have the necessary recording equipment may videotape programs from the various public broadcasting stations for later viewing during class. Copyright laws require that permission be obtained for this procedure; however, most ETV stations routinely honor such requests.

3. *Use of instructional television.* An increasing number of schools or school districts are acquiring the necessary equipment and personnel to produce their own tailor-made television presentations to be transmitted to their classrooms via cable or perhaps by producing videotapes for replay when needed by individual teachers. These closed-circuit or in-house systems are commonly termed instructional television (ITV) as distinguished from educational television, which is broadcast over the air as is regular network television. When such material comes to the teacher from a school or district studio as a telelesson or as a videotape for replay over a classroom television set, it can be handled in the classroom much like an instructional film except, of course, that there is no opportunity to stop the presentation for discussion or for the replay of crucial portions as many teachers occasionally like to do. There is the need to compensate for the smaller screen by various combinations of seating arrangements, placement of the set, or use of two or more sets.

When teacher and students have access to a total "TV chain"—that is, to a camera and recorder, with connecting set—a number of useful and creative applications become possible. For example, during the demonstration of anatomical dissections or laboratory procedures to a large audience, a closely positioned camera may be used to transmit a clear view of the proceedings into the large screen of a television set or sets. Another common use is the videotaping of particularly informative guest speakers for later replay during the school day in other sections of the same class, or perhaps, in future health classes during the next year or two. Finally, there is a whole realm of possibilities involving the use of students as television performers; these can range from a simple panel discussion to a totally student-produced dramatization of a health situation.

Laboratory activities. The feasibility and the appropriateness of conducting various laboratory demonstrations and experiments in the classroom vary considerably from school to school, depending on the availability of facilities and equipment, the philosophical orientation of the teacher and the programs, and the nature of the subject matter involved. When teacher demonstrations are presented, such as the capturing and condensing of cigarette smoke to show the tar content, the classroom procedures are similar to those used when showing a film insofar as the lead-in and the debriefing are concerned. Teachers should not necessarily tell the class specifically what they are about to see, but it is usually good to explain the general purpose of the demonstration and its relevance to the current unit of study before its presentation. During the demonstration it is usually appropriate to direct the class's attention from time to time to crucial points of observation; then after the demonstration it is well to first provide the class with an opportunity to interpret the results and draw conclusions before leading them to a structured discussion.

With a little ingenuity and reasonable access to resources, teachers can devise a number of interesting classroom experiments on health-related topics. Too often the complexity of scientific experimentation is emphasized to the neglect of its basic principles. An experiment involves nothing more than the altering of one factor in a situation while keeping all other aspects as similar to each other as possible and then observing the possible effects on the item or items of one's interest. For example, if the effect of "junk food" on health is the item of interest, a litter of young rats could be divided, placed in separate but similar cages, and provided with dissimilar diets such as plain white rice for one group and commercially prepared pellets for the other. The health status of the rats in each cage could be observed in terms of appearance, activity level, and rate of growth. Many good sources

are available that provide help with the specific details of classroom experiments.*

Community resources. A twofold advantage is commonly realized by teachers who utilize field trips, guest speakers, and other similar community resources in their teaching. The students learn not only about topic at hand, but gain specific information about their own locality and where they may obtain health information on future occasions.

The field trip. Both logistical as well as educational aspects must receive careful attention in the planning of a field trip. The common logistical tasks for most field trips include:

1. Obtaining permission or clearance from the school administration.
2. Making reservations or arrangements with the facilities or organization to be visited.
3. Making arrangements for transportation and, in some cases, meals and lodging.
4. Providing for supervisory personnel in the form of other teachers or parent volunteers.
5. Arranging for the release of the students from any other classes that will be missed.
6. Obtaining written parental permission for each individual student and informing the parent of the exact itinerary.
7. Providing clear instructions to the students as to meeting times and locations, and any necessary restrictions or rules for the trip.
8. Reviewing school policies and establishing contingency plans for such problems as illness or injury en route, inclement weather, and missing students.

From an educational standpoint the general task where field trips are involved is to

---

*See, for example, Morholt, E., Brandwein, P. F., and Joseph, A.: *A sourcebook for the biological sciences,* ed. 2, New York, 1966, Harcourt Brace Jovanovich, Inc.

take the steps necessary to reap the fullest possible benefits from this highly effective but relatively expensive teaching device. This requires effective planning not only for the trip itself but for the related educational activities before and after the trip. For example, a field trip to a mental hospital might provide the focal point for a unit on mental illness for a senior high school. With the approaching trip as an added incentive, the students could be encouraged to become as informed as possible on mental illness and its treatment prior to the trip. In many cases it would also be useful to organize the students into investigative teams with each one concentrating on a particular phase of the hospital's operation. Upon their return to the classroom, the various subgroups could report their observations to the full class. The students' observations could also be incorporated into any written reports or other assignments that were completed during the remaining portion of the unit.

The small group field trip. In many situations the small group field trip can yield most of the educational benefits of the large group trip with only a fraction of the bother and expense. This technique consists of recruiting a small group of well-motivated students to visit a community facility on their own time and then report their observations back to the total class. Many community organizations that might refuse to allow a visit by 25 or 35 partially interested students may welcome a smaller group of three or four students who seem genuinely concerned about the problems with which the community facility deals. Students are usually charged with the responsibility of reporting back to the class, and very often they can be encouraged to take pictures, perhaps tape record interviews, gather brochures, and otherwise embellish their reports.

Resource speakers. Whereas field trips take the students to the community, the resource speaker represents an effort to bring the community into the classroom. Such persons have the advantage of being

new to their audience and of speaking on a narrow range of topics, which enables them to master their subject matter. Consequently, even a mediocre speaker in terms of techniques of presentation can usually provide the student with a worthwhile experience, and a clever speaker can yield an outstanding one. Unfortunately, poor speakers who have little ability to reach their audience sometimes get into the classroom despite the efforts of teachers to screen their selections. In some cases the teachers can intervene as a moderator and turn the speech into a question and answer session, which often serves to get the presentation in line with student interests. Some other more routine considerations are:

Wherever possible, the selection of resource speakers should be restricted to those who have demonstrated the ability to communicate with the age and maturity level of the students involved.

Generally, resource speakers are more useful during the second half of a unit of study after the students have gained some general knowledge of the topic involved.

It is often helpful to provide the speaker with a general description of his prospective audience, particularly as to their background in the topic and their general responsiveness to discussion techniques. Speakers typically assume that their audience knows nothing about the topic and occasionally waste time on elementary information that the students have already covered.

Students gain more benefit from a classroom presentation with opportunities for discussion and interaction as compared with assembly-type settings.

Techniques for the affective domain. Teachers have traditionally devoted more attention (at least more systematic attention) to such cognitive outcomes in the classroom as the ability to remember facts, to apply them to new situations, to use facts and understanding in the analysis of situations, and to perform similar tasks that are basically intellectual in nature rather than emotional. In other words, they have been concerned with thinking and not feeling. Of course, many teachers in the past have been aware of the importance of student attitudes and values; they have felt a responsibility in this area and have devised ways of coping with this responsibility. For the most part, however, these actions have been viewed as something peripheral to the teacher's main job of inculcating knowledge and teaching young people how to think. More recently, there have been strong efforts to develop relatively precise categories and terminology so that many of the random, intuitive strategies good teachers have been using for years can now be shared, evaluated, and planned as a systematic part of the school curriculum.*

As noted earlier in this chapter, it is somewhat of a misnomer to label certain teaching techniques affective and others cognitive, because any classroom activity contains both elements to some degree. Every item of content brought to the students' attention is about something (cognitive) and tends to take on connotations of being good, bad, highly important, or trivial (affective). Therefore, all teaching techniques are both affective and cognitive in nature, but certain of these techniques tend to be more clearly identified with one or the other of the two common domains of classroom outcomes.

Perhaps the most important consideration regarding the use of affective teaching devices is the need for teachers to clearly decide what they are trying to accomplish in the areas of attitudes, values, beliefs, and personal behavior. One of the most popular points of view in this regard is that espoused by advocates of the general technique of values clarification.† The basic

purpose of this approach is to bring attitudes and values out into the open so that students can review, examine, and compare their respective positions and perhaps make favorable changes or modify their behavior to conform with their values. An attempt is made to create an open and non-judgmental atmosphere in which each student is the final authority in the assessment of his or her own values and merely uses the group, and perhaps the teacher, as a sounding board. This approach has much to recommend it as long as teachers bear in mind that it is impossible for people in the same classroom to avoid influencing one another's value structure even when they try very hard not to do so. Also, some small degree of influence is probably desirable. It is possible that when the teacher and the group both try to avoid having any influence at all on the values of individual students, they will probably influence students' values in something close to the optimal degree.

The affective discussion. Under the proper conditions, such phenomena as attitudes, values, and personal feelings can be discussed and examined in a relatively normal discussion format either as a total class or within small groups. Proper conditions in this case include, first, an atmosphere of openness and trust within the class and, second, the leading or focusing of the discussion topic or topics on affective material. The first of these conditions in particular is not easy to achieve, and the difficulty of this task varies considerably from class to class. Occasionally particular classes appear to represent a happy combination of personalities wherein mutual confidence and trust occur early in the school term; however, in the normal case it often requires the use of some of the more highly structured values clarification techniques to reach this desirable state.

Values clarification. Sidney Simon and his associates* in their book *Values Clari-*

---

*For an example of one of the more influential of these efforts see Krathwohl, D. R., Bloom, B. S., and Masia, B. B.: *Taxonomy of educational objectives, handbook II: affective domain,* New York, 1964, David McKay Co., Inc.
†For a thorough discussion of the theory of this approach, see Raths, L., Harmin, M., and Simon, S.: *Values and teaching,* Columbus, Ohio, 1966, Charles E. Merrill Publishing Co.

*Simon, S. B., Howe, L. W., and Kirschenbaum, H.: *Values clarification,* New York, 1972, Hart Publishing Co., Inc., pp. 38-40, 116-119, 308-310.

fication describe 79 specific classroom strategies and, in addition, advise teachers to modify those presented and develop their own unique techniques to meet special needs. Basically these techniques involve first presenting students with an issue or situation that normally evokes differences of opinion, then providing them with an opportunity to make their personal choice or position known to themselves and the group. A sampling of these techniques as adapted to health education are provided below.

VALUES CONTINUUM. This technique is used to provide students with the opportunity to graphically display their position on an issue and compare their position with that of other members of the class. The teacher draws a line on the board to represent a scale of opinions and characterizes the extreme positions; a continuum on the legal control of drugs might look like the one shown below.

| |_____|_____|_____|_____| |

Liberal Lou
All drugs available to
   everyone

Repressive Raymond
No drugs allowed
   regardless of the
   circumstances

On this scale students who supported the status quo might locate themselves in the middle; those who would legalize marijuana would be slightly to the left, whereas modern prohibitionists would place themselves to the right. Once all those who desire to take a stand have placed their names on a scale, the various positions are discussed in an effort to explore and understand them. In an interesting variation, the continuum with the student's names in place is left posted in the classroom throughout a unit of study so that students can change their positions should their personal views be changed.

EPITAPH. Despite its title this technique is focused on life rather than death as students are asked to express in a few words how they would best like to be remembered. Students who make a conscientious effort will tend to reveal to themselves and to others the main aspect or aspects of their lives about which they are most proud. In some cases, of course, students will describe characteristics they hope to acquire in the remaining years of their life. Some efforts also may be "off beat" of self-effacing but nonetheless valuable in revealing something of each student's self-concept. One cautionary word is offered by those experienced in the use of this technique; occasionally a particularly superstitious student may feel that participation in this activity might somehow hasten the day of his or her own death. As with all values clarification techniques, the teacher must be sensitive to such personal reactions and allow students who feel unduly threatened to "pass."

VALUES VOTING. In what is perhaps the simplest of the values clarification techniques for most teachers to use, the teacher simply asks the class a series of questions pertinent to a particular issue. The students respond to each question by raising their hand for "yes," making a "thumbs down" gesture for no, folding their arms for "no opinion," and simply making no sign if they choose to pass. The teacher also votes but withholds his or her signal until a split second after the class has responded. A short series of up to ten questions usually produces optimal results in student involvement in the issue and readiness for a more systematic discussion of its major aspects. Some examples that could be appropriate are:

Do you believe that everyone in the world has a right to an adequate diet?

Would you give up meat 1 day per week to help the world food supply?

Would you donate money to prevent famine in countries that refused to try to control their birth rate?

Dramatizations. Another way to deal with affective-oriented content is by use of role playing or playlets. Students who have had little experience with either of these activities may at first tend to respond to the amateurish acting efforts of their classmates rather than to the content of the dramatization, but this will soon pass after the first few instances of use. Many variations of these techniques exist; however, an overview of their basic elements will enable the average teacher to get started.

Teachers often ask students to think of how it would feel to be in someone else's shoes. *Role playing* goes one step further and asks them to act as if they were someone else as a means of gaining more insight into the motives and feelings of the person they are portraying. Also, their audience (in this case, the remainder of the class) is provided with a concrete situation to which they can relate and analyze. This is accomplished by providing the participating students with a brief description of the character of their role and the situation in which it is to be played. Usually two or more such role players interact, and the teacher stops the action occasionally for discussion and terminates the activity when he or she feels the main points have been made. It is usually best to select relatively stable, middle of the road students rather than those unduly introverted or extroverted when initiating this technique with a new group. Another way to get started is to divide the class into small groups of four or five and ask various pairs to role play before the remaining two or three members. Once the students have acquired a little confidence in this technique, the majority will be willing to participate before the total class.

In most cases it is not wise to ask students to portray roles too close to any possible real/life problems, such as taking the role of a daughter of an alcoholic when the student is indeed living in that situation. This procedure is sometimes used by psychotherapists (in which case the technique becomes psychodrama), but it is inappropriate for most classrooms. Even with precautions, individual students may on rare occasions become too emotionally involved in a role and require some sympathetic support and a chance to calm down before proceeding to their next class or activity.

In the *playlet* technique the teacher trades off the spontaneity of role playing for the more predictable results that can be obtained when students are provided with specific lines and behavior to portray to the class. The playlets in some cases are available from commercial sources; innovative teachers can write their own playlets to meet specific educational objectives; and in perhaps the most creative alternative, students can be encouraged to do the writing.

QUESTIONS FOR STUDY AND DISCUSSION

1. Compare those teaching techniques located near the top of Dale's cone of experience with those near the bottom in terms of their relative usefulness in the classroom.
2. Distinguish between cognitive and affective objectives and discuss the selection of appropriate teaching techniques for each.
3. Compare the relative effectiveness of student-centered versus teacher-centered teaching techniques.
4. Identify and discuss the basic factors necessary for a good classroom discussion.
5. Describe various sets of circumstances that justify the use of the lecture technique.
6. Discuss the procedures necessary to ensure that the use of a sound film, filmstrip, or slide-tape presentation will result in a meaningful learning experience.
7. Discuss the relative advantages and disadvantages of overhead projector use as compared with other techniques of visual presentation.
8. Discuss the role of television in modern health education in terms of the potential offered by commercial, ETV, and ITV applications.
9. Compare the relative advantages of the whole-class versus the small-group field trip as applied to various teaching situations.
10. Describe the basic process of values clarification in terms of its purpose and the common features included in various specific techniques.
11. Distinguish between the relative usefulness of role playing and playlets in various teaching situations.

REFERENCES

Armsey, J. W., and Dahl, N. C.: *An inquiry into the uses of instructional technology,* New York, 1973, Ford Foundation.

Brown, J. W., Lewis, R. B., and Harcleroad, F. F.: *AV instruction: media and methods,* ed. 3, New York, 1969, McGraw-Hill, Inc.

Dale, E.: *Audiovisual methods in teaching,* ed. 3, New York, 1969, Holt, Rinehart and Winston, Inc.

Epstein, C.: *Affective subjects in the classroom: exploring race, sex, and drugs,* Scranton, Pa., 1972, Intext Educational Publishers.

Fraenkel, J. R.: *Helping students think and value: strategies for teaching the social studies,* Englewood Cliffs, N.J., 1973, Prentice-Hall, Inc.

Mayshark, C., and Foster, R. A.: *Health education in secondary schools,* St. Louis, 1972, The C. V. Mosby Co.

Morholt, E., Brandwein, P. F., and Joseph, A.:
A sourcebook for the biological sciences, ed. 2,
New York, 1966, Harcourt Brace Jovanovich,
Inc.

Read, D. A., and Greene, W. H.: *Creative teaching
in health,* ed. 2, New York, 1974, Macmillan,
Inc.

Simon, S. B., Howe, L. W., and Kirschenbaum,
H.: *Values clarification,* New York, 1972, Hart
Publishing Co., Inc.

Wurman, R. S., editor: *Yellow pages of learning
resources,* Philadelphia, 1972, Group for Environmental Education, Inc.

CHAPTER 8 ❧ Selection and acquisition of instructional media

An ideal teaching situation was once described as "a talented teacher seated on one end of a log and an apt pupil on the other." However appealing this simplistic description may be in these days of conflicting educational theories, exotic technology, and soaring school budgets, the fact remains that few teachers or pupils are equipped to function well under such conditions even if a one-to-one teacher-pupil ratio somehow became feasible. Modern, efficient teaching requires the use of a variety of activities other than sitting and listening as well as a variety of materials in the form of books, films, filmstrips, audiotapes, still pictures, and other such items. The proper selection and acquisition of this latter category of teaching tools, commonly referred to as educational media, are complex and demanding tasks that are crucial to any program's effectiveness.

PROPER ROLE OF MEDIA

The use of media in teaching was once a simple matter that began with an assignment in a textbook and ended with the viewing of a 16-mm sound film with little occurring in between other than the occasional use of the chalkboard. All this was changed by the Sputnik space race syndrome of the 1960's wherein technology was seen as the answer to all problems ranging from national security to domestic illiteracy. The combination of this common point of view with a vast infusion of federal money into the nation's schools via such legislation as the National Defense Education Act stimulated a proliferation of new audiovisual devices and ambitious applications of existing devices. During this period language learning labs, instructional television, and a variety of relatively exotic teaching machines be-

came common classroom items. During the heyday of enthusiasm for this general approach many teachers feared that they would be relegated to a mere baby-sitting role as educational technology took over most of their teaching functions.

Promises and problems. These fears proved to be largely unfounded as the educational technology movement encountered more than the usual number of growing pains. Schools found it easier to buy equipment than to provide or encourage teachers to acquire the training necessary for its proper use. The manufacturers likewise found it easier to sell these new items than to provide the high degree of service and maintenance needed to handle the many problems arising from the combination of sophisticated machinery and partially trained operators. Meanwhile, no one seemed capable of providing the new films, tapes, programs, and other such items needed to bring these new pieces of equipment to life; as expressed in the new jargon of educational technology, the "hardware" was always ahead of the "software."

Fortunately, the growth of educational media seems to have worked its way through this awkward stage. Partially because of a newfound respect for the human element in teaching and partially because of tight budgets, schools have become more discriminating in their purchase of equipment. Also, virtually a whole new industry was established to fill the software void, with the result that educational technology is coming into its own as an important teaching tool rather than as some electronic substitute for the teacher. Vestiges of the old problems and negative attitudes still remain, however, and account for many of the frustrations and misuses that commonly occur as teachers seek to realize the rich potential offered by the proper use of educational media. The machines still occasionally break down, software suitable for many specific topics still does not exist, and it is still often hard to acquire at the proper time. For the most part, however, these problems can be overcome to yield benefits in the classroom that can be achieved in no other way.

Real benefits of media. In a broad sense, young people are exposed to media every day in the form of real-life experiences. Some teachers tend to take the position that in a field such as health, which is so involved with everyday life, the proper role of the teacher is to help students discuss and sort out these experiences rather than to bombard them with new stimuli through the use of classroom media. Although this position is valid to a certain point, there comes a time when it is necessary to introduce some new experiences into this system of classroom interaction so that both teachers and students can transcend the limits of their immediate environment. Carefully selected media can do this and more. Stanton Oates* lists ten reasons for media use; five that seem particularly appropriate to health teaching are presented here.

1. *They provide a common background.* All of the members of a class have the same experience or starting point for learning new concepts. An "alcoholic," for example, in the mind of a student with abstinent parents might be anyone who takes a drink, whereas other students whose parents use alcohol might restrict their definition of alcoholics to skid row inhabitants. A series of case histories presented on film or in written form can modify these extreme views and provide a common basis for discussion.

2. *They catch and hold attention.* Teachers seeking to impress students with the importance of serious bleeding,

stoppage of breathing, and poisoning as the three most urgent first-aid situations may fail if they rely on a verbal presentation alone. However, the support of a vivid series of overhead transparencies will not only provide a visual image to aid retention but also focus the students' attention on the lesson rather than on the view out the window or the actions of a nearby classmate.

3. *Students can see and hear events remote in time and space.* The television or movie camera can bring the sights and sounds of the emergency ward, the scientist's laboratory, other related settings of the present, and (through suitable re-creation) dramatic events of the past.

4. *Action can be slowed down or speeded up.* Time lapse photography can condense the weeks and months required for the insidious growth of cancer or the miraculous transformation of an egg into a mature organism into a few minutes of time; similarly, the beating of a heart or the wink of an eyelid can be slowed for ready observation.

5. *They stimulate interest and provide motivation.* Hungry and starving people can no longer be regarded as mere statistics when the students can look into their eyes. Dramatic portrayals of situations involving love, hate, pleasure, and disappointment can add the affective dimension necessary to convey the full reality of health situations or concepts.

In addition, media can also be used by the health educator to enable students to view very large and very small objects, simplify various processes through animation, reduce instructional time, provide for individual differences, or provide remedial help. Although many of the benefits or reasons for media use seem obvious or self-explanatory, the basic practice of selecting media to accomplish a specific purpose merits strong emphasis in light of the too common tendency among some teachers to

*Oates, S. C.: *Instructional materials handbook,* Dubuque, Ia., 1971, Kendall/Hunt Publishing Co., pp. 1-2.

use a film, pamphlet, or whatever simply because it happens to be available. These media abusers have caused many other teachers to overreact in the opposite direction and refuse to use anything beyond a textbook and a few worksheets. These extremes can be avoided by first determining one's specific objectives and then reviewing them in light of the available media possibilities. A medium is then placed in its proper role as a support rather than as a detriment to the learning experience.

OVERVIEW OF MEDIA

At least three major preconditions must exist before the full benefits of media can be realized. The first is the teacher's general awareness of the nature and purpose of specific categories of media so that a review of media possibilities becomes a habitual part of the daily planning process. The overview presented in this section is designed to help develop this necessary awareness. The second precondition consists of the specific skills involved in matching media to objectives and integrating media smoothly and effectively into the ongoing activities of the classroom. Finally, there is the challenging logistical task of acquiring or gaining access to suitable media. This task is deceptively simple in theory but frustratingly complex in practice. It will be covered later in the chapter in some detail after an overview of the basic types of media has been given.

Textbooks. The quality of health textbooks appears to be steadily improving to the point that a number of worthwhile series are available for the elementary grades as well as a number of individual selections for the junior and senior high school levels. The general coverage of nutrition, personal hygiene, and the basic structure and functioning of the body is particularly good in the better texts. Of lesser quality, at least in our opinion, is the treatment of the more value-laden areas such as alcohol and drugs, sexuality, and mental health, which tend to be excessively traditional, bland, sketchy, or otherwise hampered by the efforts of publishers to please a wide variety of com-

munity tastes. For these and other reasons the conscientious teacher will usually find individual parts of any text to be of little or no use. Despite these limitations, however, the textbook remains an exceedingly useful classroom tool because of its comprehensiveness and its convenience. A further advantage is found in the many teaching suggestions and source lists that are commonly provided in the teacher's edition of most textbooks.

Supplementary books, periodicals, and pamphlets. Although other media and activities may provide more vivid experiences, books and magazines are unexcelled in their ability to provide detailed information on a wide range of topics at a relatively low cost. The logical repository for most supplementary books and magazines is the school library or instructional materials center. For this reason it is essential that health teachers fully exercise whatever voice they may have in the selection of new titles for such facilities. Within the classroom, pamphlets and booklets on special subjects may often be obtained and distributed to the students to fill in the voids and inappropriate coverage that are occasionally found in even the best of texts. Also, the presence of *Today's Health* and/or other similar publications contributes to the general atmosphere of a health education classroom and provides a good source of current information.

Audiocassettes. Through the medium of relatively inexpensive, commercially prepared audiocassettes, students can hear experts in many health-related fields discussing their specialties in their own words. When properly used in short presentations that are interspersed with discussion and other alternate activities, such cassettes can be used in whole class activities. With the use of individual earphones, cassettes are highly valuable for individual study in the classroom or library carrels. Perhaps even more useful is the variety of possible uses for locally recorded material. Guest speakers may be taped for later study for the benefit of students not present during the original ap-

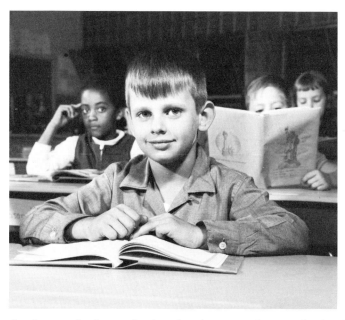

Fig. 8-1. A well-written textbook can stimulate thought and produce genuine involvement with subject matter.

pearance, and students working on assignments may go out into the community and tape interviews for classroom use. Teachers may tape the directions for special optional assignments that individual students may select and may also tape any unusually complex general assignments for students who are unable to be present for the original explanation.

Charts, graphs, and posters. A wide variety of health-related charts may find useful applications in the classroom, such as anatomical charts that show the basic structure of cells, tissues, organs, and organ systems; organizational charts that show the interrelationships among given components, such as the divisions of a public health department or present and past relatives on a "family" genealogical tree; and flow charts that show the sequence of operations involved in some complex process, such as the transmission of an infectious disease involving an intermediate host. Graphs are useful in the presentation of data in concise form and commonly appear as line graphs, bar graphs, or circular or pie graphs. Posters

incorporate various combinations of eye-catching illustrations and slogans to present an idea at a single glance. These have instructional value, particularly in reinforcing ideas that should not be ignored. In addition, attractive posters can help establish the identity and add to the attractiveness of classrooms where health teaching takes place.

These graphic items tend to be abused by some teachers who rely on them to add a bit of interest to their daily lectures or recitation-type discussions; however, they can add much to a program when properly used, not only to introduce new topics, but to follow up, review, and generally aid in the process of leisurely digesting information originally presented in more vivid media as sound films, dissection activities, or field trips. Charts and graphs can serve to make a wide variety of detailed information readily available for instant use when questions arise during wide-ranging class discussion. Although these items are commonly available from a variety of commercial sources, an additional advantage is gained through the experience of the construction process when they are student prepared.

Still pictures, photographs, and filmstrips. Whether they are artist renditions or photographs, still pictures are among the more versatile of teaching tools. They can be mounted and displayed on bulletin boards, used for individual study, or used to illustrate points in oral presentations either directly or through the use of the opaque projector. Many teachers find it very worthwhile to develop their own file as they collect suitable pictures from both magazines and commercial sources. Appropriate mounting by use of rubber cement and laminate processes can add greatly to both the ease of handling and the effectiveness of the display. Assistance in the application of these techniques is often available from school media specialists or librarians.

With the rapid increase in the popularity of photography, many teachers are combining this interesting hobby with their professional responsibilities as they incorporate their own photographs into their teaching. Also, many students (particularly at the secondary level but also at the elementary level) can be encouraged to use the camera as a tool to support their written and oral assignments. The popular 2 × 2 slide that is produced by the 35-mm camera has obvious applications, particularly when instructors focus on community organizations and resources. Such slide shows may be arranged in proper sequence and stored in convenient, albeit somewhat bulky, magazines for ease of handling and ready accessibility. Many schools are combining the advantages of lower processing costs, tailor-made enlargements, and special effects with the development of a new instructional facility by operating their own darkrooms.

Filmstrips offer a number of unique advantages that are sometimes overlooked in the modern trend toward ever more exotic media. Many teachers find the silent filmstrip more adaptable to a variety of needs because they can provide their own narrations, skip over sections of marginal importance to the lesson at hand, and discuss at some length those particularly relevant frames. Another attractive feature of the filmstrip is its convenience. A strip of standard 35-mm film that is 3 to 6 feet long can carry 24 to 48 still pictures and can be projected from a small, portable projector. Many teachers who happen to be serious amateur photographers often make their own filmstrips. Also both elementary pupils and secondary students as well as teachers can make interesting filmstrips by drawing on clear film with felt-tipped pens.

Sound filmstrips and slide tapes. The added convenience of the tape cassettes over the older phonograph record has enabled the sound filmstrip to come into its own in recent years. The slide tape is identical in function to the sound filmstrip but involves a slide magazine (2 × 2) rather than a strip of film for its visual component. Many schools find that much of their audiovisual budget is better spent on the direct purchase of a broad selection of sound filmstrips or slide tapes than on the purchase or rental of conventional motion picture films. Purchase of motion picture films is often impractical because of their higher cost, and film rental usually involves the inconvenience of planning requests several weeks or months in advance, the frustration of delayed delivery, and the continual expense of rental fees and handling expenses. With a moderate degree of creativity, teacher-photographers find it worthwhile to produce their own slide-tape shows, as do some of the more ambitious students in the completion of term projects.

Motion pictures. As we noted earlier, the use of motion pictures often involves heavy expenses and/or significant inconvenience; however, this medium also offers certain unique advantages that account in large part for its continued popularity among teachers. They present activities taking place, things in action. They bring events from other parts of the world to the classroom. They are often more instructional than field trips because the films present only the things the student should see and do not confuse them with unimportant details; moreover, they are certainly more convenient and less expensive than field trips. Documentary films present complicated laboratory demonstrations that are too difficult, expensive, or dangerous to arrange for the lecture period. The eye of the camera can be at the most desirable place, and thus when the picture is projected, the whole class sees the demonstration from an ideal vantage point. The camera can look through the fluoroscope and record such physiological activities as the contractions of the stomach and the beating of the heart.

Slow motion analyzes rapid movement. Stop motion speeds up an activity, such as the growth of bacteria, which is too slow to watch through the microscope. Films using animation illustrate processes that are not visible, such as the exchange of gases or dissolved substances between the blood and the tissue cells.

Dramatic films can re-create historical events and reach students on the emotional level to add the essential affective component to various health concepts and issues. Films for these purposes must be selected with special care, however, because of the fragile nature of dramatic impressions. Amateurish acting or outdated (or otherwise inappropriate) situations will seldom produce the desired student responses.

Silent films are making a comeback in the form of 8-mm loop films housed in convenient cassettes. Unfortunately, the selection at this writing is still very restricted insofar as health topics are concerned. The conventional silent film, although considered old-fashioned by many, should not be overlooked; it does offer certain special advantages. It may be stopped at any time, leaving a picture on the screen for class discussion. For example, a motion picture of the heart in action may be stopped on the screen to discuss structure or sequential processes such as the filling of the heart chambers,

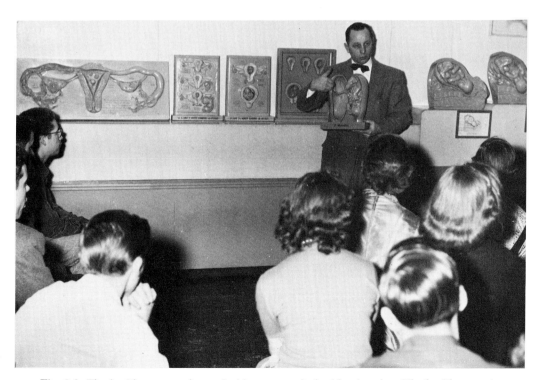

Fig. 8-2. The health museum is a valuable resource in health education. The health presentation above is illustrated by the use of anatomical models.

and the action of the valves may be stopped at any point to discuss and clarify the various steps involved.

Silent films, like most other media, also lend themselves to teacher or student production. Visits to water-treatment plants, food-processing plants, and health-related facilities may be filmed for later use in class. Sound films may also be produced by the amateur, but the cost tends to be prohibitive in most school situations.

Models. Anatomical models give a better understanding of actual size and structure than word descriptions or drawings. Like charts, they are used in health teaching to show relationships of health significance. Models, for example, give the student a clear understanding of the eustachian tube as the avenue of middle ear infection, the delicacy of the middle ear and inner ear, and innumerable other structures in their relationships to health and disease. Many models are made so that they can be taken apart and reassembled.

Perhaps the most famous model is the transparent woman, which can be seen in many health museums. This model is nearly life size and is made of plastic. It is equipped with an electric lighting system that illuminates one system of organs after another as a voice recording describes the model.

Artificial resuscitation may be effectively taught by use of a child-size model designed to respond in a way similar to a live subject in regard to chest movement and exhalation as resuscitation is administered. Although somewhat expensive, this teaching aid seems extremely worthwhile in view of the obvious importance of the skill involved.

Videotapes and cassettes. As described in the preceding chapter, classroom television presentations can serve many of the same purposes as motion pictures. Most schools, however, find that the use of commercially prepared videotapes or cassettes have thus far offered few advantages over conventional sound films. Consequently, the selection of such tapes tend to be quite limited. From a materials standpoint, the best sources appear to be local studio productions and, after permission is obtained, the taping of programs broadcast by public service networks off the air for later use in the classroom.

Exhibits. Exhibits may be made by the teacher or the students, or they may be borrowed, rented, or purchased from health agencies or other sources in the community. They provide an opportunity for students to construct models, collect specimens, or create materials. They utilize visual learning and often bring the community into the school.

School-made exhibits deserve careful planning including carefully selected materials and close attention to space needs and lighting. Design, color, and lettering must serve to bring out the central theme effectively. It may be desirable to set up the exhibit in the classroom if it is going to be used for work periods and with discussion groups. An exhibit that is large and carefully prepared may be made available to the other classes in the school building and shown to visitors, perhaps with student guides to provide narrations. There are key spots in the building where exhibits may be effectively displayed. For example, an exhibit on foods and nutrition may be located in the lunchroom, while exhibits in other fields such as school safety or first aid may be presented in a corridor or in the school auditorium at the time of a parent-teacher meeting in the building.

Objects and specimens. Many real objects, often termed "realia," can be brought to class to provide the experiences of seeing, touching, or handling in the study of an object. Primary school children may become acquainted with individual fruits and vegetables at a fruit and vegetable party. A real meal can be set up in the classroom. Different kinds of cloth can be seen and felt, as can various items of clothing. Pupils may learn to read the thermometer as they study temperature. Different kinds of plants may be brought to school or pets may be kept. Older students may obtain bacterial cultures and grow common bacteria.

Maps. Outline maps or maps showing limited geographical detail may be used to demonstrate many health situations. A spot map of the neighborhood or state can be made to show the distribution of disease in time of epidemic. A neighborhood map can show the exact location of an accident. State or national maps can be made to show areas of food production, concentrations of population, or which states have specific laws or regulations.

Flash cards. These usually consist of words or pictures on cardboard and can be flashed by hand for quick identification or for memory drills; the answers are commonly written on the back, thus facilitating student-to-student use. They have been used in health education for drill in the study of word meanings and for strengthening the immediate recognition of foods with different nutritional values as well as for the study of harmful insects, poison ivy, and other poisonous plants. They can help to distinguish quickly the differences between harmless and poisonous snakes or poisonous and edible mushrooms in situations where this knowledge is important.

Flip charts. The flip chart is a device made of large sheets of heavy paper that are bound together at the top and mounted upon an easel, which allows the sheets to be turned readily. It may be made by pupils as they study a topic to show, for example, a series of safety situations, community health activities, different food groups, or other relationships.

Cartoons. Just as political cartoonists use humor and satire to provoke thought and discussion of serious topics, health-related cartoons may be brought to class by the teacher or pupils to stimulate interest in health topics. They are especially enjoyed by pupils of the intermediate grades. Constructive discussion may be developed while

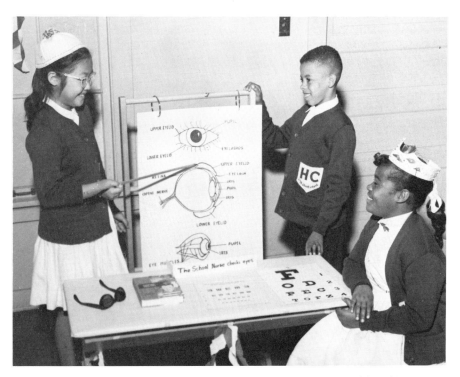

Fig. 8-3. Flip charts are relatively simple but highly useful teaching aids.

bringing out the facts in the situation, thus contributing to education and not merely to entertainment.

Chalkboards, flannel boards, magnetic boards, and overhead transparencies. Chalkboards that are colored for effective contrast and are sufficiently abrasive to take chalk well, and yet are sufficiently smooth and impermeable for ease of cleaning, retain their popularity as a useful medium for the presentation of visual impressions. They are used not only for word lists but also for diagrams, charts, graphs, and sketches. Chalkboards are usually located at the front of and at one side of the classroom, but smaller chalkboards can serve as the center of a teaching nook or corner for small group instruction.

A flannel board is made by covering a sheet of masonite or similar material with flannel cloth. Flannel figure cutouts or pictures mounted on a card with sandpaper backing will stick to the surface of the flannel. The ease with which it can be put up and taken down makes the flannel board an interesting device for the presentation of health ideas, either directly or in connection with class discussion. Other materials that can be attached to a flannel or felt surface include blotters, corduroy, velvet, and cotton. Although most popular at the elementary level, the flannel board is useful at all levels of instruction. It is particularly valuable in illustrating a series of events or activities in a discussion period. Pupils may go to the flannel board and change the illustrations as needed.

Flannel boards with suitable components provide a good method for presenting and discussing balanced meals, the basic food groups, the production and distribution of milk, seasonal clothing needs, the units of anatomical structure, the health facilities of the community, and the routes through which communicable diseases are transmitted.

Magnetic boards are similar in purpose and use to flannel boards. They are metal sheets to which either magnetic pieces or materials attached to magnets will adhere.

Some magnetic boards are covered with a thin layer of oilcloth or other material which will not hinder the use of the magnet.

Overhead transparencies are similar to flannel boards and magnetic boards in their purpose as aids to oral presentations, but they generally offer more important advantages in most teaching situations. They provide large, vivid images that can be more detailed and realistic. They can handle printed text in a better fashion and lend themselves to a wide variety of creative production techniques (see pp. 99-100). Overhead transparencies do, however, require the use of a special projector and screen, thus sacrificing some of the intimacy that is desirable in some small group discussions such as with kindergarten or primary schoolchildren; in these particular situations the flannel board may be more effective.

Bulletin boards. The general purpose classroom is often equipped with a bulletin board or tack board made of pressed fibers, soft wood, or self-healing cork. Plastic wall coverings are sometimes used to provide a washable bulletin board surface. The classroom bulletin board provides a suitable place for a variety of visual materials. Items may be posted by pupils and teachers for their current interest, or the bulletin board may be devoted to an extensive series of clippings, pictures, charts, maps, and grafts related to a unit of study in health in which the children are engaged. Bulletin boards in corridors, cafeterias, libraries, and other rooms may be used to carry health messages. Those in the health service suite or the the gymnasium more commonly carry bulletins of health advice or health schedules, in contrast to the displays that are provided and serviced frequently on the bulletin boards of classrooms and corridors.

An interesting variation of the conventional bulletin board is the hook-and-loop board, which is covered with special fabric with minute but strong loops incorporated into its weave. Moderately sized items such as dishes, tools, or scientific apparatus can be mounted for display by use of special tape with a strong adhesive on one side and small burr-like hooks on the other. This technique enables relatively large three-dimensional objects to be conveniently arranged and yet securely mounted.*

Workbooks and scrapbooks. Workbooks have been successfully used in the development of units of instruction and in the solving of health problems both in elementary and secondary schools. Many classes in the elementary school have had a successful experience in keeping a class scrapbook in which health activities have been used as exchange material among teachers of the same grade. Each scrapbook carries the name of the class and teacher who produced it.

The health museum. Another excellent resource for health education is the health museum. Both health museums and special health exhibits in general museums are becoming more numerous. In a few places, traveling health exhibits may be brought to the individual school. A field trip to special exhibits is of value, assuming of course that the exhibits are well arranged, adapted to the age levels of the students, and related to the program of study. Students need to be prepared in advance for the exhibits that they are to study. The museum lesson should be directed toward definite objectives rather than to superficial observation of whatever exhibits may be found upon arrival. Discussion and review of the museum trip following its completion are especially important.

The Cleveland Health Museum† is a source for the purchase, rental, or loan of exhibits. Teachers will find that their local art museums, museums of natural history, science museums, or children's museums may have loan exhibits or will arrange field trips on topics in the health course.

SELECTION PROCESS

Thus far in this chapter, health teachers have been advised to become aware of media possibilities by familiarizing themselves with the various categories in terms of their advantages, disadvantages, and general features. Once this has been accomplished, teachers must next look to the requirements of the curriculum within which they are teaching in order to determine the specific tasks that must be accomplished in the classroom. As presented in Chapter 5, behavioral objectives (statements that describe the desired learner behavior in specific terms) represent a very effective way to express these classroom tasks. As each behavioral objective is reviewed, media needs may become apparent.

Planning sequence.* As they plan for instruction, many experienced teachers develop habitual patterns or sequences, which serve to improve their efficiency. Although each teacher must develop the approach that serves him or her best, many find that the following steps work quite well.

1. *Review each behavioral objective and visualize the type of learning experiences that the students need for its attainment.* For instance, if the objective states that students must "review three different advertisements for a single type of health product and select the one that appears least deceptive," then it seems clear that the students must (1) gain access to the advertisements and (2) have the opportunity to develop suitable criteria for judging deception.

2. *Review possible activities and/or media presentations that will provide the needed experiences.* A wide variety of possibilities exist for the accomplishment of the first part of the objective. Students may be asked to bring in magazine advertisements for specified products; the teacher might have 2 × 2 slides made of such advertisements where facilities were available; or certain students could make a tape recording of radio advertisements as extra credit assignments. The second aspect might be achieved by use of pamphlets from govern-

*Oates, S. C.: *Instructional materials handbook,* p. 18.
†8911 Euclid Ave., Cleveland, Oh. 44106.

*The content in this section is based on Allen, W. J.: Media stimulus and types of learning, Audiovisual instruction, Jan. 1967.

ment agencies or consumer organizations, a suitable film on the topic, or perhaps an assignment in the textbook.

3. *From this group of possibilities, select the optimal learning activities and/or media presentations in terms of effectiveness, efficiency in terms of time and expense, and availability of material and equipment.* Many factors should be considered in this selection process. In some cases the learning task might be best accomplished by role playing, values clarification, or some other nonmedia-oriented activity. If it is early in a new unit of study, media with high stimulus value such as an attractive motion picture may be justified as a motivational device, even though it may be time-consuming and may carry a high rental fee. Later on in a unit in which the students have developed a high degree of interest in the content, a pamphlet or other reading assignment might convey the necessary information more effectively than a lengthy film, which at this point might tend to destroy the class's momentum. A smoothly narrated slide tape with beautiful woodland scenes and pleasant background music might be an ideal choice if the objective calls for the "development of an appreciation for the natural environment," but within the same area of study a more cognitive task such as "describing the basic steps of the nitrogen cycle" might be better accomplished with a set of teacher-produced overhead transparencies, which would permit the interspersing of discussions and variations in the pace of the presentation to accommodate the needs of different individuals and classes.

These three steps, in addition to their practical value in the media selection process, illustrate at least two major generalizations concerning media use. First, the objective must determine the media; the media should not determine the objective. Second, situational factors such as availability of equipment, cost of materials, size of class, time allotted, and the general ability and attitude of students must also enter into the media selection process. Implicit in

this second point is the dynamic nature of media selection. Curricula are revised; objectives are modified; situational factors change; old materials become dated; and new materials and new media technology constantly evolve. Consequently, the conscientious teacher must remain continually aware of these changes in program, situation, and media availability.

Criteria for selection. In addition to selecting from among the various categories of media (motion pictures versus slide tapes, for example), teachers usually must choose from among individual items within the same category. Such situations commonly occur both as teachers make selections for immediate classroom use from among available alternatives in the school or district media library and when the teacher is provided the opportunity to make selections and recommendations for new acquisitions for these facilities. Erickson and Curl* provide twelve criteria to guide this selection task as follows:

1. Is the content useful and important to the learner?
2. Will it be interesting to students?
3. Is there a direct relationship to a specific objective or problem-solving activity?
4. How will the format and presentation treatment affect the organization and sequence of learner activities?
5. Is the material authentic, typical, and up-to-date?
6. Have facts and concepts been checked for accuracy? Are the producers expert in the subject matter, or have they employed competent consultants?
7. Do the content and presentation meet contemporary standards of good taste?
8. If [the subject is] controversial, are both sides given equal emphasis? Should they be?
9. Is bias or propaganda evident? If so, how should students deal with it?
10. Is technical quality satisfactory? Are images clear? Narration or dialog intelligible? Color, motion, and special effects used authentically and creatively?
11. Do content and structure reveal careful planning by the producer?

*Reprinted with permission of Macmillan Publishing Co., Inc. from *Fundamentals of teaching with audiovisual technology,* ed. 2, by Erickson, C. W. H., and Curl, D. H., pp. 166-167. Copyright © 1972 by Carlton W. H. Erickson and David H. Curl.

12. Has the material actually been validated or tested with learners? If so, who performed the evaluation? Under what conditions? What were the characteristics of the students? How successful were the results?

Individual teachers will undoubtedly choose to assign higher or lower priorities to each of these twelve criteria, particularly as they apply to different types of media. In any event, it seems clear that their proper application requires a thorough and careful review or previewing of any item prior to its acceptance or rejection. When it is feasible, the teacher's own field trial with a representative group or class of local students can be very helpful. The teacher must beware of producer claims that the material has been field tested. As one authority noted, such procedures may be poorly done to produce a sales gimmick. "Most often, no one looks at the results of these evaluations. Producers and purchasers alike are content to know that 'at least the stuff was tested.' "* The key to good media production is the use of field-testing results in the actual shaping of the final product. Even in those relatively few instances wherein this costly process is thoroughly applied, the results my not be valid for student populations that vary in any important respect from the original trial group. These considerations underscore the importance of each teacher's need to make careful selections.

Teacher production. Many teachers find that one of the best methods of obtaining good educational materials is to produce them themselves. There are many advantages to this practice, the most important of which is the closer tailoring of the materials to the specific needs of the situation. The relative depth or complexity, the length, the editorial bias, and the emphasis or organization of the material can be controlled, and usually the content and examples presented can be based on the local community rather than on some generalized, hypo-

thetical situation as is the usual case with commercially produced material. Although the task often requires considerable time and effort on the part of teachers who choose this approach, once the materials have been produced they will generally provide several terms of service. The production process also yields useful by-products in the form of the teacher's increased knowledge and understanding of the subject matter involved. The time spent in the creation of overhead transparencies or a slide-tape presentation, for example, seems guaranteed to do more for one's professional growth than an equal amount of time spent pouring over media guides in the often frustrating task of locating good professionally produced materials.

The local production of educational materials is often more feasible than one might suspect. Most directors of instructional materials centers will provide the material and expert assistance to teachers who show any interest in this task, and most are very happy to do so. Even in the absence of such direct help, much can be done through reliance on one of several good media textbooks that are on the market.* Also, teachers who return to the campus for graduate work during evening or summer sessions are well advised to consider a media production course as one of their electives. Although it is sometimes difficult for teachers to find the courage or ambition to begin their own production, once started they usually find that the task becomes easier and the results more professional as they gain experience. Few teachers, of course, will be able to meet all their media needs through their own effort, but most will find themselves to be one of their best and most reliable sources of educational materials.

ACQUISITION PROCESS

Each year dozens, or more likely hundreds, of new health-related books, films,

*Komoski, P. K.: 50,000 educational consumers can't be wrong—but who's listening? Audiovisual Instruction, Sept. 1971.

*For one of the better examples see Kemp, J. E.: *Planning and producing audiovisual materials,* ed. 3, New York, 1975, Thomas Y. Crowell Co., Inc.

tapes, posters, models, and other educational materials are produced and made available by various commercial firms, voluntary health agencies, and government organizations. The abundance of this material tends to be overwhelming and somewhat frustrating to the individual health educator, because the relatively few items appropriate for any given situation tend to be lost among the shoddily produced, biased, overpriced, or otherwise unacceptable items. However, the temptation to abandon the search must be resisted; many very good materials are produced that can greatly add to program effectiveness, although the search does present a challenging task.

Local sources. The way to tap available resources most easily and effectively is to turn to possible sources of aid in the order of their availability. Health teachers will often find that many materials are available within their own schools and communities.

Instructional materials center. To an ever-increasing degree, schools are combining their collection of print and nonprint materials in a single facility referred to as the IMC. Teachers who are new to a school will usually find the IMC director, or perhaps the audiovisual coordinator where the older pattern prevails, to be a prime source of information and assistance in regard to materials that are available within the school building itself or that may be obtained on short notice from any media center that the school district may maintain. Such persons may also provide sources and procedures for borrowing or renting materials from outside sources.

Supervisory or administrative personnel. Many school systems provide health education supervisors, coordinators, or resource teachers whose responsibilities center on the assisting of teachers of health at the secondary and/or elementary levels. Such persons are usually aware of health education materials that are available locally. Also, they may control the budget for the purchase or rental of needed materials.

Local health agencies. Public health de-partments, local offices of voluntary health agencies, and other health-related agencies or organizations such as water departments and power companies almost always will provide pamphlets and other literature on topics within their areas of concern and in many cases will provide useful films on a free loan basis. They also, of course, may make resource speakers available. Often these materials and services may be obtained merely by phoning in the request.

Remote sources. Once the search for edu-cational materials is widened beyond the teacher's local community, the number of possible sources becomes almost endless. Because of the intrinsic importance and the extremely broad scope of health as a field of study, a great many organizations and agencies of widely varying origins produce and distribute health materials either for profit, for motives related to advertising or public relations, as a public service, or as a public responsibility. These include:

1. International agencies such as the World Health Organization
2. Federal agencies such as the U.S. Public Health Service
3. State and regional agencies such as state health departments
4. Voluntary health organizations such as the American Cancer Society
5. Professional organizations such as the American Medical Society
6. Trade associations such as the National Dairy Council
7. Insurance companies such as the Metropolitan Life Insurance Company
8. Health-related business corporations such as drug companies and toothpaste manufacturers
9. Commercial producers of educational materials

Although some individual sources within these various classifications will be found to be much more useful than others, no group should be categorically ruled out. Many business firms or trade associations produce instructional films that include little more than a credit line in the way of advertising content and whose bias parallels that of the health education program as in the case of films advocating the promotion of better sewage treatment, regular dental care, or similar courses of action. Conversely, material from some supposedly unbiased source such as a federal agency is always subject to the author's or producer's personal views and in some cases may be a blatant propaganda piece designed to whitewash the agency's own basic inefficiency in carrying out its public responsibilities. Thus, while no source should be ruled out, no source should be automatically accepted as objective and authoritative.

Writing for materials. Procedures for the actual ordering or requesting of materials that involve the expenditure of money vary considerably among individual schools or school systems. The final approval of such orders usually must come from the IMC director or some designated school administrator. However, individual teachers may often solicit many free and inexpensive materials from the aforementioned sources on their own initiative. Specific means of locating the current address of sources and their specific offerings will be covered later in this chapter. Once this necessary information has been obtained, care is needed to properly place the order or request if the best service is to be obtained. The following suggestions generally apply to this task:

Write on school letterhead stationery, showing clearly the name and school address (including zip code) of the requestor. Letters written by students should be countersigned by the teacher.

Write only one letter for an entire group rather than having each student in a class write an individual letter.

Request only the number of items actually needed, within the limits imposed by distributors. Sponsors recommend that teachers request one copy of an item for careful review prior to asking for it in classroom quantities.

Specify kinds of materials and information desired; describe clearly the field of interest and grade level of the class with whom they will be used.

Inform the producer of how the materials were used and how effective they were.

Give suggestions for improving them.*

One additional hint: when there is a choice involved, it is usually wise to first phone or write local or regional rather than national or international offices. This often saves time and reduces the risk of the mishandling of requests, which in most organizations are channeled to local outlets when they are received at the national headquarters.

Locating sources. One of the best ways to keep abreast of the availability of new instructional materials is to regularly read the reviews provided in the regular features of a number of the health-related and general education journals. Perhaps the most useful of these to teachers of health education are those found in the "New Aids for Instruction" section that usually appears several times a year as a feature of the *Journal of School Health* and the "Resources" section of *Health Education*. Incidentally, most specialists in the field of health education will find it well worth their while to join the organizations that publish these journals. Elementary school teachers will find the "Reviews" section of *Instructor* magazine very helpful in addition to the two health journals. These and the corresponding section of similar journals and magazines generally provide a brief description and/or evaluation of the instructional items together with the current address of the source.

The task of systematically searching out materials for a given topic or purpose is somewhat more complicated whether the need is for free and inexpensive items or for the purchase or rental of more costly materials. Advertisements as found in the various professional journals or that may come to teachers unsolicited through the mail should not be discounted as a selection aid. All materials must be reviewed for

---

*By permission from Brown, J. W., Lewis, R. B., and Harcleroad, F. F.: *AV instruction: media and methods,* ed. 4, New York, 1973, McGraw-Hill, Inc., p. 393.

bias regardless of source; therefore, items accompanied by a hard-sell sales effort should not be automatically rejected. In most cases, however, the use of the many general guides to educational materials will be found to be more helpful. These well-organized and generally well-updated catalogs are designed to bring some order to this sometimes chaotic media world; many of these guides can usually be found in the instructional materials or audiovisual centers of schools or school districts and in the libraries of most colleges or universities with teacher-training programs. Some of those that are particularly relevant to health education are as follows*:

Educator's Guide to Free Health, Physical Education, and Recreation Materials. Provides comprehensive information about current free materials of use to health educators, physical educators, and recreation personnel. Available from Educator's Progress Service, P.O. Box 497, Randolph, Wis. 53956; $8.00.

Free [Holiday Material . . . Pictures . . . Posters . . . Teaching Aids]; Free and Inexpensive Pictures for the Classroom; Free Travel Posters; Free Pictures; Holiday Material for Use in Classrooms. Materials listed are for elementary grades through high school and for nearly every field of interest. Colorful pictures available help in building a file on a wide variety of subjects. Available from Bruce Miller Publications, P.O. Box 369, Riverside, Calif. 92502; $.50 per list.

Monthly Catalog of U.S. Government Publications. All government publications are entered in the *Monthly Catalog;* sixty-five thousand different titles are included under subject or title. Available from the Superintendent of Documents, U.S. Government Printing Office, North Capitol and H St., N.W. Washington, D.C. 20401; $7.00 per year; $.75 per copy.

National Center for Audio Tapes Catalog. The 1,200 tapes included in this catalog cover the school curriculum from elementary through college level. Available from National Center for Audio Tapes, University of Colorado, Room 320, Stadium Building, Boulder, Colo. 80302; $4.50.

---

*Based on information provided in Perkins, F. L.: *Book and non-book media: annotated guide to selection aids for educational materials,* Urbana, Ill., 1972, National Council of Teachers of English, pp. 97, 114, 171, 172, 179, 186, 209, 212, 255. Further information on these and other selection aids may be found in this excellent source.

National Directory of Safety Films. Provides a listing of safety films to be used in accident prevention programs. Available from National Safety Council, 425 North Michigan Ave., Chicago, Ill. 60611; $3.50 each; 10 or more copies, $2.10 each.

New Educational Materials. Includes classified guides to books, films, recordings, multi-media kits, filmstrips, transparencies, teaching-learning games, professional guides, posters, study prints, tapes, laboratory kits, puzzles, charts and maps, resource articles; products for prekindergarten through grade 12. Available from Citation Press, Scholastic Magazines, Inc., 50 West 44th St., New York, N.Y. 10036; $3.75 (1970 cost).

NICEM Media Indexes; individual catalogs entitled *Index to 8mm Educational Motion Cartridges (Film Loops); Index to Overhead Transparencies; Index to 16mm Educational Film; Index to 35mm Educational Filmstrips.* Material is derived from a computer-based index system of audiovisual materials, and the subject categories used represent a wide cross section of those used in many individual catalogs. Available from National Information Center for Educational Media (NICEM), R. R. Bowker Company, 1180 Avenue of the Americas, New York, N.Y. 10036; $1.50 per catalog.

Reading Ladders for Human Relations. Purpose is to make it possible to offer children the right books at the right time, books that will help open up children's understanding and sensitivity to their problems and the problems of others. Available from American Council on Education, One Dupont Circle, Washington, D.C. 20036; write for price.

Recommended Reading about Children and Family Life. Subject headings include family planning, family life, the middle years (6 to 12), sex education and development, reading and television, and school problems and the family. Available from Child Study Association of America, Inc., Publications Department, 9 East 89th St., New York, N.Y. 10028; $2.50.

U.S. Government Films: A Catalog of Motion Pictures and Filmstrips. Subject headings covered include such things as agriculture, health and medical, human relations, physical fitness, and safety. Available from National Audiovisual Center, National Archives and Records Service, Washington, D.C. 20409; catalog free.

Vertical File Index. A selected list of pamphlets, some of which are frankly propaganda and biased in viewpoint. There are numerous excellent free or inexpensive materials for current reference and also current ephemeral printed material that cannot be found elsewhere. Available from The H. W. Wilson Company, 950 University Ave., Bronx, N.Y. 10452; $8.00, U.S. and Canada; $10 elsewhere.

QUESTIONS FOR STUDY AND DISCUSSION

1. "The hardware is always ahead of the softwear." Discuss the meaning and the factors responsible for this statement.
2. Describe at least five specific reasons or purposes for the use of educational media.
3. Discuss the nature of and the motivations for some of the more common examples of media abuse.
4. Discuss the relative advantages and disadvantages of at least four commonly used types of educational media.
5. Describe the basic steps involved in planning for the selection of specific media items for specific lessons or educational tasks.
6. Discuss at least six criteria commonly used for judging the quality of educational materials.
7. What factors should be considered as one assesses the claims of media producers that their work has been field tested?
8. Discuss the advantages and general feasibility of the teacher production of educational materials.
9. What sources of educational media are commonly available in the teacher's own school or community?
10. What are the general categories of agencies or organizations that commonly provide health-related educational materials? What type of biases might be incorporated into the materials provided by specific categories of these sources?
11. What are the recommended procedures for writing for free and inexpensive materials?
12. What general procedures should be followed in the search for sources of educational materials located outside one's school or community?

REFERENCES

Allen, W. J.: Media stimulus and types of learning, Audiovisual Instruction, Jan. 1967.

Brown, J. W., Lewis, R. B., and Harcleroad, E. F.: *AV instruction: media and methods,* ed. 4, New York, 1973, McGraw-Hill, Inc.

Chisholm, M. E.: *Media indexes and review sources,* College Park, Maryland, 1972, University of Maryland.

Dale, E.: *Audiovisual methods in teaching,* ed 3, New York, 1969, Holt, Rinehart & Winston, Inc.

Erickson, C. W. H., and Curl, D. H.: *Fundamentals of teaching with audiovisual technology,* ed. 2, New York, 1972, Macmillan, Inc.

Kemp, J. E.: *Planning and producing audiovisual materials,* ed. 3, Scranton, Pa., 1975, Chandler Publishing Co.

Komoski, P. K.: 50,000 educational consumers can't be wrong—but who's listening? Audiovisual instruction, Sept. 1971.

Miller, L. G.: *Ready-made bulletin boards for elementary schools,* New York, 1974, Citation Press.

Oates, S. C.: *Instructional materials handbook,* Dubuque, Ia., 1971, Kendall/Hunt Publishing Co.

Perkins, F. L.: *Book and non-book media: annotated guides to selection aids for educational materials,* Urbana, Ill., 1972, National Council of Teachers of English.

Rufsvold, M. I., and Guss, C.: *Guides to educational media,* ed. 3, Chicago, 1971, American Library Association.

PART FOUR

School health services

CHAPTER 9 ❧ Objectives, health appraisal, referral, counseling, and follow-up

OBJECTIVES

The ultimate and highest goal of school health services is to *promote positive health* among students and staff. If this goal were reached, the result would be a completely well population functioning at peak physical, mental, and social efficiency. Desirable as it is, such a state of being is pretty much beyond our ability either to achieve fully or to identify completely and measure. Evidence and common sense lead us to believe that positive health is promoted by regular exercise, optimal nutrition, and a safe and pleasing physical and social environment. The occurrence of expected growth and development in children and the achievement of work goals and job satisfaction by adults serve as indicators of progress toward positive health. It is part of the business of school health services to promote positive health and to measure it as best they can.

A less ambitious aim of school health services is the *primary prevention* of disease occurrence. Present knowledge makes this goal more achievable and measurable than positive health, but complete success eludes us. Scurvy can be completely prevented by diets that provide adequate amounts of vitamin C. Tuberculosis can be partially prevented by detecting and treating carriers of the disease organism. Common disorders of visual acuity are not preventable with present knowledge. However, school and community health services have succeeded in preventing the occurrence of many other diseases wholly or in part, and successes are well documented. As knowledge of disease causation is increased through research, the further development and application of primary prevention can be expected.

Where primary prevention partially or completely fails, it is often possible to identify probable cases of disease at an early stage and treat them in some way so that damage or discomfort to the individual or society is prevented or minimized. This is referred to as *secondary prevention*. Early detection and treatment go together. It is a futile exercise to detect probable disease if no remedial treatment or other action is available. Early detection and educational or counseling types of treatment are functions performed by school health services. Definitive diagnosis and medical types of treatment are traditionally the joint responsibility of families and the community at large.

When secondary prevention fails and disease recovery is neither spontaneous nor complete (as is the case in certain types of hearing loss), habilitation or rehabilitation measures are often helpful. Such *tertiary prevention* seeks to improve physical, mental, and social function to the greatest extent possible. Habilitation and rehabilitation processes include counseling, school management, and special education services, all of which are legitimate school health services functions. Other processes, such as surgical and vocational rehabilitation, are conducted under community auspices.

In general, health promotion, primary prevention, the detection phase of secondary prevention, and in-school aspects of tertiary prevention constitute the primary aims of school health. Even though definitive medical and surgical treatments are not as yet provided in schools, school health services do provide emergency care and referral to appropriate sources.

The remainder of this chapter is devoted to description and discussion of selected traditional and innovative school health services and program segments designed to meet the aims of school health services. Other services, together with roles and relationships of individuals involved in the provision of school health services, are discussed in Chapter 10. Applications of health services, health education, and healthful school living to specific health problems of children and youth are presented in detail in Part Six.

HEALTH APPRAISAL

Health appraisal is the process of determining the health status of individuals and of the school population as a whole. Most authorities agree that both positive and negative health status variables should be evaluated. In practice, however, attention is still primarily directed to the identification of specific health defects. A number of techniques are used to gather a variety of health status data. These data are collected and preserved in the form of health records. The recorded evidence provides the basis for appraising health status, which in turn is used in decision making with respect to individual counseling and follow-up, the identification of school health program needs, and the evaluation of program success. In the following subsections, commonly used data-gathering techniques are described and discussed.

Health histories. A health history of each individual is usually taken prior to or as part of medical health examinations. A form such as the one shown in Fig. 9-1 is used to obtain health history data. Although the specific information requested varies with the maturity of the group for which the form is designed, it includes: (1) identifying personal information, (2) a history of past or present diseases or health problems of significance, (3) the individual's status with

respect to required or recommended immunizations, (4) family information, and (5) health-related behavior.

Such information is useful not only as part of the ultimate record to determine health status but also as a guide to the medical examiner since it may suggest some modification of the standard examination procedure. For example, a history of frequent sore throats or of scarlet fever may have caused rheumatic fever, which may exist even though it is not checked on a health history.

The health history form may be completed by parents for their children, by older pupils or employees for themselves, or by a health service staff person acting as interviewer. The advantages of completion by parents or pupils include the sense of involvement that active participation provides. If the form is completed at home, the employee, parent, or pupil may have access to a baby book or immunization record forms that may increase the accuracy of the responses given. Disadvantages include the fact that some parents and pupils may be non-English speaking, functionally illiterate, or may simply fail to understand some of the specific questions or instructions. For example, a 7- or 8-year-old normally lisps because the primary baby front teeth have been shed, but a parent may record this as a speech defect.

Use of staff members as health history interviewers is costly in time and thus in money, but a trained interviewer can probe when the respondent seems uncertain. Bilingual staff interviewers can be chosen for service in schools where they are needed. It is generally agreed that volunteers should never be used as health history interviewers because of the danger that potentially embarrassing information (bedwetting, for example) may not be kept in confidence as it should be.

Health histories provide notoriously unreliable data even when they are completed by skilled interviewers. One report revealed frequent inconsistencies between surviving family members and death certificates with

HEALTH HISTORY FORM*

Dear parent: Your answers to the following questions will help the school to meet your child's needs in planning his school program and provide valuable information for our school records. Please fill out the answers and bring this form with you or send it with your child.

School.. Room no......................

Date..

Name.. Address.................................... Phone....................

Birthplace.................................. Birthdate................................... Grade....................

Family doctor............................. Address.................................... Phone....................

Date of last visit...................................

Please check any of the following conditions that your child has had (give age and date):

Asthma............................	German measles................	Fainting—when?...............
Eczema............................	Heart disease...................	Recent bed wetting...........
Hayfever..........................	Hernia (rupture)..............	Growing pains..................
Chorea.............................	Measles...........................	Operations—what?............
Diabetes...........................	Mumps.............................	
Diphtheria........................	Poliomyelitis....................	Accidents—what?..............
Ears, running....................	Rheumatic fever...............	
Epilepsy (convulsions)........	Scarlet fever....................	Other serious illness, what?...
Frequent colds (how often)...	Speech defect...................	
Frequent coughs (how often)...	Tuberculosis—self.............	
Frequent headaches (how often)...	Tuberculosis—family..........	
Frequent nosebleeds (how often)...	Wears glasses...................	
Frequent sorethroat (how often)...	Tires easily?....................	

Has the child been immunized against the following?

	No	Yes	If yes, give date or dates
Diphtheria................			
Tetanus (lockjaw).......			
Whooping cough..........			
Smallpox..................			
Poliomyelitis.............			
Others.....................			

Family history:

	Yes	No	Health condition
Who lives in the home?..			
Father.....................			
Mother....................			
Brothers—ages...........			
Sisters—ages.............			
Others.....................			

Health habits:

How much milk every day?..
Any food allergies?..
What does child eat for breakfast?.............................
Usual bedtime on school nights?................................
Give any other health information you feel we should have..
....
....
....
....

....
Signature of parent

*Prepared by the Health Records Committee of the School Health Section of the American Public Health Association.

Fig. 9-1

respect to cause of death.* The data provided should therefore be confirmed by further questioning or by another source, such as by medical examination, before costly or time-consuming action is recommended or taken.

Attempts to create checklists of health symptoms that might be of value to the medical examiner and that can be administered either as part of the health history or independently of it have not been entirely successful. Stine and associates† compared the usefulness of two such forms (Alexiou's and Levine's). Alexiou's form was too lengthy for use with adolescents and identified an excessive number of students as having problems that were not confirmed by examination. On the other hand, Levine's short form failed to identify an excessive number of health problems that upon examination were found to exist.

Medical health examinations. At regular intervals health examinations of apparently well children and school staff members are required by law or by local school board policy in many states and districts and recommended in most others. If properly organized and conducted, they can be useful educational and counseling experiences. Most authorities assume that health examinations are a useful screening device to detect health problems, although this assumption has been questioned.

Timing. It is generally recommended that each child and employee be examined at time of entry into the school system. Most authorities agree that student athletes should be examined annually and that other students should be examined at least three other times during their school lives, usually at or about the time of entrance to the fourth, seventh, and tenth grades, depending

on how the local schools are organized. Practices with respect to reexamination of employees vary with the state and district.

When routine medical health examinations of school children were introduced around 1900 and for many years thereafter, annual examinations were assumed to be the ideal and were required by law in many states. Physician shortages during World Wars I and II were accompanied by reductions in the number of examinations required. Studies by Yankauer* and by Rogers and Reese† during the 1950's and 1960's led to the conclusion that periodic reexaminations of children have little value in detecting health defects. Thus, the present standard of four examinations appears to represent a compromise between the assumed ideal, research findings, and shortages of health personnel.

Nevertheless, preschool or school entrance examinations are highly desirable, especially in areas where adequate routine preschool-age health care is unavailable or neglected. Head Start medical examinations showed that over one third of these preschool entrants had uncorrected medical defects.‡ Adjustment to school life is difficult enough without the unnecessary burden of visual defects, diseased tonsils, poor nutrition, or other handicaps. It is desirable to schedule preschool examinations during the summer prior to school entrance so that there will be time for the correction of defects before school starts in the fall. Other new students and employees are usually examined as they enter the local school system.

Source and location. It is generally agreed that the medical health examination

---

*Napier, J. A., and others: Limitations of morbidity and mortality data obtained from family histories: a report from the Tecumseh community health study, American J. Public Health **62**:30-35, Jan. 1972.
†Stine, O. C., and others: Two health questionnaires for adolescents, J. Sch. Health **44**:136-139, March 1974.

*Yankauer, A., and Lawrence, R. A.: A study of periodic school medical examinations. I, methodology and initial findings, Am. J. Public Health **45**:71-78, Jan. 1955; Yankauer, A., and others: A study of periodic school medical examinations. II, The annual increment of new defects, Am. J. Public Health **46**:1553-1562, June 1956.
†Rogers, K. D., and Reese, G.: Health studies: presumably normal high school students, Am. J. Dis. Child. **108**:572-600, Dec. 1964.
‡Anderson, E.: Commitment to child health, Am. J. Nurs. **67**:2076, Sept. 1967.

should be conducted by and at the individual's own personal source of medical care. This policy has several advantages. First, the source of care is likely already to know the individual and to have relevant information about his or her present condition and health history on record. Second, resources for indicated laboratory tests are more likely to be available at the source of care than at school. Third, restraints against disrobing and examination of genitalia are less likely to be operative at the source of care. Fourth, relationships with the source of care and assumption of parental and individual responsibility may be enhanced. Finally, and perhaps most important, the source of care is in a position to immediately provide needed immunizations and to begin definitive diagnosis and treatment of defects if indicated.

Disadvantages are also associated with examination by and at the source of care. Many individuals still have no usual source of care. Such examinations usually cost more money, which families of many children can ill afford. The source of care may be inappropriate (such as a chiropractor) or incompetent. Examination of apparently healthy children is costly in terms of pro-

fessional time, which may be better spent in providing care to those with known health problems. The examination and the resulting report to the school are likely to be sketchy or incomplete.

Examinations given in school are free of direct charge to the family but costly to taxpayers generally. As is the case with examinations by source of care, they dilute the ability of health care professionals to meet urgent community needs. Quality can be controlled through careful selection of examiners, provision of adequate time (about 15 to 30 minutes per child), and careful orientation of examiners with respect to the nature of the examination desired. However, prohibitions against complete disrobing and examination of genitalia still exist in many communities, and access to desirable laboratory tests is usually lacking. The resulting report to the school is more likely to be complete and useful than is a report from a typical source of care, however.

Nature and scope. The examination should be as thorough and comprehensive as possible, but not diagnostically exhaustive. The examination begins with a review of the health history of the individual, in-

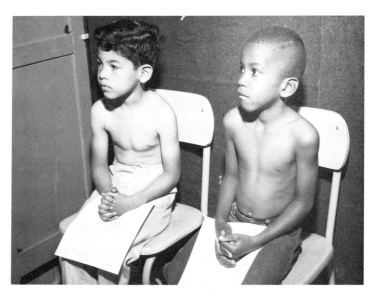

Fig. 9-2. Waiting for examination. (Courtesy Los Angeles School Districts.)

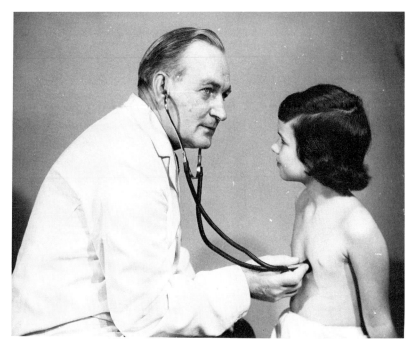

Fig. 9-3. Medical health examination.

cluding records of screening test findings and health observations by teachers, nurses, and parents.

Such examinations usually include systematic appraisal of organs and systems, as indicated on the form in Fig. 9-4. The detection of cases of communicable disease is not a primary purpose of medical health examinations, because infections tend to come and go. Coincidental discovery of infections may occur and should be noted and followed, however. Procedures are modified as indicated by available health history and record information. The examiner's findings and recommendations, based on what he or she sees, hears, and feels, are desirably recorded in a form useful and understandable to teachers and counselors as well as to another health professional.

If the examination is conducted in school, it is considered desirable to have each elementary-age and preschool examinee accompanied by a parent, the teacher, and school nurse (who may serve either as examiner if qualified as a practitioner, or as

recorder and assistant, if not). No nonprofessional other than the parent should ever be present. For secondary students, parents and teachers should be excluded. If these and only these relevant individuals and the examinee attend, an appropriate and productive discussion of findings and next steps can occur. Although time is limited so that detailed individualized education is rarely feasible, discussion should include reference to some positive aspect of the examinee's health as well as to defects that require attention. A written report should be made to parents (see Fig. 9-5).

The attitude of pupils and parents toward the examination, and thus their motivation to follow through on recommendations, is determined in part by the personalities and professional relationship of the professional who is present as well as by the apparent thoroughness of the examination and reasonableness of the recommendations. A warm and quiet examination room, the presence of appropriate equipment and furnishings, a private place to disrobe and dress, and provision of an examination gar-

Last name   First   Middle   Mo._____Day_____Yr._____
                                                            Birthdate

Physician's record of examinations

Date	Grade	Eyes	Ears	Tonsils	Mouth Breath.	Teeth	Gums	Glands	Organ.	Funct.	Lungs	Hernia	Other	Genitalia	Nervous system	Nutrition	Posture	Feet	Other	Skin, scalp	Other	Name of Physician
				Nose-throat					*Heart*			*Abdomen*					*Orthopedic*					

0—Normal, no defect
x—Slight defect, keep under observation
xx—Defect recommended for treatment
xxx—Gross defect, immediate attention urged
Circle defect symbol when corrected

G1—Wearing glasses
(xx)—Defect cured
T—Under treatment
I—Irremediable

Physicians' comments, recommendations, physical education assignments

Nurse's follow-up notes and home call records

Fig. 9-4. Health examination form.

Form 33.112—70M—1/66

LOS ANGELES CITY SCHOOLS
Health Services Branch — Auxiliary Services Division

REPORT OF HEALTH AND DEVELOPMENT EXAMINATION

School _____   _____ Date

Dear Parent:

During the physical examination of _____

the following was found: _____

_____

_____

_____

_____

You may or may not be aware of this condition. If it is attended to, we believe
your child will be helped, and we advise you to seek professional care. If you
are financially unable to meet such expense and are eligible for clinic care,
assistance may be obtained by consulting the school nurse.

Children's teeth should be examined periodically by a dentist, as only plainly
visible dental decay is noted on this examination.

Please sign and detach the note below and return it to the school.

Yours very truly,

School Physician _____ M.D.

Principal _____

N.B. The school physician's next day at school is _____,
please make appointment if desired. The school nurse is at school

on _____ . School telephone number _____

· ·

To the Principal of _____ School: Room _____

I have received notice of the school physician's examination

of _____

_____ I will have the condition cared for privately.

_____ I will consult with the school nurse.

_____
Signature of Parent or Guardian

Fig. 9-5

ment all contribute to formation of positive attitudes toward the process.

Medical examinations of staff personnel. These examinations arouse the sometimes justified suspicion that the results may be used as a basis for denying or terminating employment. Cases known to these authors include one teacher who was denied employment because of obesity even though the excess weight was obviously the result of large muscles and not of fat. Another teacher who lost his vision as a result of diabetes was discharged and regained his job only after a series of court battles.*

As was noted earlier, routine examination is a poor way of discovering cases of communicable diseases, and it is not much more useful in detecting mental illness. Screening tests and observation are more reliable.

Communicable diseases such as tuberculosis, which can be transmitted by in-school contact to other employees or to children, should of course be discovered and the individual excluded during the period of communicability. Persons with mental illnesses that interfere with job effectiveness should either be excluded or relocated to another more suitable position pending recovery. Many defects discovered will be correctable. Some may require job reassignment, but denial or termination of employment without consideration of its effects on the employee and of possible alternatives is no more justified in education than it is in business or industry.

If examinations are designed and used primarily to identify health problems in need of correction, and if personnel policies and fringe benefits are designed to allay hardships, then employee entrance and periodic examinations become benefits, not threats, especially after 40 years of age. Much of the threat is also removed when examinations are conducted by the employee's own usual source of health care rather than by board of education examiners. Some school sys-

tems, however, choose to maintain a quite complete service for the pre- and periodic examination and health counseling of employees.

Question of value and alternatives. In a perceptive and well-reasoned paper, Eisner and Oglesby* conclude that few previously undetected and treatable health problems are discovered by the routine medical examination of apparently well schoolchildren. They view routine health assessments by a child's usual source of care as an important part of continuing health supervision but *not* as a basic school procedure for those children under outside supervision. They propose the substitution of a selected battery of screening tests plus health observation of children by teachers as a reasonable and effective substitute for in-school periodic health examinations. Medical examiners in the school would provide diagnostic examinations for children selected by observation and tests. Entrance examinations, however, that are performed by either the school or source of care should be continued.

Other possible alternatives include the substitution of qualified nurse practitioners for physicians as examiners and the limitation of the scope of in-school routine examinations to a search for those few conditions not discoverable by observation or presently administered and available screening tests.

The statutory need for school athletic examinations on an annual basis remains, and at least one athletically relevant type of defect—hernia—remains outside the ability of tests and teacher observation to detect. In addition, Fiedler† reports that 63% of the supposedly healthy female adolescents (age 11 to 17 years) examined in a New York family planning service showed undiagnosed medical conditions (mainly gynecological disease and malnutrition) requir-

---

*Associated Press: Blind teacher wins fight to get job back, The Evening Bulletin, Philadelphia, Aug. 17, 1974.

*Eisner, V., and Oglesby, A.: Health assessment of school children. I, physical examinations, J. Sch. Health **41**:239-242, May 1971.
†Fiedler, D.: Pathology in the "healthy" female teen-ager, Am. J. Public Health **63**:962-965, Nov. 1973.

ing treatment. Also, the need for specialized examination of selected children and young people for certification and reevaluation as candidates for special education programs still remains.

Thus, much work remains for in-school medical examiners without wasting time and money in the rediscovery of previously detected problems through frequent reexamination after school entry.

Dental health examinations. Authorities in preventive dentistry recommend that every child have a dental examination at the age of 3 and thereafter as frequently as is advised by the dentist, usually twice each year. Although a sizable decline in the prevalence of cavities has taken place in communities served by fluoridated water supplies, almost all children surveyed elsewhere have been found to be in need of dental care. Fulfillment of the basic care needs of all of today's students is beyond the ability of the present number of dental professionals.

The need for dental health examinations of children and youth fortunate enough to be receiving adequate continuing dental care should obviously be filled by the practitioner or clinic that serves them. An effective motivating device, called the Malden Plan for its city of origin in Massachusetts, was devised by Turner many years ago. Under this plan, a two-part form is presented to each child. The first part of the form is a communication to the parents informing them of the child's need for continuing dental care. The second part is a report of the child's dental health status to be completed by the dentist and returned to the school. If distribution and collection of the form are accompanied by a planned program of health education directed to parents and students and by follow-up contacts as needed, the Malden Plan will effectively stimulate continuing dental examinations and care.

For the unfortunate child who is confronted by impassable parental, economic, geographical, or racial barriers to continuing dental care, the Malden Plan form only

adds insult to injury. In-school examinations that result in referrals for unattainable care do the same and, in addition, only waste scarce dental personnel. Unless some sort of care is available, such children are no worse for remaining unexamined. The professional time required is better spent in providing preventive services such as oral hygiene instruction and prophylaxis. Inspection is a normal part of such services and requires little additional time.

In-school dental health inspections or examinations are usually limited to inspection with a mirror and explorer. They rarely if ever include x-rays, which are essential in a complete examinatiton, and are therefore more properly referred to as inspections. If performed under standardized lighting conditions with standard equipment and if the findings are systematically recorded, such inspections can be useful in evaluating school population dental health status as a means of program evaluation. For this purpose, inspection of a systematically selected random sample of the school population or of all pupils in selected grades will suffice. Inspection of every pupil is neither necessary nor desirable.

Health observations. Health observation is a process conducted by teachers, parents, nurses, and others in which the observer seeks to identify any complaint or sign of appearance or behavior that may indicate a physical, mental, or social health problem. Students sometimes observe what they perceive to be health problems that they themselves have and report them. The process is carried out continuously and informally. The basic criteria for identifying possible trouble are:

1. Is this individual like his or her normal healthy self today?
2. Is this individual like other normal healthy individuals of his or her sex, race, and stage of growth and development?

If the answer is no to either question, something *may* be amiss. Thus, observations are primarily based on a knowledge of the individual observed plus a knowledge of normal child growth and development. Any valid knowledge that the observer possesses of specific complaints or signs of appearance or behavior associated with specific health problems affecting the observed population increases the validity of health observation. The end result of observation is not diagnosis but a determination that the individual observed may have a health problem in need of attention.

As such, some confirmation of the validity of an observation is usually desirable before an implication leading to action is drawn from it. Observations by teachers, for example, may be confirmed by a nursing inspection, and the nurse or nurse and teacher together may then determine what further actions are indicated. This practice is based upon a demonstration project that was conducted in the Astoria section of New York City about 1940. The study showed that eight out of ten children who were referred by teachers trained in health observation, acting with the guidance and advice of a nurse in a teacher-nurse conference, actually had health problems requiring professional attention.*

Most authorities state that all observations should be included in the permanent health record. In our opinion, observations should be permanently recorded only after some evidence of validity and significance is obtained. Otherwise, valid and significant record entries may be lost in the clutter of transient or meaningless observations.

Years ago teacher observation was formalized and routinized. Teachers were provided with checklists that they used to conduct a morning inspection of each child, quietly seated, for clean fingernails as well as for signs of illness. The process has since been abandoned for good reasons. A child who looks and feels well in the morning can develop a case of measles by midafternoon. Dirty fingernails are as often a sign of industriousness as of lack of cleanliness, and

certain orthopedic problems, apparent when the child is active, are hidden in a sitting position.

Used rightly and based on sound knowledge, health observation is one of the most useful of the health appraisal techniques. It is particularly useful in the early detection of acute illnesses, injuries that a child may attempt to hide, orthopedic problems, and emotional disturbances. Eisner and Oglesby* conclude that teacher observation together with teacher-nurse conferences is generally superior to either medical examinations or health inventories (histories) as practical detection devices.

Screening tests. Lessler has proposed a broad definition and set of objectives for screening testing. He states, "Screening is the acquiring of preliminary information about characteristics which may be significant to the health, education, or well-being of the individual, and which are relevant to his life tasks. The means of data collection must be appropriate and reasonable with regard to the economics of time, money and resources for dealing with large numbers of people."† He suggests that the objectives include:

1. Provision of information "to those who work with the child relevant to his life tasks."
2. Utilization of screening information "to promote growth and positive development, . . . provide follow-up diagnostic services, . . . [and] to provide treatment or remediation. . ."
3. Utilization of data for research.
4. Utilization of data for primary prevention (for example, as a basis for health education).

These statements may be construed as applying to health observations and self-referrals as well as to the devices tradi-

---

*Nyswander, D. B.: *Solving school health problems,* New York, 1942, Commonwealth Fund, p. 34.

---

*Eisner V., and Oglesby, A.: Health assessment of children. VIII, the unexpected health defect, J. Sch. Health **42**:348-350, June 1972.
†Lessler, K.: Health and educational screening of school-age children: definition and objectives, Am. J. Public Health **62**:191-198, Feb. 1972.

tionally viewed as screening tests. Schools traditionally include screening tests for visual and auditory acuity, and tuberculin skin tests; their traditional purposes were the first two listed by Lessler. Our traditional conception of them is that they are not diagnostic in character but are intended only to "sort out apparently well persons who probably have a disease from those who probably do not."*

Accuracy. In addition to being cheaply, quickly, and easily administered preferably by nonprofessionals or volunteers who require little training, a useful screening test should be highly reliable and valid. That is, it should ideally be *sensitive* enough to classify as "positive" *all* of those who actually have the disease or condition sought, and it should be *specific* enough to classify as positive *only* those who have it. Underreferrals may cost those thus given false reassurance their continued health. Overreferrals are costly in time, money, and worry. But few tests are 100% sensitive and specific.

The sensitivity and specificity and the under- or overreferrals falsely identified by a screening test can be measured quantitatively. Let us suppose that a new screening test for "disease X" has been developed. Let us further suppose that disease X is chronic and that it has been determined by accurate but complex diagnostic techniques to affect 5% of the school population. We administer the new screening test to a school population of 1,000 and find that 950 students are identified as negative by the test and that 50, or the expected 5% are identified as positive. The test arrives at the correct percentage, but we still do not know if all 5% identified by the test actually have the disease.

To find out, we submit the 5% who were screened positive to the complex diagnostic procedure and compare the diagnoses with

Table 9-1. Screening test results for disease X by diagnosis

Screening test results	Diagnosis for disease X Diseased	No disease	Total
Positive	(a) 30	(b) 20	(a+b) 50
Negative	(c) 20	(d) 930	(c+d) 950
Total	(a+c) 50	(b+d) 950	(a+b+ 1,000 c+d)

the screening test findings in a 2 × 2 table as in Table 9-1. (Cells b and c will rarely be equal in real situations. Cells c and d are estimated from prior knowledge of prevalence.)

Both the screening test and the diagnostic procedure identify 50 individuals as having disease X, but they are not all the same individuals. Likewise, the two procedures do not identify the same 950 individuals as free of disease X. If they did, the b and c cells of the table would contain no cases and the screening test would be perfect.

Sensitivity, or the ability of the test to correctly identify those who have disease X, is computed by the formula:

$$Sensitivity = \frac{a}{a+c} \times 100 = \frac{30}{50} \times 100 = 60\%$$

Specificity, or the ability of the test to correctly identify those free of disease X, is computed by the formula*:

$$Specificity = \frac{d}{b+d} \times 100 = \frac{930}{950} \times 100 = 97.9\%$$

The percentage of overreferral is computed by the formula:

$$Overreferral = \frac{b}{a+b} \times 100 = \frac{20}{50} \times 100 = 40.0\%$$

The percentage of underreferral is computed by the formula:

$$Underreferral = \frac{c}{c+d} \times 100 = \frac{20}{950} \times 100 = 2.1\%$$

*Commission on Chronic Illness: *Chronic illness in the United States, vol. 1, prevention of chronic illness,* Cambridge, Mass., 1957, Harvard University Press.

*Adapted from Grant, J. A.: Quantitative evaluation of a screening program, Am. J. Public Health **64:**66-71, 1974.

The new test is thus highly specific but not very sensitive. It overrefers a high proportion and underrefers relatively few. The high percentage of overreferrals may possibly be reduced by using a test-retest procedure. That is, those who are screened positive the first time are retested. If they are screened positive on retesting, they are referred, but if they are screened negative on retesting, they are not. Such a procedure tends to reduce specificity and results in more underreferrals, but it will save time and money for those overreferred and will result in better public relations for the school health program.

Since errors in mechanics or testing procedures can also result in poor test results, it is important to use carefully calibrated test equipment and to administer tests under favorable and standardized conditions. For example, a noisy environment can invalidate hearing testing results, as can an audiometer that emits sounds that are of a different pitch or intensity from those dialed by the tester.

Test statistics are also affected by the population tested. Kindergarteners may be unable to recognize the letters on the vision test chart used for literate adults. If the prevalence of a disease is higher in adults than in children, then the validity and reliability of the test will be different in the two groups. You can assure yourself that this is so by changing the data in Table 9-1 to show a 20% prevalence of disease X instead of 5% and then reevaluating specificity and sensitivity.

Interpretation and education. The fact that screening tests yield over- and under-referrals makes it mandatory that the meaning of the results obtained be correctly interpreted to the individuals tested and to parents. A positive screening test result indicates a need for diagnosis. Whether or not treatment is required depends on the diagnostic examiner's conclusions. Children who fail (are screened positive) on visual acuity screening and their parents should be informed that a professional (diagnostic) eye examination is needed. They should *not* be told that a child needs glasses.

As in the case of routine medical health examinations, routine screening tests can and should have an educational purpose. The experience of being tested is not necessarily educative in itself, but the experience can initiate or culminate classroom education about the health problem in question. Interpretation of the meaining of screening test results can be stressed both in the classroom and as part of the health counseling and referral process.

Assessing health status. Information collected and recorded from health histories, examinations, observations, and screening tests must be interpreted in order to assess the health status of an individual. A list of dates of immunizations must be processed through either a knowledgeable mind or a properly programmed computer to determine what other immunizations are to be recommended and when. The bits of information available from various sources, which by themselves must always be regarded as only more or less reliable and valid, acquire greater reliability and validity if they tend to be mutually consistent. Such assessments are made possible by the individual health records in which health appraisal and other types of information are gathered.

HEALTH RECORDS

Means: threat or goal? Adequate, accessible, and continuous health records are needed not only for assessment of the health status of individuals, but also for follow-up and health counseling, emergency care, disease control, and the school management and guidance of exceptional children and young people. In addition, data compiled from permanent health records as well as from the temporary working records of school health professionals are useful in conducting research and in describing, evaluating, and thus improving the school health services program.

It is apparent that records are meant to be used as means by which the goal of school health services—the improvement and promotion of health—can be better achieved. Some school health professionals mistake or accept complete and accurate records as the goal and then work toward this end, to the neglect of the individuals the records represent. Some parents and employees view health records as a threat —as potentially incriminating or embarrassing evidence that is available for use against them.

Nature of health records. Health records fall into two categories: work records and individual health records. The former are temporary and are used to keep track of work in progress and to compile reports of work progress. The latter are permanent records.

Work records are kept on various forms by school health professionals. Examples include class lists of individuals screened that indicate the individual test results and whether or not each individual was referred. Another example is a record of contacts and progress made in attempting to secure indicated health services for individuals. Such records provide data needed for making periodic reports of work completed. Data from them are also summarized and transferred to individual health records. Their precise nature varies from school to school.

Individual health records are intrinsically more important than work records and tend to be more time-consuming and threatening to the individual. An example is the school health record proposed for use or adaptation by school systems in the United States by the Health Records Committee of the School Health Section of the American Public Health Association (Fig. 9-6). In some schools certain individual work records such as health history and health examination reports are filed as part of the individual school health record. In others these data are transferred to the record form to avoid clutter.

A time-saving national shorthand for use with such records has evolved to indicate the severity of a defect and to report its correction. "O" means no defect, or a normal finding; "X" means a minor defect that should be kept under surveillance; "XX" means a defect that requires attention but

is not considered urgent; and "XXX" means a condition that demands immediate attention. When corrections have been completed, the X or X's are encircled, such as ⊗⊗. "T" is used to indicate a defect under treatment, and "I" is used to denote defect that is irremediable.

One characteristic of individual health records is that the data come from various sources, such as health histories, medical and dental examinations, screening test reports, observations, and disease occurrences. This fact increases the possibility that vital information may be lost or misrecorded in the process of transferring data from work records to permanent individual records.

Storage and access. A recurring issue is where records should be filed and who should have access to them. In some schools they are filed in the central office, where they are more or less available to all concerned professionals. In other schools they are kept in the guidance or pupil personnel office or are filed in the classroom or homeroom. It is generally agreed that all those and only those professionally involved with a student should have access to his or her individual record. It is also agreed that health records should be filed with academic and guidance records, because each of these parts contributes to an understanding of the whole individual.

Health needs may be hidden away when records are filed, and some device is needed to show which students need attention and what progress is being made. In some elementary schools a notebook or card file is kept in each teacher's desk into which both teacher and nurse record corrections and other developments as they occur. In some secondary schools a follow-up card is kept in the hands of the homeroom teachers. In other school systems such records are maintained by the nurse and may be kept in the central office where they are available for reference by guidance workers and teachers. Nurses may keep similar records in their own offices. While this latter option makes records more accessible to the nurse, to whom these records are of greatest concern,

SCHOOL HEALTH RECORD*

.... M ☐ F ☐   Mo.....................Day.....................Yr.....................

| Last name | First | Middle | Sex | Birthdate | | Birthplace |

Addresses   Home phone   Schools   Rm. (pencil)

Parent or guardian...Business address...Phone................
Father's occupation...Mother's occupation..Phone................
Family physician...Address...Phone................
Family status: F.......................M.......................Bro. No.................Ages.................Sis. No.............Ages................

Personal history, illnesses, operations

	Date or check		Date or check
Accidents		Mumps	
Allergy		Operation	
Chorea		Poliomyelitis	
Diabetes		Rheumatic fever	
Ear infection		Speech defect	
Epilepsy		Tuberculosis—Self	
German measles		Tuberculosis—Family	
Headaches		Upper respiratory	
Heart disease		Others	
Hernia		Others	
Measles		Others	

Immunization history

	Basic	Booster	Booster
Diphtheria.....			
Tetanus.....			
Whooping cough..			
Polio.........			

	Date	Result	Date	Result
Smallpox....				
Tuberculin...				
Chest X-ray..				

Teacher or nurse observations and tests

Date	Grade	Height	Weight	Vision Without Glasses R	Vision Without Glasses L	Vision With Glasses R	Vision With Glasses L	Plus sphere	Speech	Behavior	Scholarship	Attendance	Hearing Date	Hearing R	Hearing L	Dental record Date	Obv. decay	Cleaning	Gums	Irreg. teeth

Date	Teachers', principals', or coordinators' notes (please initial)

*Prepared by the Health Records Committee of the School Health Section of the American Public Health Association.

Fig. 9-6

this location makes access more difficult for other concerned professionals. Multiple systems also increase the time and effort required in record keeping.

Time and effort reduction. In a study of nursing time spent in various functions rated according to priority by an expert jury, Lowis* concluded that Los Angeles school nurses spent a third of their time in record keeping, a proportion unwarranted by the relatively low priority assigned to record keeping as a nursing function.

We have already stated that universally used and accepted *recording shorthand* saves time. Acceptance of the principle that *only the unusual should be recorded* can also reduce time and effort. In most schools every student enrolled in certain grades is administered certain screening tests, and if the youngster is absent when a test is given, the test is administered later. A majority of screening test results are usually normal (negative). Under these conditions, neither the fact of screening nor a negative result need be recorded.

Utilization of a *systems approach* to school health records was reported by Gaskins to reduce record-keeping time by half. In the Darien, Connecticut schools, all input data are referenced to a particular health problem (such as visual acuity), and each possible problem is assigned a code number. The date of each new bit of information about a given problem and person is also recorded. A strip form that precisely matches the record form is used by medical examiners to report findings. The strip is simply attached to the records form so that it is aligned with other information about the same problem.† Such an approach is suitable either for written or for computerized systems.

Nationwide adoption of a *single record*

system together with a policy that a photocopy or computer printout of each *record moves with the individual from school system to school system* has enormous potential for saving time and effort not only in recording but also in negating the necessity of repeating a recent examination. It seems unlikely, however, that the required unanimity of action by all state and local school systems will occur.

Adoption of the practice of *recording only relevant and significant information* could effect considerable economy. Success of such a policy depends on a degree of judgmental wisdom that few of us possess and fewer still practice. However, the development of some useful guidelines may result from future research. Such guidelines are important not only to efficiency but to threat reduction and computerization of records as well.

Threat reduction. *Education U.S.A.** cites a proposed amendment to the Elementary and Secondary Education Act and a critical report of the National Committee for Citizens in Education as evidence that school record-keeping procedures are under attack. The amendment, since passed, opens school records to inspection by parents and students and provides that they may submit corrections. Such legislation, buttressed by court decisions upholding the individual's right to privacy and to have access to recorded information about oneself, is an obvious trend. Also a trend is the inclusion of the right of employees to review their own records and to comment about adverse information as part of collective-bargaining agreements.

Opening records to the individuals involved is in itself a threat-reducing action. One logical effect of such action will be to cause professionals to record only information that is truly useful to the school or that does not invade individual privacy.

Hyman and Schreiber† suggest that out-

---

*Lowis, E. R.: An appraisal of the amount of time spent on functions by Los Angeles City school nurses, J. Sch. Health **39**:254-257, April 1969.
†Gaskins, J. A.: A systems form of school health records, School Management **4**(4):32-33, April 1973.

---

*Education U.S.A. **16**(40):223, 1974.
†Hyman, J., and Schreiber, K.: The school psychologist as child advocate, Children Today **3**(2): 21-23, Feb. 1974.

dated material, especially that of sensitive nature, be destroyed periodically.

A decision to computerize individual records carries with it a threat to privacy, which should be considered. The threat arises more out of the big brother mystique associated with computers than out of fact. It is fairly easy for an unauthorized person to invade a file and copy a written report, even if the file is locked. Technical competence not only in computer operation but also with respect to the local system and codes in use is required to invade, copy, and interpret a computer file. Nevertheless, the threat exists and is forceful to those who perceive it as such.

Computerization of records. Reported experience indicates that computerization of health records yields no reduction in the time required to make entries of information. The advantages lie in the small space required for storage of punch cards or magnetic tape, and in the rapidity and accuracy with which data can be retrieved, ordered, and analyzed.

For example, students who require special attention (such as follow-ups of defects, immunizations, obesity control) can be readily identified and listed. Form letters (which can be individualized) can quickly be printed, addressed, and mailed to parents to secure their consent for immunizations and screening tests. If height and weight are recorded by date, individual growth curves and norms can be quickly and accurately printed. High accident locations and activities can quickly be identified. Accurate and up-to-date group data can be computed for evaluation purposes.*

Computerization is costly primarily in terms of the difficult, logical thought by all involved that must go into the development of the system and in terms of the technological expertise required. Most school systems, particularly larger ones, already have available the necessary equipment and technical personnel. Therefore, initial costs can be recovered rather quickly in terms of the decreased human time and error that goes into the retrieval, ordering, and analysis of data.

TRIAGE

As applied in school health work, triage is the process of deciding whether to do nothing except reassure an individual or watchfully wait, retain complete management of the case within a school setting, or refer it to an outside source or sources of health care. The decision is based on an informal cost-benefits analysis and may involve the individual and/or the parent. Reassurance and watchful waiting are often appropriate in the case of minor bumps or bruises. Deep or dirty cuts warrant referral to a source of care, while soap and a bandage applied at school suffices for small clean ones. Since orthodontia is costly, the decision to make such a referral must involve the parent in determining whether the cost to the family is outweighed by the benefits of treatment.

Triage decisions, therefore, culminate the health appraisal process and are the first step in the process of solving health problems.

SOLVING HEALTH PROBLEMS

It does no good to discover a health problem unless something helpful is done about it. What helpful actions are possible and the probability of success depends on the problem, the nature of the affected individual and his or her family, the resources available and policies and practices in the school and the community, and the approaches and techniques used in the referral, health counseling, and follow-up processes.

The problem and referral. As was indicated in the discussion of triage, it is useful to know something of the present state of medical knowledge and treatment capability concerning a given health problem before referral or health counseling is undertaken.

---

*Schneeweiss, S.: The computer in school health services, J. Sch. Health **40**:145-149, March 1970; Stennett, R. G., and others: Exploring the possibilities of computerized student health records, J. Sch. Health **41**:59-64, Feb. 1971.

Definitive medical diagnosis, which may not be available in school, may be needed to differentiate between a remediable or irremediable defect. If a cure is not presently available for a given disease, treatment to relieve symptoms or to support function during the course of the disease may be possible. There are some problems for which referral to a source of medical care is not appropriate.

Medical treatment is not the only helpful action possible. Group or individual health education or counseling or some adjustment of the school curriculum or routine is often useful either cojointly with medical treatment or without it. Still other kinds of problems are best solved by social or physical changes or by individual or family action, again with or without concurrent medical treatment. For some of these, referral to a social agency may be appropriate.

In the latter chapters of this book specific helpful actions for specific health problems are discussed. More likely than not, however, the range of possible helpful actions will have been expanded by the time this book appears in print, and some actions that now appear to be helpful will be proven not to be so. Updated information that is obtained through critical reading of current scientific literature and through continuing education courses is essential to the school health professional.

The individual, the family, and referral techniques. In a study of medical and dental referrals among Los Angeles public schoolchildren, it was found that care was most likely to be obtained by Jewish, white Protestant, Asian, Spanish surname, black, and white Catholic children, in that order. As might be expected, low social rank status was associated with lower rates of referral completion, while strong family ties were associated with high completion.*

In a later Los Angeles study of referral completion success that was achieved as a result of the efforts of a variety of agencies in a low-income ethnic minority community, such individual and family variables as sex, age, ethnicity, occupation, possession of a Medicare or Medicaid card, lack of transportation, lack of a baby-sitter, lack of money, or limited English were *not* found to be associated with whether or not referral was completed. Instead, actions by the referring agency were found to influence whether or not the consumers followed through.*

From these two studies it may be inferred that if society makes it possible for those in need of health care to cross ethnic and economic barriers, they will do so if given the kind of assistance that health counseling and referral can provide.

Of the two studies cited above, the most recent identified two specific referral techniques that were successful in improving referral completion by those referred. The first is for the referring agency to give the consumer a specific appointment with the source of care. The second is for the referring agency to give the consumer the name of a person to contact at the source of care. Together these two procedures may provide both the motivation to follow through and a commitment to act.†

The earlier study among Los Angeles schoolchildren also showed that a written referral notice plus a telephone call or other personal contact has optimal impact on referral completion. Such contacts are more effective if they are personalized and if they are made by two different persons (such as the school nurse and the teacher).‡ Three or more such contacts were not significantly more effective than two.

*Cauffman, J. G., and others: Health care of school children: variations among ethnic groups, J. Sch. Health **39:**296-304, May 1969.

*Cauffman, J. G., and others: A study of health referral patterns. IV, factors related to referral outcomes, Am. J. Public Health **64:**351-356, April 1974.
†Cauffman, J. G., and others: Am. J. Public Health **64:**351-356, April 1974.
‡Cauffman, J. G., Warburton, E. O., and Shultz, C. S.: Health care of school children: effective referral patterns, Am. J. Public Health **60:**1904-1909, Dec. 1970.

If a referral is deemed necessary when a medical health examination is held at school with the parent present, the referral can be made at that time. An appointment can be made by phone with a staff person at the source of care if this type of assistance seems desirable. A written or telephoned second contact can be made later if necessary. If the referral results from a screening test, the first contact will usually be written, but a personalized letter is more likely to be effective than an impersonal printed form. Experience indicates that a mailed letter is more likely to reach the parents than one sent home with a student, particularly if the student is past the third or fourth grade. Communications from school so often spell trouble to students that they tend to fail to deliver them.

School policy and practice should provide for excused absence to secure health care. This is helpful not only to the students and parents but to overloaded providers of care as well. In many instances examinations and treatment procedures are better conducted in the early part of the day when the individual is rested.

Health counseling: principles and techniques. Concepts of counseling range from that of a knowledgeable person giving advice and guidance to another, to a mutual exchange of ideas, to the development of a plan or scheme of action. Counseling can occur on either a one-to-one or group basis. The simple act of referral, even though it involves no more than the sending of a form letter to parents to advise them that the test results indicate that their child needs a professional examination, is counseling.

Counseling also goes beyond such simplistic approaches to include far more complex interactions if these are necessary. It includes a wide variety of approaches and techniques and operates under guiding sets of principles that vary somewhat with the counselor's philosophical orientation. The approach, for example, may be humanistic, one based on warmth and sympathetic understanding, or it may be behavioristic, in which rewards and punishments are used to modify individual habits and practices. All authorities seem to agree on one guiding principle; effective counseling is nonjudgmental. Guilt feelings about pregnancy or venereal disease do nothing to solve the problem; they only make a solution less likely.

Kelly* has suggested a flexible approach. He views some problems as the result of an individual's undesirable attitudes, values, and behavior, and others as arising out of the individual's environment. He suggests that the counseling process cannot be regarded as a series of steps to be followed like a recipe but as a variety of possible actions that may be utilized or not, depending on the nature of the client and his or her problem.

The counselor, Kelly states, may work with the client personally and/or through significant others in the client's life (peers or teachers, for example). The process of helping may involve the use of a variety of techniques, the first of which might be *problem exploration,* if the problem is not clear-cut and apparent. Here counselors may use one-to-one discussion with clients, testing, classroom observation, and referrals to other appripriate professionals for help. Or they may interview others, such as parents, teachers, and friends, to obtain information about the client. A next step might be that of helping the client in *understanding the problem.* This may involve assessment of the personal and environmental interactions that have resulted in the problem, but the emphasis is on the present situation. Present emphasis is essential, because preoccupation with the past can lead to guilt judgments, which seldom if ever help solve the problem. It may also be useful to arrive at an understanding of the problem with those significant others who may help the client in solving his or her problem.

The final step is that of *action planning,* or deciding what to do about the problem.

---

*Kelly, E. W., Jr.: Counseling focus: success not process, School Counselor 20:375-381, 1973.

Planning may involve changes that clients can make in their own behavior, changes that need the reinforcement provided by behavior modification techniques, or changes that are brought about by the understanding and help of significant others. Environmental changes such as a curriculum change or other changes in the client's school, home, or peer group environments may also be appropriate.

There can, of course, be no guarantee that the action plan first selected will work. A high probability of success, simplicity, and low cost (in terms of time, money, and effort) are useful guidelines in selection of an action plan. Action planning implies that logical modifications may be made as action proceeds and that if the first plan fails, another is selected and tried.

One innovative approach is that of peer counseling. The behavior of all of us is influenced by the behavior and attitudes of our peers, and such influence can be as desirable as it is sometimes undesirable. A report in *Nations Schools** describes a formal program developed in the Palo Alto, California secondary school by Varenhorst. Peer counselors are volunteer students who receive a 12-week training course. Clients are referred by teachers or others or come in on their own initiative. The peer counselors deal with such problems as shyness, unpopularity, or depression of the kind that is a reasonable outgrowth of client's situation, but they refer clients who have deep problems such as heavy drug use or irrational behavior to professionals. Program guidelines stress the importance of strong commitment by peer counselors, a strict training schedule, and informality of the program itself. Those who have problems themselves often make the most effective counselors.

Others, including school health professionals, do counseling. Unfortunately, many who do it are not prepared for the task, unlike the counseling and guidance professionals and the prepared peer counselors who were described above. Formal course-work in counseling, including a practicum experience, is an important part of the preparation of school health professionals.

Volpe* has called attention to many similarities between physical and health education and counseling and guidance. Among these are the concern of both fields for the same topics, the emphasis that each places on total development, and the rapport that both seek to develop with students.

Health care for children of indigent families. The major source of payment for health care of children of poor families in the United States at this writing is Medicaid, which was enacted as Title XIX of the 1965 amendments to the Social Security Act. Medicaid is essentially a federal-state welfare program. The states must provide certain basic services (medical diagnostic and treatment services, and hospital care) to recipients of Aid to Families with Dependent Children and other federally defined classes of needy persons such as those who are blind or disabled. States are permitted to broaden eligibility standards to conform to their own definitions of what needy or indigent means, and they may provide other services in addition to those federally specified. Thus, both eligibility requirements and the range of services provided vary significantly from state to state.

A significant preventive segment was added to Medicaid with the enactment of a 1967 amendment that established the Early and Periodic Screening, Diagnosis, and Treatment Program (EPSDT). Under this program Medicaid children and youth under the age of 21 became eligible to receive periodic screening tests and health examinations together with follow-up treatment services if indicated. The program includes outreach activities that are designed to bring eligible children and youth into the program. The battery of screening tests that may be administered is impressive. It may include de-

---

*Nations Schools **92**(5):40-41, 1973.

*Volpe, N. P.: Counseling: its relationship to physical and health education, The School Guidance Worker **28**:41-44, Sept.-Oct. 1973.

velopmental testing of preschoolers, a hemoglobin or hematocrit test for anemia, a test for lead poisoning, sickle cell anemia testing of black youngsters, and vision and hearing screening. Some tests are administered routinely at specified ages; others are administered to selected individuals only at the request of the examining physician. In addition, routine immunizations are administered.

Medicaid and the associated EPSDT have provided adequate and sometimes excellent health care to many infants, children, and young people, but numerous difficulties and deficiencies exist. For example, many families whose incomes fail to meet the state definitions of poor, but who are clearly unable to meet the costs of the basic necessities of life, are left out of the program. A Medicaid card carries with it a poverty stigma that may cause providers to treat eligible persons less than humanely. Many physicians simply refuse to accept Medicaid patients. Those who do accept them find themselves enmeshed in a plethora of forms and other bureaucratic red tape and are inadequately compensated for the services that they do provide. The high standards required of EPSDT providers, as well as the inadequate compensation, has made it impossible to implement this valuable service in many locations. School health services usually find it impossible to offer EPSDT, because they would only be compensated for services to Medicaid-eligible youngsters and cannot offer the program to all.

Nurses and other school health service professionals have traditionally begged funds from service clubs and other organizations to provide health care for needy children. Funds available from such sources are not only inadequate, but the begging process is time-consuming and often degrading. Some organizations, for example, insist that information about the recipients, which should be confidential, be made available to them in order that they might judge which cases are worthy and which are not.

The ultimate solution, if one is found at all, is believed by many to be some form of compulsory national health insurance, perhaps combined with a reorganization of the present system of organizing and delivering health care. However, care must be taken that changes do not create new problems that are worse than those they were designed to solve.

Assessing outcomes. An important aspect of referral and counseling involves follow-up procedures to determine whether the actions recommended or agreed upon have in fact been taken and to determine the extent to which these actions have successfully cured or ameliorated the problem.

The best evidence of action completion is probably a reappraisal of the individual's health status by means of a repeat examination or screening test. Observation is sometimes useful, as of a student who is referred to an eye doctor and then appears in school with glasses, or of the improved behavior of a student after counseling.

Written reports from outside sources of diagnosis and treatment are extremely useful but are sometimes difficult to obtain. Some physicians refuse to supply such information at all on the grounds of the confidentiality of the physician-patient relationship. Most will do so if a form that includes a release statement signed by the parent is provided by the school. Effective school nurses and physicians usually build relationships with nonschool sources of care, which permit them to obtain useful follow-up information by telephone.

A nonstructured interview with the student or parent can also be used to determine referral completion, but students and parents tend to tell school staff members what the staff members wish to hear; thus such interview reports are not always valid.

Follow-up of actions recommended within the school is also important. School inter-staff communication systems never operate as effectively as they should, and a special curriculum or other adjustment for a student is not infrequently stymied by red tape or bureaucratic inaction. In addition, the student who requires special class placement one year may not require it the next.

QUESTIONS FOR STUDY
AND DISCUSSION

1. What are the objectives of school health services? What is meant by promotion of positive health, and primary, secondary, and tertiary prevention?
2. What is meant by health appraisal? Why is it useful to determine the health status of school populations as well as the health status of individuals?
3. What is meant by health histories, and what are the advantages and disadvantages of this appraisal technique?
4. What is meant by a medical health examination? What current recommendations with respect to timing, source and location, the nature and scope of such examinations, and their application to school staff members are presented in the text? Which of these recommendations are disputable, and why?
5. What are the values of medical health examinations, and what alternatives are proposed? Given the present availability and accessibility of medical care, what directions should be taken with respect to health examinations?
6. What are the relative advantages and disadvantages of dental health examinations conducted in school and under the Malden Plan? What procedure is recommended for assessing school population dental health status?
7. What is meant by health observation? How can the validity of observations be improved? How does health observation differ today from previous practice?
8. What has been our traditional concept of the nature and purposes of screening tests, and how has Lessler proposed that the concept be broadened?
9. How is the accuracy of screening tests determined? What problems are associated with overreferral and with underreferral? What are some of the ways in which test accuracy can be improved?
10. What are some right ways and wrong ways in which you might interpret the results of a hearing screening test to a student or a parent?
11. What health screening test did you last receive as a high school student? Did the experience contribute to health education objectives, and why? In what specific ways might this experience have been made more educative?
12. What valid purposes are served by health records? What disadvantages result from keeping school health records?
13. How do working records and individual ones differ in purpose and relative importance?
14. How can the usefulness, cost in time, and the threat posed by recording to individuals each be improved?
15. List the advantages and disadvantages of opening an individual's health record to the employee, the student, and the parent.
16. List the advantages and disadvantages of record computerizations.
17. What is meant by triage, and what are its implications in practice?
18. How should the nature of a health problem influence referral practice?
19. How should the nature of the individual referred and his or her family influence referral techniques?
20. What referral techniques and practices improve referral completion?
21. What are some of the varied activities that may be construed as health counseling?
22. What quality is most important in a counselor, and why?
23. Describe the counseling approach explicated by Kelly. What is meant by peer counseling, and what are its advantages and disadvantages?
24. What means are presently available for financing health care for children of indigent families? What problems are associated with these means?
25. List methods proposed for assessing the outcomes of referral and counseling. Evaluate the relative validity of each method.

REFERENCES

Anderson, C. L.: *School health practice,* ed. 5, St. Louis, 1972, The C. V. Mosby Co.
Mayshark, C., and Shaw, D. D.: *Administration of school health programs,* St. Louis, 1967, The C. V. Mosby Co.
Miller, D. F.: *School health programs: their basis in law,* Cranbury. N.J., 1972, A. S. Barnes & Co., Inc.
National Education Association and the American Medical Association Joint Committee: *School health services,* Washington, D.C., and Chicago, 1964, NEA and AMA.
Nemir, A.: *The school health program,* ed. 3, Philadelphia, 1970, W. B. Saunders Co.
Wheatley, G. M., and Hallock, G. T.: *Health observation of school children,* ed. 3, New York, 1965, McGraw-Hill Inc.
Wilner, D. M., Walkley, R. P., and Goerke, L. S.: *Introduction to public health,* ed. 6, New York, 1973, Macmillan, Inc.

CHAPTER 10

❧ Exceptional children,
emergency care, services to
environment and instruction,
and staff roles and relationships

This chapter is devoted to school health services other than those where the major purpose is to assess health status and to refer and counsel those with defects. School services for *exceptional children* are those primarily aimed at tertiary prevention through the habilitation or rehabilitation of handicapping defects. *Emergency care* services provide early care and appropriate referral for those who become ill or injured at school. In providing services to the *environment and instruction,* school health service professionals lend their expertise to health promotion and primary prevention activities. Finally, health service *staff roles and relationships,* an area that can now best be described as being in a state of flux, are discussed.

SERVING EXCEPTIONAL CHILDREN

The concept. Exceptional children may be defined as all those who deviate from the average range of function to such an extent that either they themselves have difficulty or they create it for others in situations designed for those within the average range. The exceptional group thus includes those who are exceptionally creative or gifted as well as those with extreme physical, mental, emotional, or social disabilities. Planning school buildings and curricula to meet the need of as wide a range of average as possible and educating and hiring staff members who are tolerant of individual differences decrease the numbers of exceptional children.

Identification. Health appraisal procedures serve to identify exceptional children as such, but determination of the appropriate school placement and management of an exceptional child also depends on appraisal of his or her academic ability and social and emotional development. These determinations are best made cooperatively by educators, guidance and psychological specialists, and health professionals. When the individual's total status has been appraised, it is desirable to hold a team case conference and to make a decision about appropriate school placement and management. The individual or a parent may be involved in the decision-making process, but most frequently the decision is made by the specialists involved and approved by the administrative hierarchy. The parent and the individual are then informed of the decision. It is helpful to include an explanation of the evidence and rationale that underlie the decision.

Placement. The prevailing philosophy holds that an exceptional child should be placed in a regular classroom in a regular school if at all possible. A good general rule to follow is to do so and then see how things go before considering other solutions. The rationale behind the philosophy includes the belief that the exceptional child needs to learn to cope with average people in an average world and that average persons need to learn to get along with those who are exceptional. Such placement also avoids labeling children abnormal, which tends to encourage greater dependence on others than is necessary. The cost of edu-

149

cating exceptional and average children integrally is considerably less than the cost of educating the two groups separately. Furthermore, segregated education, which is inherently unequal, tends to produce segregated subcultures, as has occurred among deaf-mutes.

If regular class placement in a regular school proves inadequate, it is sometimes possible to make it adequate by providing consultant help and special devices and materials for the teacher. Consultant help may be provided by an itinerant special educator who visits and works with a number of teachers and schools. Devices and materials such as magnifying lenses and large-type books for the partially sighted may either be brought by the itinerant teacher or maintained in a resource room within each school where they are needed. If a disability prevents useful participation in a given subject, another activity can be substituted if the school and curriculum are flexible enough to do so. Such types of assistance provide the exceptional child with needed assistance and avoid the problems of segregation.

Some exceptional children will still re-

quire the extra help provided by their own special teachers, classrooms, equipment, and curricula. Therefore, some school systems place one or more special education classrooms in a regular school building. This plan permits associations with average peers and participation to the extent feasible in regular school activities.

Separate special schools are maintained by some school systems. Here, therapists and the special equipment and facilities they need to give physical, occupational, speech, or other therapies can also be located. Some authorities feel, however, that such rehabilitative treatment should be provided by community agencies other than the school. On the other hand, special schools are often able to provide the full range of services required by those with multiple handicaps. Several small districts can provide a single special school jointly or through the intermediate (county or regional) school district. The few exceptional children found in each small district can thus be served.

Those who are confined to their homes or in hospitals temporarily or permanently can be served by a homebound special teacher. Such service may be supplemented

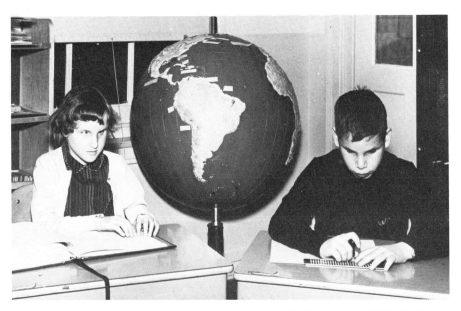

Fig. 10-1. Special education for the blind. (Courtesy School District of Philadelphia.)

by special telephone contact between the youngster and his or her classroom at school.

Placement in a residential school is now generally regarded as the alternative of last resort. Such institutions are designed primarily to serve the blind, deaf, or those with extreme mental retardation.

Health and rehabilitation services. Health services to exceptional children should not end with special education placement. Annual reappraisal of their health, social, and educational status will result in reassignment of many of them in the direction of either more normal or more specialized school placement. In addition, they need the same immunizations, emergency care services, and guidance and counseling as other children do. Some students will require the administration of prescribed

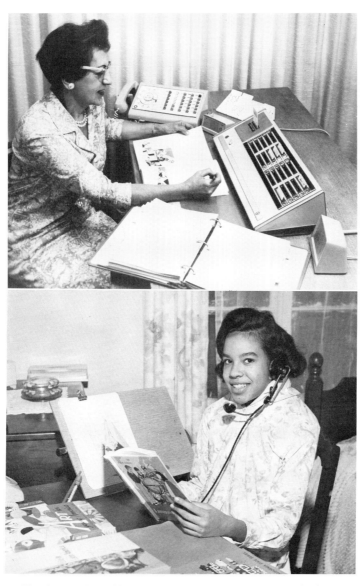

Fig. 10-2. Teleteaching. (Courtesy Los Angeles School Districts.)

medications during school hours by the local health service. State law may or may not govern policy. A sensible policy includes requirement of a written, signed statement from the prescribing practitioner, which states diagnosis, names the medication, and specifies times, method, and amount of medication to be administered. There should also be a signed statement from the parent requesting that the medication be given as prescribed. The medication should be kept in a locked cabinet and a record kept of each dose given.

At about age 16, young people whose disabilities present a probable employment handicap should be referred to the local office or to a representative of the state vocational rehabilitation service. In some states this service operates as a wing of the state department of education, but this provides no guarantee of automatic referral. Vocationally disabled students include individuals with such disorders as diabetes and epilepsy, and they are almost always placed in regular school classrooms. (Students with such disorders are handicapped more by social stigma and prejudice than by their physical health problems.) This invaluable federal-state service provides testing and counseling to select a suitable vocational goal and any treatment or special training (including college) that is required to reach that goal. The cost of this service to the federal government is more than offset by the increased income taxes paid by those who receive the service as well as by savings in welfare costs.

EMERGENCY CARE

Minor illnesses and injuries are common occurrences in schools. Those that are serious occur frequently enough that every experienced teacher has at least one experience that he or she would prefer to forget. Minor or serious, emergency care of sick or injured students and staff members is a responsibility of the school and one that is better and more easily fulfilled if a well-planned set of procedures and appropriate supplies and facilities are available.

The concept. What constitutes appropriate emergency care varies with the circumstances. Its purposes are to provide such care as is needed to preserve life and prevent further damage, to prepare the victim for and arrange transportation if need be, to notify the family as soon as possible and provide comfort and reassurance to them and the patient, and to see that the patient is promptly placed under the care of the family or a source of care designated by them if necessary. Lack of availability of parents or a source of definitive care, however, exerts pressure on the school to provide treatment in some cases. If such pressures prevail, adjustments will have to be made in the law, the competence of school health personnel, and in the facilities, equipment, and supplies provided.

The emergency care plan, supplies, and facilities desirable for any given school or school district must in any event be locally determined. Factors to be considered include existing state and local laws, regulations and policies, the availability of trained medical or first-aid personnel in the school, and the presence and quality of community ambulance and hospital emergency services. Good emergency care planning results from the involvement of administrators, teachers, school health professionals, representatives of available community resources, and representative students and parents.

Planning elements. Elements of a suitable plan are presented and discussed below.

In-school sources of care. Some schools restrict the provision of in-school emergency care to school health professionals (nurses or physicians). Since the vast majority of injuries that occur are minor, such a policy results in considerable waste of both professional and student time. A preferable alternative is to provide first-aid training and supplies to many or all teachers and other staff members and to utilize health professionals only for care of illnesses and major injuries. Regardless of school policy, teachers and others have a legal obligation to render first aid whenever necessary and should therefore be trained and equipped to do so.

Provision of standing orders. Such orders should be in a form that all concerned can find and read easily (see exemplary list in Appendix B). Some schools print such orders on flip charts, which are then hung next to first-aid kits on walls in classrooms and in other strategic locations. The front page of the chart lists emergency telephone numbers. Each succeeding page, which is a little longer than the one preceding, headlines one type of emergency at the bottom where it is visible. The text above the headline lists precise steps to be taken for that emergency in chronological order. In communities where emergency services are inadequate, consideration should be given to the inclusion of provisions for the relief of pain.

Selection of approved supplies. Because of the school's limited role, this selection usually need not be extensive. It should, however, be complete enough to provide for anticipated emergencies according to standing orders. If first-aid kits are to be placed in various areas about the school, specific lists for specific locations may be desirable (such as in regular classrooms, gyms, laboratories, and health rooms). The health-room list will be somewhat more extensive if a physician or nurse is on the school staff, and less extensive if good quality ambulance and hospital emergency service is near.

Some of the items that might be included in a regular classroom kit include:

1. An antiseptic of expert local choice, such as a soap or isopropyl (rubbing) alcohol. Ethyl alcohol, 70%, is a good antiseptic, but it has the disadvantage of being drinkable. Benzalkonium chloride or related quaternary ammonium compounds are also useful.
2. Applicators for cleansing wounds.
3. A variety of bandages, including nonmedicated adhesive strip bandages, butterfly bandages, 1- and 2-inch rolls of bandages, and various sizes of gauze pads. Butterfly bandages, used to bring the edges of small clean cuts together, promote healing.
4. Adhesive tape of various sizes.
5. Blunt bandage scissors.
6. Ice bag.
7. Tweezers.

Other possibly useful items can be derived from the first-aid procedures offered in Appendix B. There is considerable disagreement with respect to appropriate supplies and procedures; thus, it is best to be guided by local expert opinion.

There should be no oral medications in first-aid kits, and nonmedicated bandages are preferred if for no reason other than that someone is likely to be allergic to any selected medications.

In small schools blankets, stretchers, and splints should be kept in a central place such as the health room, and in large schools they should be kept in other strategic locations, such as gyms.

Maintenance of kits. A plan whereby kits are kept clean and properly filled by selected and instructed student monitors has proven successful in many schools where kits are placed in classrooms and other locations. The health service staff is primarily responsible for the maintenance of supplies in the health room and other special locations.

Facilities for rest and isolation. Facilities for individuals awaiting transportation or under observation for a suspected communicable disease must be provided. Cots should be screened from one another and provisions included for observation by the staff person in charge. The facility should be designed and equipment and supplies selected with the needs in mind of those suffering from such common complaints as nausea, vomiting, and diarrhea.

Individual emergency information. At least once a year each student and staff member should be given an individual emergency information card to complete. At a minimum the student card should provide:

The name, home and business addresses,

and phone numbers of both parents and a nearby surrogate

The name and telephone number of the usual source of medical care

The name of the preferred hospital or hospitals (usually the affiliation[s] of the source of care)

It is helpful also to list the date of the last tetanus shot, any medication allergies, and any significant chronic medical disorders such as diabetes.

Development of a plan for reporting. The most important reason for systematically reporting school accidents is to provide data useful in controlling future accidents through improved safety education, and school environmental and policy changes. A persistent myth is that accident reports provide legal protection; they provide evidence, not protection. If an accident results in legal action, a report is useful in establishing what the circumstances were and who did or did not do what. Original reports should be kept on file indefinitely, because in many states minors can sue on their own behalf upon reaching adulthood.

Developing an accident reporting plan involves the definition of what a reportable accident is; the development or selection of a report form; determination of who is responsible for reporting accidents and who is to receive, process, and file the reports; and a procedure for analyzing the data and disseminating the useful information thus obtained.

One useful definition of a reportable accident is any accident that occurs under school jurisdiction that results in either the utilization of nonschool medical care or in a school absence of one-half day or more. Excellent reporting and summary forms can be obtained from the National Safety Council. Reporting policies and procedures are best determined locally. Except in very small districts where the amount of data permits easy hand tabulation, useful summary data and statistics can best be derived by encoding and keypunching data on cards or tape for counter-sorter or computer processing. Such procedures reveal high-acci-

dent schools, locations, and activities where accident control activities are most needed.

Apparent occurrences of reportable communicable diseases, especially of outbreaks, should be reported as they occur to public health authorities according to locally prearranged policies and procedures.

Follow-up. Sympathetic and friendly telephone calls and visits from school staff following an accident demonstrates the human interest of the school. Such calls are not only good manners but are good public relations as well. Those to whom goodwill is thus demonstrated may be less inclined to consult an attorney than might otherwise be the case.

Insurance. Many if not most schools offer group accident insurance to students and staff members who wish to buy it. Such insurance is something of a nuisance for schools to handle, but the cost is low and the public relations value can be high. Care must be taken to select an underwriter with a reputation for prompt and full payment of justified claims. Two studies have shown that subscribers to school accident insurance were more likely to obtain follow-up medical evaluation and care than nonsubscribers.* The development of adequate compulsory national health insurance would probably make such plans unnecessary.

SERVICES TO THE ENVIRONMENT AND INSTRUCTION

A safe and healthful school environment is everyone's business and therefore often tends to be neglected. In the absence of a school environmental health specialist, school health service professionals often are assigned or assume some responsibility for health aspects of the environment. Although the professional preparation of nurses, phy-

---

*Podesta, V. J.: A study of the actuarial experience of student accident insurance programs of selected New Jersey school districts, unpublished doctoral dissertation, Rutgers University, 1962; Chmielewski, M. B.: Factors associated with the frequency of reportable injuries in a junior high school, unpublished master's degree project, Temple University, 1974.

sicians, and other medical specialists provides some knowledge of environmental health, it by no means makes them experts. Nevertheless, their encounters with sick and injured individuals in the school often enable them to observe and report the existence of hazards in need of correction. Their expert knowledge of the nature of handicapping conditions enables them to be of assistance in planning a school environment in which those with disabilities are better able to function. The potential contributions of health service staff members to school plant planning are often overlooked by school administrators. These contributions include not only the identification of specifications for design and equipment of health service facilities but also of other facilities that affect general health and safety throughout the building.

Health service professionals may or may not also be competent health educators by preparation, but their knowledge of the subject matter equips them to serve the health education aspect of the school program in several useful ways. One such function, that of providing health information to school personnel with a view to protecting and promoting staff health, is usually either performed by service professionals or not at all. To this end, service professionals may supply the teacher's lounge with relevant literature, drop information informally in the course of casual conversations, or plan and conduct formal group sessions. They may offer and interpret to the staff those screening tests and immunizations that are relevant to adults. They may provide health counseling and information to staff members on request, particularly in respect to the wise choice and use of available health products and service.

School health educators are often more well prepared in respect to educational objectives and methods than they are in regard to current content. Health service professionals are therefore often called upon to evaluate texts and other instructional material from the standpoint of factual accuracy and to serve as visiting resource persons when topics calling for extensive health knowledge arise in the classroom. Their expert knowledge and their experience in dealing with locally and currently important problems of children and youth equip them to assist in the selection of health education objectives and content.

Although health service professionals are sometimes used as primary classroom health educators, such use should be discouraged for at least four reasons. First, they are not usually well enough acquainted with the students to function efficiently. Second, unless they are also professionally prepared as teachers, they often do a poor job of it. Third, unless they are certified or licensed as teachers, such service can arouse animosities on the part of teaching colleagues. Fourth, if given on a regular basis, such service robs time from the health service functions and thus arouses resentment on the part of health service colleagues who must take up the load. On the other hand, if the health professional has the requisite preparation, certification, and time allocation, some regular classroom teaching can enrich the educational experience of students and enhance the relationships of the health service professional with both students and teachers.

ROLES AND RELATIONSHIPS

In his poem *Mending Wall,* Robert Frost wrote, "Good fences make good neighbors," and "Something there is that doesn't love a wall." We have seen that a fence of law and custom that excludes definitive diagnosis and treatment has been erected around school health service program functions, leaving those functions to other health care providers in the community. The fence makes it possible for school health services to function more or less in harmony with physicians and dentists in private practice. It has been suggested that the school may be forced to expand its functions to include the more complete treatment of minor illnesses and injuries. Changing attitudes toward pregnant students logically lead to the provision of pregnancy testing, contraception services, abortion counseling, prenatal care and the like either by the school or by a cooperative relationship with some other agency. Such forces do not love existing walls and may breech them. New fences must then be built if health service workers are to be good neighbors. Like walls or fences that run along real estate property lines, their nature and placement must be agreed to by neighbors.

School physicians and dentists: endangered species? By reason of their long and rigorous education and their superior earning capacity, school physicians and dentists have long perched atop the hierarchy of school health service professionals. Some serve as full-time and others as part-time school employees. Some school districts manage to get along with one or neither of them or with such service as may be supplied by volunteers from the community.

It is not uncommon, especially in large districts, for a physician, and at times a dentist, to serve as administrator of the school health service or total school health program. Yet there is nothing in their usual professional preparation that provides administrative competency. Years ago hospital boards learned from experience that good physicians often made incompetent administrators and turned instead to nonphysician administrators who are especially trained for the role. School dentists and physicians by reason of their professional status and affiliations are, however, ideally suited to develop cooperative relationships between the schools and individual or organized professionals, health departments, and other community health agencies and groups.

Schell,* an active public health officer and school physician, analyzed the primary responsibilities of each of the principal school health tasks and responsibilities and identified only one area—presport examinations and athletic injury care—in which he considered service by a school physician alone

to be essential. Presumably, even this function could ably be served by a school nurse practitioner or by a well-prepared athletic trainer. Current tendencies toward the demasculinization of athletics and the defeminization of nursing should remove sexual barriers to such substitutions.

Schell's analysis yielded ten other areas in which school physicians share responsibility with others:

1. Physical education and fitness programs, shared with physical educators.
2. Learning and behavioral disorders, shared with psychologists and special educators.
3. Evaluations and decisions regarding physical and mental handicaps, shared with psychologists and educators.
4. Behavioral and emotional disorders, shared with psychologists and educators.
5. Health of school personnel, shared with the personnel director.
6. Health education, shared with health educators.
7. VD, drug, or teen-age pregnancy problems, shared with nurses, psychologists, and educators.
8. Nutrition problems and lunch menus, shared with educators and dietitians.
9. Safety of school environment and buses, shared with administrators and custodians.
10. First aid and emergencies, shared with nurses, educators, and school nurse practitioners.

Schell observed that to serve these functions well, the physician's level of knowledge and concern must be increased with respect to a number of specialties, such as sports medicine, health education, learning and psychological disabilities, nutrition, and physical and special education. The physician thereby qualifies as a new species named school health consultant.*

*Schell, N. B.: School physicians: a weakening breed, J. Sch. Health **43:**45-48, Jan. 1973.

*Schell, N. B.: School physicians.

All of the above functions are served by three broad types of activity:

1. Administering medical examinations and making recommendations based on the findings (the most time-consuming of physicians' present activities).
2. Providing emergency service to athletes and some others who may be seriously injured or ill in schools.
3. Providing medical advice and guidance relative to health and health-related programs and policies of the school (perhaps the most productive and essential of physicians' activities).

Routine medical health examinations can be made by qualified nurse practitioners. A physician's higher skills may be needed for more complex diagnostic examinations, especially those required for the certification or delabeling of individual students as exceptional, and for advice to and guidance of the trainer in managing athletic injuries. Emergency service can be provided by non-physicians, as previously indicated. However, according to Lampe,* few individual school physicians are now well prepared to deal with the full range of school programs and policies for which medical advice and guidance are required. One would need to be qualified in educational psychology, health education, mental health, and learning problems, as well as general medicine.

The present functions of school dentists include:

1. Administering dental examinations and making recommendations based on the findings (the most time-consuming function served by school dentists).
2. Organizing, supervising, and assisting in preventive dental programs, including:
   a. Oral prophylaxis and fluoride applications (in communities where these services are appropriate).
   b. Mouthguard fittings for athletes.
   c. Dental health education.
   d. Provision of dental health promotion and protection advice and guidance relative to school policies and programs.
3. In some communities, providing restorative or other treatment services in school or community clinics.

The school dental health examinations or inspections and most if not all preventive dental functions can be conducted just as well by dental hygienists as by dentists. Whether or not dental treatment beyond first-aid measures is justified at all as a school service should be carefully considered in each community. Such a venture is illegal in some states, usually expensive beyond belief, and rarely if ever successful in adequately meeting dental needs.

Thus, the most time-consuming functions of school physicians and dentists can be fulfilled adequately by others, usually by school nurse practitioners and dental hygienists. Such a solution is economical in view of the high cost of physician and dentist time. It has worked effectively in a number of communities. It saves dentist and physician time for the diagnostic and treatment functions that are desperately needed by the total community.

One remaining needed school physician-dentist function is that of advice and guidance to policy and program. Bryan* observed that the organization and use of a medical and dental advisory board are growing and apparently successful trends. Relevant specialties are represented on such a board. The board's function is advisory only; it does not adopt policies or implement programs. Such a board could also serve as liaison agent between the schools and professionals in the community.

The need for specialized or diagnostic examinations of individuals beyond the competency of the nurse practitioner, such as for special education placement, can be

---

*Lampe, J. M.: The school physician of the future, J. Sch. Health **42:**197-201, April 1972.

*Bryan, D. S.: *School nursing in transition,* St. Louis, 1973, The C. V. Mosby Co., p. 173.

resolved either by use of the individual's specialist source of care or by use of a panel of specialist medical examiners who might serve on a fee basis. Such examinations can be conducted either on a mass clinic or individual basis and either in the school setting or in the examiner's own facility. Availability of the appropriate facilities and equipment is an important consideration.

An alternative solution is that of employing a single school health consultant with advanced preparation, as suggested by Schell and Lampe. Such a solution might be better suited to the needs of smaller communities where a full range of needed specialists does not exist. The consultant could meet the need for both program and policy advice and for special examinations.

School nurses. Functions of nurses in schools vary with the expectations of administrators, the presence or absence of physicians and other health service specialists, the professional preparation of the individual nurse, the policies and programs in effect, and nurse-student ratios. A precise and accurate definition of school nurse roles and functions, therefore, is impossible. It is safe to say, however, that school nurses play some part in the conduct of every component of the school health service program.

In most states and communities, specialist school nurses are employed by the schools and answerable to school administrators. In fact, the school nurse is the *only* health service specialist employed in many schools. In a few localities, public health department nurses serve the schools as part of a generalized public health program. Incompetent or ignorant school administrators abound who expect nurses to remain in the school at all times for the purpose of providing emergency care and identifying malingering students. A poorly prepared health officer may be no more cognizant or appreciative than a poorly prepared school administrator of the totality of school health and health education. The public health expectation may be limited to

considerations of communicable disease control and sanitation. Fortunate is the nurse and school that have an administrator, whether school or public health, who supports and understands a complete school health program.

Nurses who are traditionally prepared to function only in a hospital setting are not totally prepared to function as modern school nurses. Such preparation does equip nurses to assist physicians in performing examinations, to determine the nursing problems presented by individual patients and their families (nursing diagnoses), to provide nursing care to the ill or injured, to observe individuals for signs of health problems, and to plan and organize their work. Although these skills are all useful in school work, school nurses are also expected at times to serve as screening technicians, teachers, counselors and social workers, and even as physicians. Depending on the roles assigned to the nurse in a given school, considerable additional preparation may be required, but the nurse whose function is limited to providing first aid and emergency care may require less preparation rather than more.

Bryan* proposes no less than twelve different classifications of school nursing positions, each of which varies from the others in both roles and preparation required. Informal in-service training, or orientation only, is required of *volunteers,* paid *health aides,* or *nurses' assistants;* these individuals may provide assistance in clerical, first-aid or other nursing functions. A *licensed vocational* or *practical nurse* could assume some independent responsibility for such functions as first aid and the administration of screening tests. A *registered professional nurse* at the baccalaureate level or less could perform similar functions and perhaps more. In situations where the school health service program functions are limited and where higher level guidance and consultation are available, these kinds of workers

*Bryan, D. S.: *School nursing in transition,* pp. 5-6.

may provide most or all of the nursing services.

Training and experience beyond the baccalaureate produces nurses who may be classified as *school-community nurses* (or *school nurse-teachers*) and *school nurse practitioners*. Nurses in these classifications are prepared to provide maximum nursing service in individual schools. The school-community or school nurse-teacher is well prepared to serve as a counselor, social worker, and educational consultant. The school nurse practitioner is prepared to administer health examinations and to provide counseling, or in other words, to assume not only the functions of a school nurse but also those of the school physician. Increasingly, such nurses enhance their competencies through continuing education, and many individual schools are served by master's degree nurses with advanced preparation in public health, health education, paramedical practice, or counseling and guidance.

All of Bryan's other classifications require master's level preparation or more. They include nurses who are prepared to serve as special program coordinators, consultants, supervisors, and administrators of nurses. They tend to serve on an area, district, or state-wide basis, or in college or university teaching. Their functions are program and staff development.

The nurses who serve at the school building level are the most important members of the school health service staff, because they are the ones who organize and provide direct health services in the school and who provide liaison between the school and parents and community services on behalf of individuals. Traditionally, school nurses organize and conduct mass immunization and screening programs and are responsible for the follow-up of health defects.

Fricke* observes that the nurse in everyday practice must be the one who determines what needs to be done, initiates appropriate planning as a member of the pupil personnel service team and other relevant groups, conducts epidemiological studies to identify problems, knows and uses communications avenues, increases his or her own effectiveness in dealing with psychosocial problems, assists classroom teachers in planning and evaluating health education, and gets involved in promoting desirable health legislation. The school nurse who is prepared to fulfill all of these roles and functions is likely to find job satisfaction and be most useful only if he or she is allowed to do so. Conversely, if school policies and practices restrict nurse roles and functions, school nurses can either fight for change or succumb to frustration.

Dental hygienists. It has been suggested that the school dental hygienist can fulfill most if not all of the previously listed roles and functions of the school dentist. Like the nurse, the dental hygienist provides direct services to individuals. The school dental hygienist's likely roles and functions include:

1. Inspecting teeth with mirror and explorer, a function which is practically equivalent to in-school examinations by a dentist.
2. Organizing and providing oral prophylaxis and topical fluoride applications where the fluoride content of the water supply is deficient.
3. Providing preventive dental health education either directly or as a resource person to the classroom teacher.
4. Providing advice and guidance in the development of school policies and practices that affect dental health.
5. Assisting in the provision of dental care in school-community clinics.

Hygienists are well prepared in the usual course of their professional preparation to fulfill all of these functions. State law may require that they be supervised by a dentist in the performance of certain treatment or preventive functions.

Dietitians, nutritionists, or home economists. Many schools have the services of a

---

*Fricke, I. B.: School nursing for the 70's, J. Sch. Health **42**:203-206, April 1972.

dietitian, nutritionist, or home economist, all of whom are professionally prepared in nutrition and food preparation. Their functions include the teaching of nutrition (if certified to do so), service as resource persons in nutrition education, and the supervision of school feeding programs. Although they may be prepared to assess nutritional practices and other indicators of nutrition status and to assist in the development of programs designed to alleviate malnutrition, such competencies are too rarely utilized.

Teachers. Teachers are primarily prepared and hired to teach, but they are also often assigned health service responsibilities. Elementary teachers are more likely and better able than secondary teachers to serve health service functions, because they serve fewer students with whom they become better acquainted. These functions may include:

1. Observation of students for signs and symptoms of health problems, and referral to health service personnel for further evaluation and indicated action. This role is of major importance, especially in the early detection of communicable diseases and in the identification of exceptional students.
2. Adjustment of the classroom routine of students with health problems.
3. Assistance in follow-up. Use of the teacher's rapport with a particular student or parent may lead to follow-up success when efforts by the nurse or others fail.
4. Administration of selected screening tests. Such activity is ordinarily a poor use of teacher time, but circumstances or policy may require it.
5. Education and/or orientation of students concerning examinations, screening tests, or other health service program components.
6. Administration of first aid for minor injuries, depending on local policies and procedures.
7. Promotion of mental health by serving as surrogate parents and informal counselors.

Health and physical education teachers and, in some states, elementary teachers receive instruction related to some or all of these functions as part of their preservice preparation. Most other teachers enter service totally unprepared, which is a deficiency that may be overcome through continuing education. Informal in-service instruction of teachers by school nurses, physicians, dentists, and dental hygienists can and often does provide useful skills and information.

Physical educators as such promote positive health through activity and physical fitness programs. They are prepared not only to identify orthopedic problems but to provide corrective training for some of them with the cooperation of an orthopedic surgeon. Their basic preparation includes health-related instruction, and some are prepared to function in dual roles as health and physical educators.

Screening technicians. In some schools, persons other than nurses or teachers administer selected health-screening tests and sometimes maintain records of testing. The nature of the screening test determines the amount of preparation and supervision required. Technicians range from volunteers with little training who work under the close supervision of a health service professional to formally prepared paid paraprofessionals who function independently. Vision and hearing–screening technicians are employed in many school systems.

Present vision-screening techniques require relatively little preparation; therefore, technicians function economically under the supervision of the school nurse. Hearing screening, particularly of the very young, is a more complex task and is often performed by audiometrists. Often in cooperation with state health departments, some universities provide formal training. Qualified audiometrists are prepared to select and calibrate testing equipment, administer a variety of tests, orient students to the purposes and procedures of the testing program, recognize and cope with the factors that may interfere with test reliability and validity, and record and maintain test data.* Interpretation of certain test data and administration of certain complex diagnostic tests are skills usually better performed by audiologists, who are master's or doctoral level professionals.

Mental health specialists. Although school physicians, nurses, and teachers are usually prepared to some extent in mental health and identify and counsel individuals with problems that might be classified within that domain, many schools employ one or more of a variety of mental health professionals. Almost all school systems employ *guidance counselors,* some of whom devote their time largely to academic or vocational counseling. Most counselors are educators with additional preparation in guiding and counseling of students who present specific problems. Those who are prepared specifically as *social workers* work in schools under a variety of job titles, including school social worker and visiting teacher. Their role is usually perceived as one of dealing with the interrelationships of an individual with parents, peers, teachers, or others. *Psychologists* are nonphysician specialists in diagnostic testing and evaluation, who sometimes conduct therapy. *Psychiatrists* are physicians with special training in the diagnosis and treatment of mental illnesses.

Actually, role relationships between these various specialist categories have become blurred. Strictures against diagnosis and treatment by nonphysicians that have traditionally been applied with respect to physical health problems have not been rigorously applied in the mental health field. The scarcity of clinical psychologists and psychiatrists, together with the high salaries that they command, has held their employment by schools to a minimum. Some localities, however, are served by community mental health centers that provide social work, psy-

chological, and psychiatric service to schools. In other schools, psychologists, and/or psychiatrists are employed on a part-time basis primarily as consultants.

A relative newcomer in some schools is the *crisis teacher,* a building-level teacher selected primarily for personal warmth and the ability to achieve rapport with students, who helps children and young people cope with immediate problems and who has ready access to consultant help from school or community mental health professionals. This new position grew out of the scarcity of mental health professionals and the resultant lengthy waiting list for service.

Directors or coordinators. Some larger and more affluent school systems employ one or more persons to administer, direct, coordinate, or supervise the school health program as a whole, or some part or parts of it, on either a full- or part-time basis. The precise title, functions, and location of such individuals within the administrative hierarchy vary with the nature and requirements of the state and local school system. In some locales, special certification requirements are in effect.

It is relatively unimportant whether the individual is a physician, nurse, educator, or any other sort of specialist. The important qualifications are that the individual possess a thorough working knowledge of all aspects of the school-community health program, an appreciation of the goals of the educational enterprise as a whole, and the ability to function as a democratic leader of all members of the school health service team. Such a person must also come to know the community, its services, and its power structure well.

Effective directors, coordinators, supervisors and those with similar titles serve to keep the ongoing program functioning smoothly, to maintain program balance, and to achieve program improvement through democratic planning and action. In doing so, much of their attention is focused on individual staff "people problems."

Trends in roles and relationships. A recent publication of the American School

---

*Based on Hearing testing of school children and guide for hearing conservation programs, Berkeley, Calif., California State Department of Public Health, undated.

Health Association* noted a number of trends in school nursing roles and relationships that are applicable to the roles and relationships of school health service workers generally. Some of these are trends toward:

1. Higher levels of preparation.
2. Health promotion as a goal.
3. Individualization of services.
4. More federal aid in funding.
5. School-community, rather than school-centered programs.
6. Utilization of auxiliary personnel (to perform less complex functions more economically).
7. Greater emphasis on the health of the whole child and appraisal rather than on diagnostic categories and specific screening tests and observations.

This publication also noted the movement away from private health care for the privileged few toward health services available to all as a matter of right. This trend is bound to have great impact on school health services. It may transfer some problems from school to community auspices.

Another particularly salient trend was also noted: the movement from separate disciplines to a team approach. This implies that physicians, nurses, and others will work more as coequals than as superiors-inferiors and that teachers, school health professionals, and community professionals will plan and work to common rather than cross purposes.

QUESTIONS FOR STUDY AND DISCUSSION

1. Can all children be legitimately considered exceptional in some way?
2. What factors should be considered in determining special education placements? Who should be involved in placement decisions?
3. If possible special education placements are viewed as a continuum, toward which end of the continuum would placement now be considered most desirable, and why?

---

*Knotts, G. R., editor: *Guidelines for the school nurse in the school health program,* Kent, Ohio, 1974, American School Health Association, pp. 26-27.

4. Should programs and facilities at the less desirable end of the placement continuum be maintained by society, and why?
5. How often should special education placements be reviewed, and why?
6. What is the role of the federal-state program of vocational rehabilitation? When should eligible students be referred to it?
7. What are the general purposes of emergency care?
8. Will desirable emergency care procedures and facilities vary or be the same in different schools, and why?
9. What are the planning elements that must be considered in developing emergency policies and procedures? What general considerations guide local planning of each element?
10. Who are the persons responsible for a safe and healthful school environment? What are the suggested roles of school health service professionals?
11. What are the suggested roles of school health professionals in health instruction?
12. Why are well-defined professional roles and relationships important?
13. Why are role and function relationships changing, and what are some of the good and bad effects of such change?
14. What roles are commonly played by school physicians and dentists? For which of these roles are physicians well and poorly professionally prepared?
15. Why are school physicians and dentists possibly endangered species? What other species might replace them, and why?
16. What roads to survival might school physicians and dentists travel?
17. What local circumstances determine the roles and functions of school nurses?
18. For what school health service roles and functions is a competent hospital nurse traditionally well and poorly prepared?
19. For what school health service functions is advanced nursing preparation required? What is the nature of such preparation?
20. What school health service roles and functions are dental hygienists expected to perform? Is the usual professional preparation of hygienists suitable for these roles?
21. What are the general roles of screening technicians? What are the advantages and disadvantages of having screening tests performed by technicians rather than by nurses or others?
22. Distinguish between various types of school mental health specialists in terms of roles, preparation, and the probable availability of each in schools.
23. What are the functions and desirable qualifications of health program directors (or administrators, coordinators, or supervisors)?
24. What are some of the trends that appear to be occurring in respect to school health services?

REFERENCES

American Academy of Pediatrics: *Report of the Committee on School Health,* Evanston, Ill., 1966, The Academy.

Anderson, C. L.: *School health practice,* ed. 5, St. Louis, 1972, The C. V. Mosby Co.

Bryan, D. L.: *School nursing in transition,* St. Louis, 1973, The C. V. Mosby Co.

Knotts, G. R., editor: *Guidelines for the school nurse in the school health program,* Kent, Oh., 1974, American School Health Association.

Mayshark, C., and Shaw, D. B.: *Administration of school health programs, its theory and practice,* St. Louis, 1967, The C. V. Mosby Co.

National Committee on School Health Policies: *Suggested school health policies,* ed. 4, Chicago, 1966, American Medical Association.

Nemir, A. C.: *The school health program,* ed. 3, Philadelphia, 1970, W. B. Saunders Co.

Wilner, D. M., Walkley, R. P., and Goerke, L. S.: *Introduction to public health,* ed. 6, New York, 1973, Macmillan, Inc.

PART FIVE

Healthful social, emotional, and physical environments

CHAPTER 11 ❧ School climate: a healthful social and emotional environment

Those of us who have observed a number of schools closely have come to recognize some schools as pleasant places in which to teach and learn, others as bearable, and still others as jail-like places from which sensible students and teachers attempt to escape by any available means. Such judgments are subjective, and not all of us would agree on which schools belong in each of the three categories. Our individual judgments are based on our own notions of what makes a good school. The physical appearance of the building and grounds together with the physical facilities available in the school would serve as one basis for judgment. Such physical factors are considered in the next chapter. The feelings associated with interpersonal and day-by-day relationships between administrators, staff, and students serve as another basis for judgment. Such feelings are associated with what is sometimes called the climate of the school or its social and emotional environment.

The physical, social, and emotional aspects of a school affect and are affected by each other. A physically attractive, comfortable, and safe school facilitates pleasant social relationships as well as teaching and learning. Maintenance of a school building and grounds in an attractive, comfortable, and safe physical condition is facilitated by a social and emotional climate that meets the needs of teachers and students for acceptance and friendship and for recognition and achievement; when individuals have positive feelings about their school, they tend to participate in its maintenance.

IMPORTANCE OF SCHOOL CLIMATE

Teachers who are in schools that are classified as having an "open climate" were compared by Ponder and Mayshark* with those in "closed climate" schools. Teachers perceive open climate schools as energetic, lively organizations, moving toward their goals, and as providing social needs satisfactions for their members. Closed climate schools are considered stagnant organizations that have apathetic members. As might be expected, teachers in open climate schools used significantly fewer sick days (an average of 3.70 per teacher) than those in closed climate schools (6.47 days). Both teachers and students, of course, use sick days because of apathy or other negative feelings as well as for physical illness.

Fox and his associates† suggest that poor school climate is associated with high student absenteeism, cliques, vandalism and theft, a high incidence of suspensions and expulsions, and a host of other ills. They view the goals of a humane climate as achievement of productivity and satisfaction by students and teachers. In a humane climate basic skills, constructive attitudes, and knowledge will be developed and expanded, values and purposes will be clarified, and processes of inquiry and problem solving will be utilized. Members will gain a sense

---

*Ponder, L. D., and Mayshark, C.: The relationship between school organizational climate and selected teacher health status indicators, J. Sch. Health **44**:122-126, March 1974.

†Fox, R. S., and others: *School climate improvement: a challenge to the school administrator,* Englewood, Colo., 1973, Phi Delta Kappa and CFK Ltd. Occasional Paper, pp. 2-5.

167

of personal worth, enjoy living and working in the school, and enjoy participation in worthwhile activities.

A HUMANE SCHOOL CLIMATE

Some climate factors identified by Fox and his coauthors* include:

Self-respect and respect for others

The ability to trust others

High morale

Opportunities for input

Continuous academic and social growth by both students and teachers

Cohesiveness; a feeling that "this is my school"

Development of improvement projects within the school

Caring; teachers and students feel that others care about them as human beings

These factors and others are viewed as being determined by qualities of the school program, processes by which the school program is carried out, and by material resources. The program determinants include (but are not limited to) opportunities for active learning, individualization of learning, varied learning environments, the cooperative determination of rules, and varied reward systems. Process determinants include problem solving, improvement of school goals, conflict identification and resolution, involvement in decision making, and effective teaching-learning strategies. Material determinants include material and school plant resources and an effective logistics system.

Garner† calls for clearing up double-bind communications in which the achievement of goals inconsistent with either required or rewarding behavior is demanded of teachers by administrators and of students by teachers. For example, some teachers expect students to tattle on their peers in violation of the rules of peer culture. He also emphasizes the importance of participating in community affairs, developing mutual trust, making fantasies the groundwork for creativity and action, integrating knowledge and feelings in teaching and learning, and caring as much for *how* learning occurs as for *what* is learned. Garner equates lack of such qualities with schizophrenic seclusiveness and withdrawal from real life, response to fantasies and hallucinations rather than to reality, and inconsistency of thoughts and feelings. He makes the point that schizophrenic schools like schizophrenic parents may communicate their illness to children.

If one accepts the prescriptions cited above, then no single individual or group can create a humane school climate. Administrators, other school staff members, students, parents, and others from the community must all be committed to and involved in school climate improvement.

SOME ISSUES THAT AFFECT SCHOOL CLIMATE

A number of recurring educational and social issues have serious implications for school climate.

Methods of reporting grades. A recent national survey of elementary report cards revealed that a majority of schools use letter grades. Some use percentage equivalents, which are usually statistically meaningless unless they refer to percentile ranks. About 14% use a trichotomized reporting system, such as satisfactory, improvement shown, or unsatisfactory, in grades 1-3; while only about 3% use dichotomies such as pass-fail, or satisfactory, and needs improvement. The investigator concluded that present systems fail to inform parents where their children stand in relation to national norms, their own ability, or mastery of required skills and concepts.*

Based on acceptance of the importance of self-motivation and the humanitarian con-

*Fox, R. S., and others: *School climate improvement*, pp. 7-17.

†Garner, H. G.: How to prevent a school from becoming schizophrenic, J. Sch. Health **42:**554-557, Nov. 1972.

*Mousely, W.: Report cards across the nation, Phi Delta Kappan **53:**436-437, March 1972.

cepts of the basic goodness and ability of the individual to make wise decisions, Van Hoven* proposes that students be graded not in relation to another's performance but on some criterion of their individual achievement. For example, the teacher might pre- and posttest students and assign grades that reflect gains in knowledge or skills rather than class rank.

In a not altogether tongue-in-cheek article, Simon and Kirschenbaum† suggest that turnabout is fair play. They propose that if students are to be graded by teachers, then teachers should be graded by students. The same reasons can be applied in both situations: to determine peer standing, to screen individuals for advancement, and to motivate improved performance. The same means of grading could be applied; namely, quizzes, exams, and term papers.

The effects of grading on students, parents, and teachers vary widely. Students who consistently earn and receive good grades are likely to feel quite good about it, but they may also be motivated to overwork or even to cheat in order to maintain an outstanding record. Students who consistently fail may come to regard themselves as incompetent and unworthy, a state that effectively blocks learning for them. Parents may react to good grades by giving extrinsic rewards or by otherwise pushing their students too fast and too far for their own good. Poor grades have been known to motivate some parents to beat their children or to attack teachers. Humane teachers worry about the effects of the grades they give.

The bases on which grades are awarded are open to criticism. Teacher-made tests and assessment of term projects may or may not be valid, reliable, and relevant to instructional objectives, and yet their emo-

tional effects range from euphoria to devastation.

A variety of systems of reporting pupil progress have been invented, reformed, abandoned, and returned to throughout the history of education. Perhaps what is needed is not new systems of reporting but new attitudes toward the ones we use, and new systems of education in which a given student may be more likely to achieve success in at least some activity. For example, we might trade off the viewpoint that everyone should be successful in almost every school subject for the attitude that failure in school subjects does not imply failure in life.

Alternative programs and curricula. Dunn and Dunn* propose that each student be placed in the school program that best suits his or her learning style. For example, a motivated student who does not require frequent movement, who is an auditory learner, and who is persistent and authority oriented is likely to do well in a traditional classroom. A motivated, responsible student who is peer-oriented, who does not need an imposed structure, and who is not bothered by the noise and movements of others, is likely to do well in an open classroom.

The Dunns feel that concentration is affected by the physical environment, the emotional framework, the sociological setting, and the student's physical self and needs, but they also note that the optimal environment varies with the individual.

Perrone† observes that open classrooms vary somewhat because the teachers and children who occupy them vary. They do share a number of common attributes. They are active places, with a variety of activities going on at the same time, and children move about and tend to be noisy. Different activities are clustered in learning areas, each of which represents a curriculum area.

---

*Van Hoven, J. B.: Reporting pupil progress: a broad rationale for new practices, Phi Delta Kappan **53**:365-366, Feb. 1972.

†Simon, S., and Kirschenbaum, H.: The ultimate grading game, Phi Delta Kappan **53**:443, March 1972.

*Dunn, R., and Dunn, K.: Learning style as a criterion for placement in alternative programs, Phi Delta Kappan **56**:275-278, Dec. 1974.

†Perrone, V.: *Open education: promise and problems,* Phi Delta Kappa Educational Foundation, 1972.

At times, all the pupils and the teachers hold planning sessions from which children emerge with plans for their separate activities. Thus, there is order and direction, but it is not obvious to the casual observer. Open classrooms demand much from teachers. They must know each child welľ and must keep track of each child's projects. Hours are spent in selecting and obtaining new materials, which must be made available in wide variety to enable children to carry out their plans.

Perrone notes that children in open classrooms do about as well and sometimes better on traditional achievement tests than those in traditional settings. Attitudes of children, parents, and teachers and school attendance seem to improve with openness. However, open education has its problems, among which are the need for time to develop it prior to its introduction, the tendency to ignore the need of children for structure, the need for support in the form of teacher training, and the problems faced by children who move from an open elementary school to a closed secondary school.

McLoughlin* states that individualization of instruction, which can occur in settings other than open classrooms, requires programs based on individual differences rather than on group similarities. He states that there must be school- or district-wide planning for it and that greater emphasis should be placed on the effectiveness of the resource materials than on teacher accountability.

Such innovations as open education at the elementary level and secondary "schools without walls" are often heralded as panaceas but fail in practice. The previously cited viewpoint of Dunn and Dunn that students should be assigned to such schools on the basis of their learning styles makes logical sense. To extend this viewpoint to include the placement of teachers on the basis of

their preferred teaching styles also makes sense.

A flexible curriculum and a wide variety of opportunities to pursue extracurricular activities are components of a desirable school climate.* Such flexibility may be somewhat more characteristic of open than closed schools, but it is possible to achieve it in both. Minicourses taught for half a term instead of a full year provide curricular flexibility. Extracurricular offerings may be broadened either through community recognition of their value and consequent willingness to reimburse those teachers and other adults who serve as leaders or by recruiting and using volunteer adult leaders.

Affective and sex education. Many authorities have come to believe that to some extent children and young people can be taught to achieve mental health, including sexual adjustment, in school. Such teaching is aimed at helping children and young people understand themselves and their relationships with others in terms of their growth and development and their emotional feelings. The processes used rely heavily on affective techniques in which feelings and values are openly explored and clarified, and techniques of coping with disturbing situations are learned. Some segments of society reject the subject matter and/or the techniques of teaching that are employed on philosophical or religious grounds. They believe that affective and sex education are prerogatives of home and/or church. However, mental health and sexual problems occur among school-age children and youth and interfere with the attainment of other educational goals irrespective of qualities of home life and religious affiliations.

There is no minimum age limit to mental health and sex problems but such problems perhaps become more acute and prevalent during adolescence. Adolescents are faced with the task of establishing their identities.

---

*McLoughlin, P. W.: Individualization of instruction vs. non-grading, Phi Delta Kappan **53**:378-381, Feb. 1972.

*Fox, R. S., and others: *School climate improvement,* p. 105.

In doing so they tend to come in conflict with parents and others who have traditionally supplied support and reassurance. It is as difficult and frustrating to be the parent of an adolescent as it is for an adolescent to be the child of an adult. Dlugokinski* suggests that schools can provide support to adolescents through group guidance courses and career orientation work experience. PTA's and similar organizations can provide support for parents through organized group discussion of adolescence and the mutual problems faced by parents.

The nature of sex education in schools is discussed in some detail elsewhere in this book. With respect to sex education as a community issue, Mooney† states that no single program can be adopted by all school systems; the cultural and social nature of the community and the extent to which teachers are prepared to assume responsibility must be considered. She points out that sex education is in fact a responsibility of *both* schools and parents. The parent's primary role is to set behavioral limits for their own children. The school can provide instructional programs based on developmental principles. It can help students and parents understand behavior and feelings, because it is easier for the school to maintain an emotionally neutral and objective stance and because it is in a better position than parents to interpret both peer and community pressures.

One recent innovation in schools has been the adoption of transcendental meditation or similar exercises as a formal or informal part of the curriculum. Bright and her coauthors‡ define transcendental meditation (TM) as a process in which progressively more subtle levels are achieved until the mind reaches a state called "bliss consciousness." They cite laboratory evidence that indicates that decreases in oxygen consumption, metabolic heart and respiratory rates, and blood pressure and muscle tenseness are associated with it. Unvalidated subjective benefits reported by meditators include decreased psychoactive drug use, better self-adjustment, and improved grades and ability to study. Lehman* notes that effects similar to those claimed for TM have been reported by various primitive medicine men, by practitioners of Yoga and biofeedback, and by users of various drugs. He fears that if it is effective, it may lead youth to comfortable acceptance of the unacceptable aspects of schools and societies.

Optimal school size. During the 1940's and 1950's a movement of the population from farms to cities and a trend toward the deliberate consolidation of small school systems into large ones occurred. Consolidation was considered desirable, because it was believed that only large schools could offered a varied curriculum and specialized pupil services. But an unfortunate side effect occurred; in the small schools that were eliminated by consolidation almost all the teachers and students knew each other, and the opportunity for any student who wished to participate in athletics, student government, or other activities was essentially unlimited by the small number of competitors for available positions. Although behavioral problems occurred, misbehavior was less likely either to occur or to remain undetected and undealt with, because everyone was aware of being watched and was usually also aware that someone cared. Big schools bred intense competition for status-bearing positions and a sense of anonymity and depersonalization that led in turn to increased behavioral problems.

A 1973 Gallup poll revealed that 57%

---

*Dlugokinski, E.: Parents, adolescents, educators, and health professionals: some core issues, J. Sch. Health **43:**636-639, Dec. 1973.

†Mooney, E.: *The school's responsibility for sex education,* Bloomington, Ind., 1974, Phi Delta Kappa Educational foundation, pp. 25-26, 33.

‡Bright, D., and others: What school physicians, nurses and health educators should know about transcendental meditation, J. Sch. Health **43:**192-194, March 1974.

---

*Lehman, D. L.: What is a good journal like the Kappan doing with a suspicious character like TM? Phi Delta Kappan **54:**624-625, May 1973.

of a national sample of the population believed that high schools today are getting too large. The median size stated by respondents for an ideal high school was 500 students. About three in every four of a group of professional educators questioned agreed.* Postman and Weingartner† believe that schools of 3,000 or 5,000 students make humanized supervision practically impossible and conclude on the basis of literature review that an ideal school size approximates 250 students.

Schoenholtz‡ describes a 128-student high school (Malta, Illinois) that succeeded in increasing curriculum offerings fourfold by the simple expedient of creating 9-week minicourses to replace the 51 year-long courses previously offered. He affirms the notion that smallness is associated with better student behavior and participation and notes the following additional advantages: effective communication, bad situations changed easily, feeling of pride in the school, lack of bureaucratic obstacles, and ease in recognizing and helping ineffective teachers.

Costly oversized schools abound in the United States and must be used despite their disadvantages. This fact of life has led to the adoption of the "school within a school" concept. Several small schools, each with its own space, faculty, and administrators, are housed in one large building. All the schools make common use of certain facilities such as the cafeteria, gymnasium, and shops.

Segregation, desegregation, and integration. Alvin Loving§ views multiethnic schools as essential to the development of a free, democratic society that values creativity and abhors racism. All children should learn the contributions of each of the many subcultures that make up the conglomerate of American society, and they do this best by rubbing shoulders.

Barbara Sizemore* differentiates between desegregation and integration. *Desegration,* which has been adopted in the United States, is an imposed condition in which the old superior-subordinate relationship between groups is maintained. *Integration* is an attribute of a free and open society, a condition that has not yet been chosen in the United States. She postulates that before integration can occur, minority groups must move through several precursor stages: (1) *separatism,* during which group identity is defined; (2) *nationalism,* during which group cohesion is developed; (3) *capitalism,* in which an ethnic base for business and jobs is created; (4) *pluralism,* during which an ethnic political power base is established; and (5) a *power* stage, in which a balance of power is achived between the former superior-subordinate groups.

Whether or not desegregation is accepted in a community or results in the kind of violent confrontation of forces that occurred in Boston in 1974 appears to depend on a number of conditions, some of which are beyond the immediate control of the schools. Robinson's† description of the Boston situation (as well as reactions observed in other communities) leads to inferences that a united front of local, state, and federal authorities, a plan that desegregates across social class as well as ethnic lines, a considerable period of advance planning that includes preparation of both the school staff and the community, and a concerted effort to solve basic problems of social and economic inequality all facilitate relatively smooth transition from segregation to desegregation.

Once desegregation occurs, how can the chances for academic success of lower-class

---

*Gallup, G. H.: Fifth annual pool of public attitudes toward education, Phi Delta Kappan **54:** 38-51, Sept. 1973.

†Postman, N., and Weingarten, C. *How to recognize a good school,* Bloomington, Ind., 1973, Phi Delta Kappa Educational Foundation, p. 37.

‡Schoenholtz, J. B.: Small schools: panacea or malignancy? Phi Delta Kappan **53:**577-578, 1972.

§Loving, A. D., Sr.: A case for multi-ethnic schools, Phi Delta Kappan **53:**279-280, Jan. 1972.

---

*Sizemore, B. A.: Is there a case for separate schools? Phi Delta Kappan **53:**181-284, Jan. 1972.

†Robinson, D. W.: School storm centers: Boston, Phi Delta Kappan **55:**262-266, Dec. 1974.

black children be improved? Johnson and Simons* offer three suggestions:

1. *Teachers need to understand (lower-class) black culture.* For example, such children are not regarded as the equals or almost equals of adults as is the case in middle-class white culture. The nonverbal communication patterns of black children are different; for example, handslapping or black handshakes.

2. *Teachers must understand (lower-class) black dialect and accept it as a legitimate system.* It operates according to a consistent set of rules. For example, if a word ends in two consonants, the second of which is c, d, k, p or t, then the last one is reduced or omitted (told = *tol*).

3. *Curriculum and teaching strategy must then be adopted to culture and dialect.* For example, teachers might allow dialect reading of standard English or might use materials prepared in dialect. In any event, it must be remembered that standard English is a second language to many lower-class pupils, black or white, and that readings based on middle-class white culture represent a foreign culture.

Compulsory school attendance. Legal requirements that all youngsters attend school up to a given age were motivated by a number of considerations, among them the abhorrent conditions under which children labored in factories prior to the twentieth century. Gradual upward extension of the legal age of leaving school was at least associated with and may have caused a considerable amount of the misbehavior that has plagued school professionals in recent years. Johnson† opposes compulsory education past junior high school for the following reasons. First, there is a greater need at this time for service workers than for workers in occupations that require extended formal schooling. Second, it is so difficult to enforce attendance laws past age 14 that it is doubtful whether attempts to do so are worthwhile. Third, expected social benefits from compulsory education have not been achieved. Brown* expresses the opinion that recent applications of the First and Fourteenth Amendments to the U.S. Constitution have made compulsory schooling unconstitutional.

Johnson, Brown and others have proposed and described a number of alternatives to compulsory school attendance. California, for example, encourages "continuation high schools" that serve dropouts and those who cannot or will not adjust to regular high school programs. These schools provide ungraded, individualized instruction, flexible schedules, no-fail grading, and curricula that emphasize remedial reading and vocational instruction. Graduates express a high degree of satisfaction and report high levels of employment.†

Whether young people are provided jobs through work-study programs or drop out of schools and find jobs on their own, they need protection against exploitation. The dangers that they may be underpaid, overworked, used to compete with union labor, or even physically or sexually abused by unscrupulous employers are real, especially in respect to those whom we label mentally retarded. Safeguards must be provided through protective legislation, including on-site inspection and provision of enforcement procedures and staff.

SOME TRADITIONAL AIDS TO SCHOOL CLIMATE

Humane climates exist in many traditional schools as a result of a number of common sense, noncontroversial practices, and the presence of humane, mentally

---

*Johnson, K. R., and Simons, H. D.: Black children and reading: what teachers need to know, Phi Delta Kappan **53**:288-290, Jan. 1972.
†Johnson, H. M.: Are compulsory attendance laws outdated?, Phi Delta Kappan **55**:226-232, Dec. 1973.

---

*Brown, B. F.: Forced schooling, Phi Delta Kappan **54**:324, Jan. 1973.
†Weber, E. J.: The dropouts who go to school, Phi Delta Kappan **53**:571-573, May 1972.

healthy teachers, administrators, children, and youths. This section is devoted to the identification and description of some of these practices and personality factors.

Practices. *The length of the school day* increases with the maturity of the students. Most school systems limit kindergartens to half-day sessions. A shortened full-day session is common in grades 1-3. A longer day is scheduled for upper elementary and secondary students. This practice recognizes the increased capacity for work and self-discipline that is acquired with average, healthy maturation, as well as the fact that a tired or bored child is likely to be a disruptive one. Practical problems presented by such considerations as bus scheduling and the importance of providing safe passage between school and home make the establishment of precise time recommendations impossible.

In this country, *homework* is rarely assigned through grade 3. The traditional self-contained classroom enables the teacher to control the amount of homework assigned throughout the upper elementary school. In some secondary schools, each weeknight is reserved for homework for specific subjects by faculty agreement or administrative edict. One night may be homework-free. Such practices make time available for needed rest, family life, and varied nonschool or school extracurricular activities.

One important consideration in the assignment of homework is a knowledge of the home environments from which students come. Neither the physical conditions prevalent in slum housing nor the social conditions in strife-ridden families, however affluent, are conducive to study. Some parents simply do not recognize and need to be reminded by the school of the importance of a comfortable, well-lighted, and private place to study, the provision of reference materials either through family ownership or public library use, and time-budgeting.

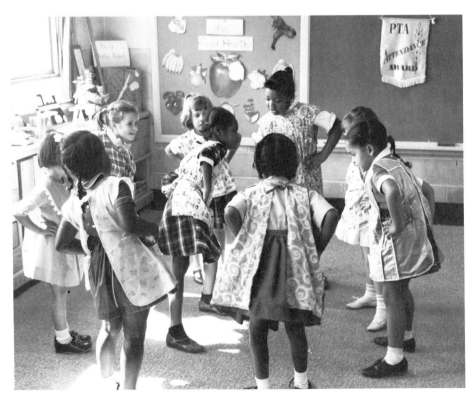

Fig. 11-1. Activity provides a change of pace.

Thoughtful teachers and schools allow ample time for makeup work and may reduce homework to the basic essentials for students who have been absent and are convalescing from an illness.

Variation in kinds of activities is recognized as important to the health and well-being of all of us, both during and after school. In humane traditional schools, teachers in elementary self-contained classrooms are free to observe the restlessness that indicates that pupils are ready for a change of activity or pace, and provide it. If playground facilities are adequate, their use may be based on this need rather than on scheduled hours. In traditional secondary schools, variation is made more difficult by class period scheduling, but it is not always impossible. It is preferable to avoid scheduling physical education just before or after lunch, and in an uncrowded building this may be possible. A minute or two during which everyone stands up and stretches can be called by the teacher. Small group discussions or projects also may provide a change of pace. A more recent development that also provides variation is modular scheduling, in which each class meets for either a long or short period as needed, rather than for a set period all week long. This plan is facilitated by the provision of library and other work-study areas that are open to any student at any time. Opportunity for social contacts and between-class toilet use can be provided to both students and teachers by extending the period between classes, but extended between-class time leads to trouble in troubled schools.

Attendance has been overemphasized in the past, largely because some states have based remuneration to local districts on average daily attendance figures rather than on enrollment or attendance data adjusted for illness. Most school districts provide a specified number of paid "sick days" for teachers. Physical illness has generally become an acceptable excuse for absence, but considerable absenteeism among both students and teachers is related to undesirable school climate factors and to social and emotional problems unrelated to school. Disturbed teachers and students may give or receive very little if they do attend school. Humane administrators and school nurses can do much to detect and alleviate such problems by asking such questions as, "Is something bothering you? Would you care to tell me about it? Is there something I can do to help?" Such an approach is much more likely to be productive than one that seeks to identify malingerers through medical observation of the supposedly sick.

In addition to the school practices cited above, there are things teachers and students can do—specific techniques—that contribute to a warm, friendly classroom climate. A classroom or a whole school, even those in old, debilitated buildings, can be made places of life and color by decorating them with products of students' work and other attractive things that teachers and students bring to school for the purpose. Pets and plants not only contribute to the climate by their presence, but help in the development of responsibility for their care. Teachers can help children feel that they are objects of interest and friendliness by greeting the children by name, making personal and positive comments about their achievements, and by exhibiting interest in their interests (early elementary grade "show and tell" sessions are one way to do this). Schools can also provide opportunity for each person to contribute successfully according to his or her abilities.

Personality factors. The quality of social interactions that occur within a school is determined in part by the mental health of its members and also affects their mental health. We have come to recognize and accept a wide range of personality differences as normal and healthy. We have also come to recognize that two perfectly normal, healthy individuals may or may not get along with each other and that the best solution in such a situation may be to separate them. In school practice, the implication is that it ought to be easy and nonthreatening to either party to transfer teachers from one school to another and students

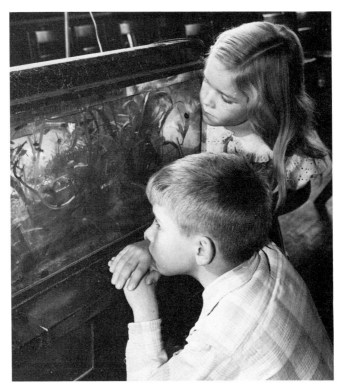

Fig. 11-2. Pets contribute to school climate.

from one class to another simply because personality differences have proven disruptive.

We have no objective definitions that validly differentiate between the mentally ill and the mentally healthy. Freud defined mental health as the ability to love and work, and this, like other definitions, is subjective. Love is a feeling, the observable manifestation of which can be hidden or faked. Work is effort expended, which may or may not result in an observable product. Mental health has also been defined as adjustment to society. However, some sick people seem to be content with and well adjusted to their environments, while others, who cause all manner of disruption, turn out to be individuals in rebellion against an unjust world.

Nevertheless, healthy individuals feel reasonably comfortable about themselves most of the time, are able to relate comfortably to most other people most of the time, and are able to cope with most of the stresses imposed by the environment in which they live. Teachers and pupils alike are constantly learning their own capabilities and limitations. They grow in understanding of their emotions and in their ability to control or express emotions in socially accepted ways. Given an adequately high ratio of successes to failures, they learn to accept both success and failure with reasonable equanimity and not to take themselves or their work too seriously.

In short, learning to be mentally healthy implies a lifetime devoted to the achievement of a number of objectives, such as: (1) developing objectivity toward one's problems, (2) improving skills in dealing with other people, (3) developing the ability to face responsibilities, (4) setting appropriate goals for one's self and others, (5) continuously broadening one's interests, (6) improving ability to schedule one's work and work one's schedule, (7) seeking constructive outlets for anger and frustration, and (8) accepting limitations that cannot be changed.

Both parents and teachers play important roles in developing the mental health of children and young people. Coopersmith's* 6-year study of 1,748 normal middle-class boys and their families, beginning at preadolescence and continuing to young manhood, reported three characteristics of parental relationship that were especially important in helping the sons to acquire the kind of self-esteem vital to the development of ambition, idealism, and a constructive program of living and successful achievement. These were (1) love (including concern, interest, and respect), (2) limited permissiveness, and (3) democracy (involving respectful if vigorous examination of opinions). (Do you think that these findings would be equally applicable to girls? Do they evoke suggestions for teacher-pupil relations as well as for parent-child relationships?)

In the promotion of an atmosphere conducive to mental health in the classroom, educators in the state of Kansas have indicated desirable teacher-pupil relationships in terms of the following advice to the teacher:

1. *Have genuine interest in children.* Love children and show a real and intelligent affection for each of them. Understand the characteristics of children at various levels of development. Seek to know their individual interests, potentialities, and problems.
2. *Respect personality.* Teach the child, not the subject matter. Realize that each child is a different person. Have respect for the dignity of the individual and show respect for the child at all times in his thinking, actions, etc. A spirit of toleration should pervade the schoolroom. Intolerance on the part of either teacher or pupils often causes damaging stress and strains.
3. *Strive to give each child a feeling of security, of belonging, and of being of value to his group.* The child must have a feeling of security and affection. The child's need for

recognition and approval must be recognized. He must feel that he is wanted in the group. The teacher should make it possible for every child to have the thrill and exhilaration of accomplishment. Teacher-pupil planning is essential. Help given when needed is important. The teacher should help the child to understand his limitations and potentialities and to take them into account in laying his plans. A distinction should be made between constructive planning and worry. The former is stimulating; the later nerve wracking and destructive. The teacher should give the child opportunities to assume partial responsibility for his actions, as much as he can assume successfully. The teacher should not break the spirit of the child by demanding of him things he cannot do.

4. *Have a sense of humor so that children will be happy and live in an atmosphere of happiness.* Laugh with the children, not at them. The teacher should not indulge in sarcasm and sharp-tongued procedure. He should strive to create an environment of happy industry.
5. *Be impartial in relations with all pupils.* An impersonal and objective attitude, as well as a constructive attitude toward offenses, should be shown. The teacher should give the children opportunity to profit from mistakes. The teacher should give social approval when aproval is merited.*

The factors listed above are qualities largely inherent in the personalities of effective parents and teachers. They cannot be put on or taken off like articles of clothing.

DISTURBED AND DISTURBING STUDENTS

Students who are upset emotionally and show it, and those who may not be disturbed but whose overt behavior patterns are disturbing to others, are disruptive of school climate and teaching-learning processes. They must be identified and dealt with for that reason. Some disturbed youngsters are not at all disturbing to others; their behavior is quiet, complacent, and compliant, but they need to be identified and helped for their own sake. Not all disturbing individuals are disturbed. Strang points out that:

most psychiatrists agree that there comes a time when the child must learn that certain behavior is

---

*Coopersmith, S.: *The antecedents of self-esteem,* San Francisco, 1968, W. H. Freeman and Co. Publishers.

*From *Health education in elementary and secondary schools,* issued jointly by the State Department of Public Instruction and the State Board of Health of Kansas, undated.

not socially acceptable and that he cannot always have what we wants when he wants. Some frustration is an inevitable part of life. Normal children need to learn to tolerate and handle a reasonable amount of inescapable frustration. In a culture demanding inhibitions, an individual who acts solely on his impulses often hurts himself and other people. Mild frustrations, obstacles on the path to a goal, call forth learning . . . are emotionally strengthening. However, serious frustrations which confront any individual with repeated failure are disintegrating.*

Regulating student behavior. Misbehavior by normal, healthy individuals is not at all uncommon, but it can be just as devastating to school climate as misbehavior that has its roots in emotional disturbance. Normal student misbehavior frequently grows out of uncertainty as to the kinds of behavior that school staff will tolerate.

Games students play. In any school, students develop ritualized games designed to test out their teachers. Those who teach students of the same subculture in which they grew up already know some or all of the games played in their school. One middle-class white game is to place an up-ended thumb tack or piece of wet gum on the teacher's chair. Teachers win if they observe the offending object before they sit down and conspicuously and disdainfully dispose of it without saying a word.

In a lower-class black game called "woofing," described by Herbert Foster, a student may walk up to a teacher and say, "I'm gonna punch you!" The winning response by the teacher is a disdainful "You're gonna punch me?" accompanied by a big laugh. Foster states that teachers have the option of refusing to play as well as playing to win, but refusal requires the ability to recognize the game as such. (This can be acquired either from painful experience or through instruction by an experienced fellow teacher.)

Foster observes that most young teachers in (lower social class) inner city schools

pass through four stages of development. In the first stage they attempt to establish friendship with students, which does not work, because what these youngsters really want is someone to discipline and teach them. The second stage is one of chaos, which results from the teacher's humiliation and lack of knowledge of what to do. The third stage is achievement of discipline, which includes self-discipline as well as the discipline of students. The final stage (which few reach) is humanism, in which the teacher is able to relax and individualize the classroom without losing control.*

Discipline, punishment, and physical intervention. There is a difference between discipline and punishment. Discipline is controlled behavior that results from training. Early in development such training is imposed by teachers and parents. Later, peers assume part of the role of training. As disciplinary training is internalized, the individual achieves self-discipline, or self-control. Punishment is simply a retaliatory reaction to misbehavior that is intended to serve as a disciplinary training function but is in fact less effective in training than are rewards for good behavior. We have come to believe that if punishment is to be effective at all, it must be administered shortly after misbehavior occurs and that it need not be excessively harsh. It must also be viewed by the recipient as justified and distasteful. (To a masochist, a spanking is pleasurable.)

To prevent a misbehaving person from injuring other people or damaging school property, physical restraint is sometimes essential. Foster proposes the use of trained interventionists for this purpose in troubled schools as an alternative to corporal punishment. The interventionist acts early in a crisis and may use physical means of restraint—not blows or kicks, but the use of noninjurious holds and pressure points.†

---

*Strang, R. Many-sided aspects of mental health, *Mental health in modern education,* fifty-fourth yearbook of the National Society for the Study of Education, part I, Chicago, 1955, University of Chicago Press, p. 36.

*Cole, R. W., Jr.: Ribbin', jivin', and playin' the dozens (an interview with Herbert Foster), Phi Delta Kappan **56:**171-175, Nov. 1974.
†Cole, R. W., Jr.: Ribbin', jivin', and playin' the dozens.

Behavior codes. Student behavior codes written by administrators and teachers usually consist of a series of statements that prescribe certain punishments and forbid a long list of misbehaviors. They are frequently so lengthy and complex that students are unable to understand or remember all the things that they are not supposed to do. Because such codes fail to include statements that define the rights of students and fail to provide due process, some of them have been successfully challenged in the courts.

An alternative proposed by Ladd* is the development of behavior codes in which: (1) many rights and powers are guaranteed to students, (2) some powers are reserved to school officials, and (3) school-imposed restrictions decrease and peer-imposed restrictions increase with grade level. Ladd notes that new state statutes may have to be enacted to permit students to regulate their own conduct in significant ways.

Recognizing the importance of local codes developed through the involvement of students and parents as well as school officials, a Phi Delta Kappa commission has developed an illustrative sample code consistent with Ladd's specifications. Some salient provisions of this code†:

1. Open records to parents or guardians and to students.
2. Require parent-student consent for any item in a student's record to be divulged to anyone other than a certified local school professional.
3. Ban unannounced mass searches of students' persons or lockers.
4. Provide limited freedom of student press, speech, and right of assembly.
5. Require due process (notice, hearings by an important officer) in cases of suspension, expulsion, or involuntary transfer.

6. Provide for the continued education of excluded students.
7. Ban corporal punishment.

Discipline in the classroom. Teachers develop and revise their techniques for maintaining control in the classroom as they learn from experience. Techniques that are useful for one teacher and one class are not necessarily useful for all. Many of the policies and procedures recommended thus far in this chapter may be useful.

Other tips to teachers on maintaining classroom control that may be helpful include*:

1. Start class promptly—before trouble starts.
2. Set behavioral standards and limits early in the term; it is easy to let up but not to tighten up later. Let students know what the standards and limits are.
3. Involve students in the development, evaluation, and revision of standards.
4. Be consistent, fair, and firm in enforcing standards.
5. Do not make too many rules.
6. Reward good behavior.
7. If you speak in a low, well-modulated voice, students are likely to listen. If you yell at them, they are likely to yell back at you.
8. Make reprimands privately, give praise openly.
9. Be well prepared for class; busy students are not likely to misbehave.
10. Asking direct questions of a misbehaving student is more likely to be productive than giving direct orders.

Helping disturbed students: identification. Early detection of emotional disorders is of paramount importance. Because of their close day-by-day contacts and emotional attachment to their child, parents may fail to recognize deviations from behavior that

---

*Ladd, E. T.: Regulating student behavior without ending up in court, Phi Delta Kappan **56:**236-242, Dec. 1974.

†Adapted from Phi Delta Kappa Commission on Administrative Behavior: A sample student code, Phi Delta Kappan **56:**236-242, Dec. 1974.

*Adapted from Stoops, E., and King-Stoops, J.: *Discipline or disaster?* Bloomington, Indiana, 1972, Phi Delta Kappa Educational Foundation, pp. 25-29. (This 38-page booklet contains many other helpful hints for teachers.)

is normal and healthy for the particular child and for the age and sex group.

Children who exhibit extreme aggressiveness, antisocial behavior, shyness, and withdrawal tendencies, or discrepancy in either direction between ability and achievement, are likely to be children in trouble. Sudden changes in the child's usual behavior, attitudes, or scholarship are other signs of disturbance.

Teachers need to understand the significance of the signs of undesirable behavior and the degree of seriousness of a problem. The attitudes and behavior that a child exhibits are ways of adjusting to his or her situation. The standards of behavior held by other adults in the youngster's environment may vary decidedly from the standards of behavior held by the teacher. Mores of families and communities vary greatly. Therefore, teacher judgments of the child must be related to cultural and family background and to total personality.

A disturbed youngster is seeking to satisfy fundamental emotional needs in ways that bring satisfaction. Teachers must, therefore, search for these needs that are not being met. However, they need to be aware that child behavior is most complex and that in more serious situations psychiatric consultation and guidance may be necessary in coming to an understanding of the child's problem. On the physical side, what seems to be the symptoms of a beginning cold may be the initial stages of measles or whooping cough. Similarly, identical forms of overt behavior may arise from widely different underlying causes. For example, hostility in a child may be due to feeling unwanted, unloved, or inadequate.

Conversely, a single, unmet emotional need may be expressed by a variety of forms of behavior. Different children may react to a single cause, such as lack of love and affection, in various ways, such as by withdrawal, by aggressiveness, by thumb sucking, or by stealing. One adolescent who fails in his or her classwork may be nonchalant and quit trying, whereas another may be deeply hurt and grow tense and worried.

A third may make the effort to discover and remedy the cause. When fundamental needs are not met, specific symptoms may disappear, only to reappear in other forms. A child may stop stealing, only to run away from home. Since a behavior pattern is not usually caused by a single factor but by many interrelated factors that have occurred in the life experience of the child, it may be helpful for the teacher or school mental health specialist to ask such questions as (1) why does this child behave in this manner, (2) what satisfaction does misbehavior tend to provide, (3) in what ways is life unsatisfactory, (4) what circumstances are causing this reaction, and (5) what can be done to help the youngster cope with his or her problem in more productive ways?

There are many opportunities within the school day and in contacts with parents for a busy teacher to study a troubled student's behavior. Four approaches that have proven helpful in understanding youngsters are: observation; informal contacts, conferences, and interviews; sociometry; and testing techniques.

Observation. As teachers learn to listen more and talk less, and to watch student behavior at work and at play, they come to understand how situations look to children and youth and what their behavior means. It is helpful for teachers to record what they see and hear at the time a significant event occurs as an aid in determining the significance of observations and in discovering patterns of relationship and change that are revealed. Such anecdotal records may serve as a conference tool both with the child and with the parents, as well as with mental health professionals who may become involved in a case. They should probably not become a part of the student's permanent record, especially since records are now open to parent-student perusal.

Informal contacts, conferences, and interviews. An informal talk with a child helps a teacher to see how things look to him or her. It is important to carry on conversations with children whenever possible—before school, at recess, at lunch time, after school. Informal conversations with parents over the telephone or upon incidental meetings in both the community and at school may give important clues to a child's behavior. Parents may be encouraged to come to school for conferences. Some school systems now have periodic conferences with parents instead of sending out report cards in the earlier grades. At such times teachers may ask specific questions that will assist in understanding the child.

Sociometry. This is a device for the study of social acceptance and relationships between children within the classroom. Children are asked to nominate other children for associates in various situations, such as seating arrangements, committees, attendance at a movie, or for a party. Only positive items should be used. The results will indicate children at the extremes of acceptance and nonacceptance, and the subgroups within the total group. Nonacceptance does not always indicate a problem; a new member of the class may simply not yet have had an opportunity to achieve a place within the group. It is common practice to place the details on a sociogram in order to view the relationships within a class in graphic form. Informal contacts and interviews can be used to follow up the sociogram and to help a teacher understand its significance. Steps can then be taken to improve the social structure of a group.

Teachers need adequate preparation in using and following up information acquired in this way. A number of manuals are now available that are of assistance to teachers.

Testing techniques. In projective tests there are no right or wrong answers. They help to give an insight into child behavior by the responses that are given to standard materials. The Rorschach test, the thematic apperception test (which is based on responses to pictures), and forms of the sentence-completion test are widely used as diagnostic tests. Olson and Wattenberg state:

In general, the most productive means of *detecting* disturbance are observation and informal contacts, conferences and interviews. *Diagnostic* testing and the interpretation of test results are best left to trained psychometrists and other formally qualified persons.*

Helping disturbed students: intervention. The resources available to provide help vary with the school and the community. Sources of help that are present in many schools or communities include understanding teachers, nurses, physicians, and clergymen. In other schools and communities one or more mental health professionals may be available. In some localities mental health professionals are employed by the schools. In others, there may be an adequately staffed and funded community health center or child guidance clinic. Appropriate referral and intervention patterns vary, therefore, with location. One technique, that of crisis intervention, can be practiced with minimal resources.

Crisis intervention. The basic concepts of crisis intervention and theory are so simple that some perceptive teachers, nurses, and others practice it without ever having been introduced to them. A fifth-grade teacher in a Philadelphia inner city school observed that one of the girls in his class appeared in tears for the afternoon session. He asked what her problem was and whether she wanted to see the school nurse, but she refused either to tell him or to accept the referral. He had no time to do more until the dismissal bell rang. At that point he informed her that he would not let her go home until she told him why she was upset. She finally told him that she had been raped on her way to school. He then discussed with her the possibility that it might be helpful to call her mother or the police, but she was too embarrassed and disturbed to take either course of action by herself. She

*Olson, W. C., and Wattenberg, W. W.: The role of the school in mental health, Mental Health in Modern Education, fifty-fourth yearbook of the National Society for the Study of Education, part II, Chicago, 1955, University of Chicago Press, p. 112.

finally consented to let the teacher call her mother to school if the teacher would stay to meet her. In the ensuing conference it was agreed to call the police, who took the girl to the hospital for treatment. Out of this experience the girl learned that she need not bear future troubles alone, that her mother and her teacher were two understanding and caring adults to whom she could turn for help. The incident also resulted in a productive class discussion, in which the pupil's anonymity was maintained, of ways in which class members could avoid attacks on the streets and ways of dealing with attacks should they occur.

Crisis intervention may be defined as the immediate actions taken by a caring person or persons when acute, short-term emotional disturbances upset an individual, family, or group, in order to alleviate the impact of the stress that produced the crisis by mobilizing appropriate action by and for those affected.

Some basic concepts of crisis theory and intervention include the following*:

1. Crisis results from the impact of an identifiable event that is new to the disturbed person, death in the family or pregnancy, for example.
2. The person in crisis is unable to cope with the disturbance successfully without help. He or she is more than worried about the problem, but less than depressed.
3. The intervener needs to be aware that:
   a. the person in crisis needs to be allowed to express his or her feelings.
   b. the intervener must often act, either with or for the person in crisis; listening is not usually enough.
   c. appropriate training, if not always essential, increases the likelihood of success.
   d. the actions taken in intervention may be complex and time-consuming and may lead not only to a solution of the presenting crisis but to the precipitation of new crises. Therefore, access to other and more highly prepared school or community personnel for referral or consultation is often an essential adjunct.
4. Ability to cope with new crises is enhanced by the resolution of previous and similar crises.
5. Following crisis intervention, the person in crisis emerges as a new person, with different perspectives or even a new life style.

Twenty-four-hour a day telephone crisis intervention services or hotlines are available in many communities, some of them designed specifically for teenagers. One such service was established by the Montgomery County, Maryland Mental Health Association.* Both paid and volunteer staff members were utilized, all of whom received preservice and continuous in-service training. Qualities sought in staff members included oral communication skills, openness and empathy, and ability to relate to the adolescent culture. Professionals, including social workers, lawyers, and physicians, were recruited to provide constantly available consultant and back-up service to the staff. Most calls received involved boy-girl relationships; others were precipitated by family conflicts, the need "just to talk," drugs, and pregnancy. Call tracing was used in such extreme emergencies as those posed by a threat of suicide.

Some schools have established standby or crisis rooms to which disturbed and disturbing children come on their own or are sent by teachers. Like the Philadelphia teacher in the case described earlier, many teachers are much too busy to provide immediate help in many instances. Blom† has described one such room that was staffed on a rotating basis by a number of teachers, the librarian, a social worker, and a nurse. Techniques developed and used depending on the case included quiet time, ventilation, limit-setting, a showing of open disapproval of a child's misbehavior, and offers of support and encouragement. The most common reasons for teacher referrals were disobedience and fighting, but many were referred because of crying or other signs of crisis. Some referrals culminated in referrals to community agencies. In some other schools, such rooms are staffed by profes-

*Adapted from Miller, C. V.: Crisis intervention and health counseling: an overview, School Health Review 1:3, 15-17, Sept. 1970.

*Montgomery County Mental Health Association: A county mental health association's hotline, School Health Review 1:3, 27-30, Sept. 1970.
†Blom, D.: A nurse's experience with a standby program in an elementary school, J. Sch. Health 41:249-253, May 1971.

sionals selected and trained specifically as interventionists.

Community mental health centers and other services. In addition to the acute problems to which crisis intervention techniques and services are addressed, a number of students present disturbed or disturbing behavior of a more chronic nature for which special education services may be provided. Some of these youngsters are classified as mentally retarded and others as emotionally disturbed. Although many in either category can be and are served by regular teachers in regular classrooms, others are better placed in special classrooms with qualified special educators. The desirable population norm for such a class is eight to ten pupils. At the secondary level, a fairly large proportion of trainable mentally retarded students can be productively involved in work-study programs. The burden on such programs was significantly increased by 1972 federal court rulings that all children are entitled to an education (Pennsylvania Association for Retarded Children versus Commonwealth of Pennsylvania, and Mills versus Board of Education).

Community mental health centers were established in many communities throughout the United States as a result of federal legislation enacted in 1963. The federal intent was that the centers would provide comprehensive mental health services, including consultation and education services to schools and other agencies aimed at mental health promotion, a 24-hour a day crisis service, and a complete range of inpatient, outpatient, and modified residential treatment and rehabilitation services. This intent has been met in some communities, and in some locales community and school services are well coordinated. In other communities either centers were never organized, or they have been unable to provide a full range of services as a result of insufficient funds and a continuing shortage of qualified professionals.

Private psychiatrists and consulting psychologists may be present in the community, but they are often too busy to accept referrals immediately. Their fees are usually beyond most families' ability to pay.

DISTURBED AND DISTURBING SCHOOL STAFF MEMBERS

School staff members sometimes exhibit disturbed and disturbing behavior. Their continued presence in the school during such periods exerts a negative influence on school climate. In one school the pupils who were taught by a disturbed teacher were observed not only to exhibit more disturbed behavior than those in other classes in the school but also to score significantly lower on standard achievement tests at the end of the semester than they did at the beginning.

Most administrators attempt to screen out disturbed applicants for staff positions by use of preemployment medical examinations (a relatively nonproductive method) and by telephone interviews with one or more individuals who know the applicant personally. School health service professionals and administrators can identify disturbed and disturbing staff members by observation, using the same general criteria as those described earlier for the observation of children, and also by noting unusual numbers of disturbed children and complaining parents who may be associated with a given staff member. Some will identify their own problems and independently seek help.

A school climate and personnel policies and practices that help make a school a good place in which to work can be expected to reduce the incidence of such cases. Humane and effective administrators, school mental health professionals, and colleagues can provide crisis intervention service for those in acute crisis. Health professionals can refer those in need of diagnostic and treatment services to appropriate sources in the community.

For the protection of children and young people it is sometimes essential that a disturbing staff member be removed from contact with them, temporarily or permanently. With the cooperation and consent of the staff member and the union, it is possible to arrange a transfer to a suitable position. When such consent and cooperation are lacking, the case may end in litigation, but this possibility does not justify failure to push the transfer through. Outright dismissal of a mentally ill person should be a solution of last resort.

QUESTIONS FOR STUDY AND DISCUSSION

1. What is meant by the concept *school climate,* or social and emotional environment?
2. Why is school climate important? What benefits can be expected from a good school climate?
3. What three broad categories of factors are identified by Fox and his associates as affecting school climate?
4. List and classify under these three broad categories each of the things mentioned in this chapter that school members (administrators, staff, students) can do to improve school climate.
5. Consider a school you have recently attended or worked in. Which of the specific climate-improving factors are present, and which are absent in that school? Would you classify that school as excellent, satisfactory, or poor in terms of climate?
6. Discuss or debate the pros and cons of one or more of the following climate-related issues:
   a. Group norms versus individual gains as a basis for grading
   b. Open versus traditional classrooms
   c. Individualized versus group instruction
   d. Flexible versus common curricula
   e. Roles of home and church versus role of school in affective and sex education
   f. Large traditional versus school within a school versus small schools
   g. Desegregation versus integration
   h. Compulsory versus optional attendance past junior high
7. What constitutes desirable practice with respect to:
   a. length of school day
   b. homework
   c. variation in kinds of activity
   d. attendance policies
8. What constitutes a healthy personality, and how is such a personality developed?
9. What personal characteristics of teachers improve classroom climate?
10. What specific actions by teachers can improve school climate?
11. Develop a series of brief statements useful in distinguishing between and dealing with student behavior that has its roots in emotional disturbance and in lack of knowledge or acceptance of school rules.
12. Differentiate between and evaluate the rela-

tive merits of discipline, punishment, and physical intervention.
13. What features distinguish useful and legal student behavior codes from those that create difficulties in terms of legality and effectiveness?
14. What are some techniques that have been proven useful and useless in maintaining classroom discipline?
15. What devices and techniques have proven useful in identifying students in emotional crises?
16. What is meant by crisis intervention? What guiding principles of theory and practice underlie this concept?
17. What is the nature and purpose of hotlines and crisis or standby rooms?
18. What services are offered by community mental health centers? Why have such centers failed to develop as intended in many localities?
19. Imagine yourself in the position of a teacher or other school staff member who is disturbed, disturbing, and aware of it. What would you do about it if you believed (a) that those in your school would treat you humanely or (b) that you would not be treated humanely?

REFERENCES
Bash, J. H.: *Effective teaching in the desegregated school,* Bloomington, Ind., 1973, Phi Delta Kappa Educational Foundation.

Disque, J.: *In between: the adolescents' struggle for independence,* Bloomington, Ind., 1973, Phi Delta Kappa Educational Foundation.

Eisner V., and Callan, L. B.: *Dimensions of school health,* Springfield, Ill., 1974, Charles C Thomas, Publisher.

Fox, R., and others: *School climate improvement: a challenge to the school administrator,* Bloomington, Ind., 1973, Phi Delta Kappa and CFK Ltd.

Henry, N. B., editor: *Mental health in modern education,* fifty-fourth yearbook of the National Society for the Study of Education, Chicago, 1955, University of Chicago Press.

Mooney, E.: *The school's responsibility for sex education,* Bloomington, Ind., 1974, Phi Delta Kappa Educational Foundation.

National Committee on School Health Policies of the National Education Association and the American Medical Association: *Suggested school health policies,* Chicago, 1966, AMA and NEA.

Perrone, V.: *Open education: promise and problems,* Bloomington, Ind., 1972, Phi Delta Kappa Educational Foundation.

Postman, N., and Weingartner, C.: *How to recognize a good school,* Bloomington, Ind., 1973, Phi Delta Kappa Educational Foundation.

Sartwell, P. E., editor: *Maxcy-Rosenau preventive medicine and public health,* ed. 10, New York, 1973, Appleton-Century-Crofts.

Stoops, E., and King-Stoops, J.: *Discipline or disaster?* Bloomington, Ind., 1972, Phi Delta Kappa Educational Foundation.

Subcommittee on Mental Health and School Health Services of the Joint Committee on Health Problems in Education of the National Education Association and the American Medical Association: *Mental health and school health services,* Washington, D. C., The Committee (undated).

Wilner, D. M., Walkley, R. P., and Goerke, L. S.: *Introduction to public health,* ed. 6, New York, 1973, Macmillan, Inc.

Wilson, C. C., and Wilson, E. A.: *Healthful school environment,* Washington, D.C., 1969, National Education Association and American Medical Association.

CHAPTER 12 ❧ A safe and healthful physical environment: school plant planning and maintenance

René Dubos* concludes that humans are so adaptable to diverse environmental conditions that we may come to tolerate insults that will destroy the quality of life. A school physical environment that is carefully planned and well maintained not only enhances the quality of life for students and staff but also helps to promote and maintain physical health. Such an environment makes it possible to teach and learn more effectively and in greater comfort than would otherwise be possible. It decreases the likelihood of infection and injury. It provides facilities for the conduct of school health service programs, for the nutrition of school members, and for physical activity. It serves as a laboratory for teaching and learning concepts of environmental health. Many of us exist in physically poor schools that could be vastly improved by exercise of ingenuity at little if any extra cost in money or environmental deterioration.

WHO IS RESPONSIBLE?

State governments and local districts share legal and moral responsibility for providing a school environment that meets minimal health and safety standards. There is usually some legal provision for review of new building plans by agencies other than the local school districts to ensure that minimum standards are met. Older buildings may or may not be inspected, and if they are, violations may or may not be corrected.

Many larger school districts employ more or less well-qualified specialists in school plant planning and maintenance. In smaller districts generalist school administrators are expected to perform these functions although they are rarely qualified to do so, and specialists in planning and maintenance rarely if ever possess the skills and knowledge of a specialist in environmental health. Typically then, environmental health and safety are concerns of everyone in the school—as they should be—but delegated as direct *responsibilities* to no one individual who is competent to assume them.

Such specialists, who usually carry the title of sanitarian or sanitary engineer, are employed by health departments and some large industries. One solution is to borrow their services. These specialists, however, usually already have as much or more work than they can reasonably be expected to handle. Callan and Rowe* have urged the employment of specialist school sanitarians on the grounds that special technical, human relations, and administrative skills are necessary for work in schools.

Modern sanitarians are specifically trained in the planning, developing, and execution of environmental programs, as well as in their traditional legal inspection and enforcement roles. School sanitarians must be able to work closely with school administrators, plant planners, maintenance specialists, and cafeteria and other school staff members. They must also be able to work with public health departments, industries,

---

*Dubos, R.: The dangers of tolerance, J. Sch. Health **44**:182-185, April 1974.

*Callan, L. B., and Rowe, D. E.: The role of the school sanitarian, J. Sch. Health **42**:360-362, June 1972.

and other nonschool organizations. Other role functions include the conduct of inspections and tests and that of teaching school staff members to function in ways that help to create and preserve a safe and healthy environment. School sanitarians are in a position to serve as advocates for optimal rather than minimal standards. Their expertise also enables them to serve as useful resource persons in environmental education.

SCHOOL PLANT PLANNING

The planning process. In far too many school districts school plant planning has been and remains a process of decision making by the board, the administrative staff, and the architect. Or worse, a standard plan and specifications totally unrelated to the available site and designed to fit an outdated curriculum are dug out of the files and submitted to contractors for bids. The result of either approach is likely to

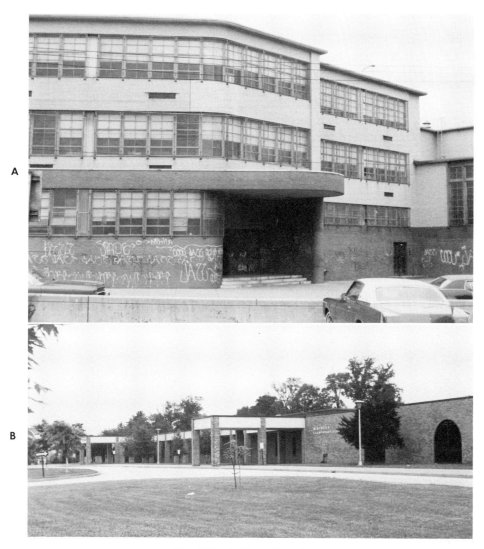

Fig. 12-1. A, Slum. **B,** Suburb.

be a school in conflict not only with its site and curriculum but with the surrounding neighborhood and its staff and students as well.

Meaningful participation in planning by teachers, students, and community representatives is likely to result in a building that is functional and that evokes a feeling of pride and ownership. Such feelings encourage future participation in building maintenance; school housekeeping is a task that requires the cooperation of all school members, not just the custodial staff.

The first step in planning the building of a new school or the rehabilitation of an old one is, therefore, the appointment of a *planning committee* that represents the teachers and students who will live and learn in it and its neighbors. In many communities schools and school sites are designed for nonschool use. Where this is the case, future community users such as the city recreation department or the public library should be included on the committee. Administrative staff members who have expert input to contribute should also be involved.

The committee's life and roles should extend from before the architect is employed until the building has been formally accepted by the local school board or other legally designated authority. The whole process will require 2 or more years to complete. The committee can assist in the selection of the architect by visiting and evaluating schools previously designed by candidates. It is essential that the architectural firm selected have regular or consulting staff specialists in such fields as acoustics, lighting, and other relevant aspects of environmental health and safety. It is almost always necessary to revise desired plans and specifications to bring costs in line with available funds. The priorities assigned to various cost-cutting proposals and possible side effects should be subjects of committee deliberation. Tours of the building by committee members during and after construction frequently result in the observation of architect or contractor errors that should be corrected before acceptance of the completed building.

A clear distinction of roles is required for orderly and efficient planning. In most states the local board of education holds the legal decision-making authority. The superintendent makes recommendations to the board and implements board decisions. The committee makes recommendations to the architect and to the superintendent and board of education. The committee's roles are to develop educational specifications, that is, descriptions of the school activities that need to be provided for, and to give advice to the architect as to styles that will or will not be pleasing to the occupants and neighbors, and to pass judgment on preliminary and final plans submitted by the architect. It is the architect's job to render floor plans and develop the specifications for materials and construction standards to be followed by the contractors.

Some considerations in planning. Intelligent planning depends on the availability of relevant information and realization of the implications of decisions made.

The school population. Declining national birth numbers indicate need for extreme caution in planning school buildings, but national figures do not necessarily reflect local trends. An annual census of all preschoolers together with estimates of in and out mobility and nonpublic school attendance permits reasonably accurate forecasts of the number of kindergarteners to be expected 5 years hence. A knowledge of the socioeconomic status and ethnicity patterns in the community is an aid to program and school use planning; in a lower-class community with a significant foreign-speaking population, more pupil personnel services will be required, and bilingual teachers may be desirable.

Available community resources. If nature trails, museums, or any other educative community resources are located in the neighborhood, they may be utilized in the school program. Such resources may be substituted for in-school resources that might otherwise be included in the educational specifications.

Will handicapped youngsters attend the school? In light of the trend toward regular

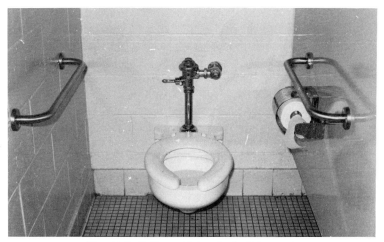

Fig. 12-2. Toilet stall for the handicapped.

school and regular classroom placement of exceptional children, the answer is probably yes. If so, physical barriers to their functioning need to be planned out of the specifications and special learning facilities planned in. For example, ramps may be substituted for steps and larger toilet stalls provided. Physical and occupational therapy centers might be provided.*

Is the school committed to traditional or open classrooms? If the commitment is to traditional classrooms, there will be fixed-walled classrooms equipped with a desk and chair and identical materials for each individual. If the classrooms are to be open, then large rooms equipped with a variety of furniture and furnishings are indicated.† Sound-absorbing carpeting is a must in open classrooms and is optional in traditional ones.

Can the school you are planning accommodate tomorrow's needs? The answer had better be yes. The circa 1970 bulge in the kindergarten-elementary population was made up of people who may be producing another such bulge around 1990, and either

or both the traditional and open classrooms may be curiosities described in history of education textbooks 10 years from now. The moral is to plan flexibility in, avoid load-bearing walls.

Site selection. Urban schools should be so located that they are accessible via public transportation and are distant from noise sources such as airports and busy freeways. Where gangs are prevalent, they should be located as nearly as possible on neutral or boundary-line turf. The probability of future development or redevelopment of the area should be considered. Adequate water supply and sewerage lines should be available.

Rural school buildings may not be accessible to a municipal water supply and sewerage system. If this is the case, a natural subsurface water supply should be on the site. The nature of the subsurface soil strata should be investigated to determine whether or not it will accommodate septic tanks and drainage fields.

The school should preferably be located on ground that is either naturally or artificially well drained and that provides space not only for physical activities but also for grass, trees, and shrubs. Filled land is to be avoided if possible because brickbats, old tires, and other junk that are buried in it tend to come to the surface in time. Sites in business districts, particularly those near honky-tonk strips, are undesirable.

---

*Molloy, L.: The handicapped child in the everyday classroom, Phi Delta Kappan **56:**337-340, Jan. 1975.

†Perley, D. T., and Martin, P. H.: An environmental perspective on educational planning, Phi Delta Kappan **56:**358-359, Jan. 1975.

A school site that is adequate in both size and all other respects is rarely obtainable in large cities. Where possible, a minimum of 10 acres is generally recommended for an elementary school, 20 acres for a junior high school, and 30 acres for a senior high school. To each such site an additional acre should be added for each 100 pupils of predicted maximum enrollment. Thus, a 200-pupil elementary school should desirably have at least a 12-acre site.

One way of acquiring sites of adequate size and quality in cities is to build schools on the corners of public parks. The school playgrounds and park recreational facilities become one. A less desirable way is to use the roof as a playground. Another possibility is to build the school underground and top it with a park-like play area.

Site development. Site development should be planned in conjunction with the building. The plan should include landscaping that is designed to reduce sunglare, provide barriers against noise, and serve as windbreaks. Play areas should be hard surfaced in part and turfed over in part. If site

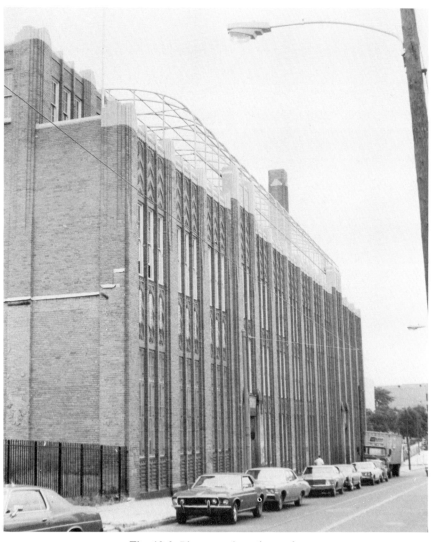

Fig. 12-3. Playground on the roof.

size permits, separate play areas and equipment should be provided for younger and older students. Equipment should be dictated by the age and interests of the users and by the objectives of the physical education programs. If a major goal is the teaching of lifetime sports, then provision for such activities as tennis should have high priority. If school bus and public transportation are provided and accessible, parking lots can and should be greatly restricted in size, especially around urban schools. Automobiles are the greatest single killer of school-aged children and young people and are the leading cause of urban air pollution; therefore, the schools should actively discourage their needless use in every conceivable way.

FACILITIES FOR HEALTH INSTRUCTION

Acceptance of health education as a valid school subject and a preplanned health curriculum are essential to planning both space and equipment for teaching and learning. A suitable location and adequate furnishings for learning are unlikely to be provided without acceptance. The curriculum, particularly its underlying philosophy and the materials and methods adopted, dictates the kind of facility and equipment needed. Recent trends in state and federal legislation appear to be supportive of both acceptance and curriculum planning.

The health education curriculum at both the elementary and secondary levels is likely to include objectives in the cognitive, affective, and action domains, and to utilize a wide variety of teaching-learning materials and methods. A desirable environment will therefore be one in which several small groups as well as a single large group can function. It will include provision for the storage and use of a variety of media, for demonstration and practice of selected health-related behaviors, and for the construction of such student products as models and posters.

At the elementary level the main focus of health instruction is likely to be the regular elementary classroom, whether it is tra-

ditional or open in nature. The instructor is likely to be a regular elementary teacher. For these reasons, those who wish to promote health education must work with elementary teachers and other subject specialists and within constraints imposed by the nature of the elementary curriculum. The interests of health education are most effectively promoted by those who show a sincere interest in and support of the aspirations of those whom they seek to influence —in this case, elementary teachers and supervisors.

At the secondary level, specialist health or health and physical educators will ordinarily have greatest independence in developing their own curriculum and in developing specifications for a facility in which it can be implemented effectively.

HEALTH SERVICE UNIT

As in the case of health education facilities, the health service unit should be planned and furnished to facilitate performance of the planned health service functions. If medical or dental examinations are to be provided in school, then provisions for them must be planned in. If examinations are to be conducted en masse and during only a few days or weeks each year, then the space planned for this purpose should be readily convertible to other purposes or functions (such as screening testing) at other times.

The need for cot rooms with adjacent toilet facilities, for facilities for emergency inspection and first aid, for individual or small-group counseling, for students awaiting service, for storage of records and supplies, and for the conduct of screening tests is universal. An adequate facility for vision screening requires a 22-foot clear path if the traditional Snellen wall chart is used. The facility for hearing testing should be soundproofed to the extent that the background noise is reduced to 10 to 20 decibels or less and desirably is partitioned into two areas—one for the audiometrist, the other for the person being tested—and with a window between. Prefabricated sound-controlled booths for hearing testing are available. The design of the unit as a whole should provide for the entrance and exit of lines of students for such purposes as mass immunizations.

Physical educators usually prefer that the health service unit be placed near the activity facilities, on the grounds that most school injuries occur there. Placement near the administrative and guidance offices, however, is preferred for at least three reasons. First, quiescence facilitates a number of health service functions, such as counseling. Second, when the nurse or other health service staff members are absent, supervision of the health unit can be assumed by clerical or administrative staff. Third, health service personnel need to interact frequently with guidance and administrative staff members in the management of problem cases. The needs of the physical activity program for supporting first-aid service can be best met by locating one or two cots, appropriate

first-aid equipment and supplies, and a lavatory within the activity complex.

SCHOOL HOUSEKEEPING

In most schools today those whose primary task it is to maintain the building and grounds in a clean, safe, and healthful condition are referred to as maintenance engineers rather than as custodians or janitors. These staff members require skills and knowledge that in some states are taught in required short courses that deal with such subjects as basic bacteriology, cleaning and sanitizing methods, pest control, and other maintenance problems.

Just as no home can be properly maintained without the cooperation of all who live there, no school can be properly maintained without the involvement of all its members. During the 1930's depression, high school students were employed with the aid of federal funds to assist custodians. One of the effects of this involvement was that

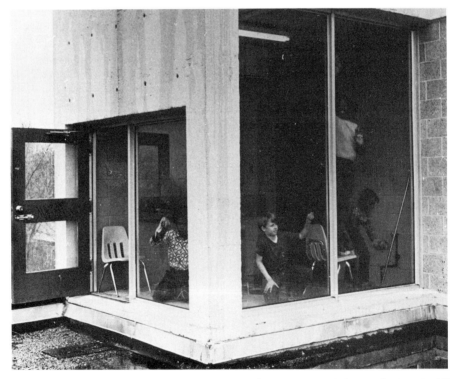

Fig. 12-4. Student involvement in school housekeeping. (Courtesy School District of Philadelphia.)

student workers littered less and exerted pressure on their peers to help keep the environment neat and clean. Union contracts discourage similar involvement today, but many schools assign students such responsibilities as picking up litter, cleaning up laboratory or shop facilities after use, and routinely inspecting the building and grounds for safety hazards. In some troubled schools where graffiti and vandalism present a problem, selected students are assigned the task of apprehending offenders, and offenders are assigned the task of cleaning up. Student groups may cover graffiti-laden walls with murals of their own design.

Periodic inspection of buildings and grounds by a sanitarian or by a member of the school health service staff also stimulates good maintenance. School environment appraisal forms are often available locally or from the state for use in making formal inspections.

School neighbors may be enlisted to help in various ways. In one school a group of parents turned out with wire pliers to twist up the sharp ends at the bottom edge of the school yard fence that had caused injuries to the feet of several youngsters. Other schools have enlisted neighbors to observe the school for occurrence of vandalism and to call police.

OTHER PLANNING AND MAINTENANCE CONSIDERATIONS

School water supply. It is rather generally assumed that water from a public supply system is safe to drink and that schools served by such supplies have little to worry about. In fact, something like one fourth of the U.S. population is served by public water supplies that fail to meet older and less stringent federal quality standards. Built-in delays make it unlikely that the provisions of the federal Safe Drinking Water Act of 1974 can be fully implemented until at least 1982. Many public supplies are drawn from sources heavily polluted by a variety of chemical wastes that the present standard treatment processes are not designed to remove. There is some ques-

tion whether present practices in the U.S. are as effective in disinfecting water of virus contaminants as they are in the case of bacteria. Treatment of water by means of ozone has been proposed as a possible solution to the virus problem.

Rural schools usually depend on subsurface water sources that are tapped by means of drilled wells equipped with pumps. If the subsoil is sandy, surface water will be naturally cleansed of bacterial contaminants as it is filtered through the sand on its way down to the pool tapped by the well. Soluble chemical pollutants are not removed that way, however. If the subsurface strata include a layer of limestone, as they do in many parts of Kentucky, the source is likely to be contaminated. Water runs through limestone in the form of underground rivers. These rivers are capable of carrying fecal material to the well from sources many miles away.

If a well is used, it should be so located, constructed, and maintained that it is not in danger of pollution from nearby cesspools, septic tanks, underground drains, or surface runoff. Once water enters a building, it may be contaminated by two coexisting means called cross-connection and back-siphonage, respectively.

Cross-connections are direct connections between a drinking water supply pipe and waste water. They are created in several ways. Plumbers may unwittingly install a fixture or pipe that directly connects one carrying contaminated water with one carrying drinking water. Improperly constructed plumbing fixtures may be used. One example of this is the old-fashioned drinking fountain with a bubbler in the center of the bowl, the top of which is below the level of the bowl rim. If the drain of such a fountain is clogged (by wads of gum, waste paper, and the like), the waste water may rise in the bowl until it covers the bubbler opening. Cross-connection also results from the common practice among science teachers and students of connecting a rubber hose to the laboratory sink outlet. This hose may be allowed to fall in the sink bowl along with waste water hoses from apparatus. Leaks may develop in pipes that occur in locations that permit waste water to seep out of a waste pipe leak into a leak in a drinking water pipe.

In the event that higher water pressure is maintained at all times in drinking water supply pipes than in pipes carrying sewage or contaminated water supplies, then contaminated water is unlikely to enter the drinking water supply. Whenever water pressure in the drinking water pipe is lower than the pressure in the contaminated source to which it is cross-connected, waste material will be sucked into the drinking water pipe. This phenomenon is called back-siphonage.

The likelihood of simultaneous occurrence of cross-connections and back-siphonage can be reduced or practically eliminated in several ways. Drinking and contaminated water pipes can be color coded. Drinking water pipes can be positioned

above and away from waste pipes with an air gap between. A firm policy that all plumbing repairs be made by a licensed plumber should be followed. The water quality should be tested periodically both at its source and at each point of use by a sanitarian who has access to the services of a public health laboratory. Periodic field surveys can be done, again by a qualified school or public health sanitarian, for observable defects in any part of the water supply, distribution, or waste water systems of the school. Protection is afforded new and remodeled schools by writing into the plumbing specifications provision for new piping and fixtures that conform to or exceed present local and state sanitary standards.

Such standards usually call for several specific protections against cross-connection and back-siphonage. One is the use of modern sanitary drinking fountains. These emit an angular jet of water from a head equipped with a guard to prevent attempts to suck water from it at times of low pressure, and which is located at one side of

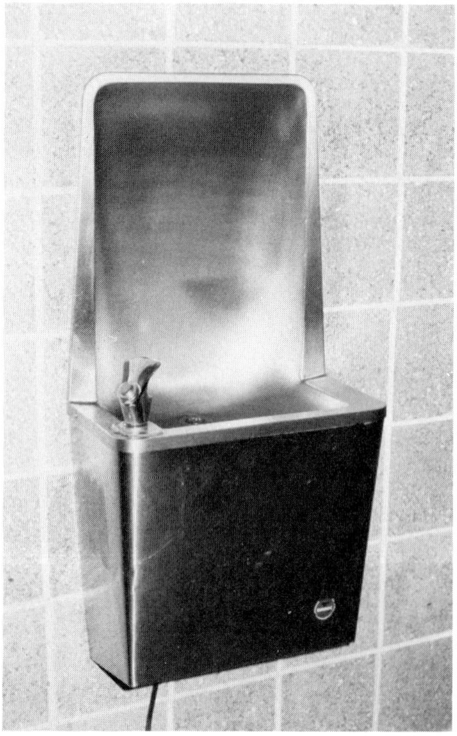

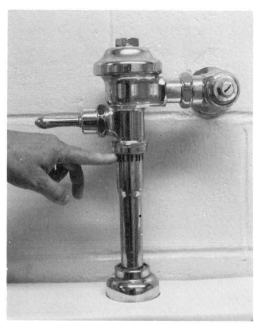

Fig. 12-5. A sanitary drinking fountain.

Fig. 12-6. Vacuum breaker installed just below a flush-o-meter valve on a toilet fixture.

and above the bowl rim so that it will not be contaminated when the drain is clogged. The water jet is emitted at an angle to prevent the ingestion of droplets of spittle left by a previous user.

The supply pipes of sanitary toilets and urinals are required to be equipped with check valves, which permit water to run out of but not into the supply pipe opening. Any valve will develop leaks in time, however. Such supply pipes are therefore also equipped with vacuum breakers, which are essentially short sections of pipe with holes around the circumference. Positive water pressure holds a flexible gasket in place against the holes to prevent leaks. If the pressure outside the supply pipe exceeds that inside, the gasket is sucked away from the holes. This breaks the back-siphonage and thereby prevents contamination of the supply pipe. These devices should also be installed in laboratory sink outlets, although we have never seen one so equipped. To control water wastage by playful students and still assure adequate flushing, modern toilets and urinals are generally equipped with flush-o-meter valves that emit a measured amount of water and then automatically shut off, even though the handle is held down.

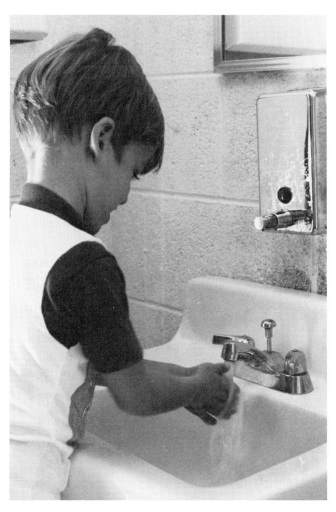

Fig. 12-7. A kindergarten classroom lavatory. (Courtesy David Spilver.)

Drinking fountain, handwashing, and toilet facilities. Drinking fountains are customarily installed in corridors. Their location in gymnasiums and classrooms, especially those used by early elementary and handicapped students, should also be considered. Classroom installations in socially disrupted schools eliminate one excuse for leaving the classroom and creating trouble. Wherever they are located, they create a safety hazard that can be reduced by placing them in wall recesses, They should be designed for easy cleaning and should be cleaned more than once daily with safe cleaning agents. The American preference for cold or at least cool water has resulted in the installation of cooling systems. These cost money to operate as well as to install and are not essential to health, but they do stimulate desirably higher levels of water consumption.

Minimum handwashing facilities should provide an opportunity for all school members to wash their hands before meals, after going to the toilet, and at other times when necessary, with a reasonable expenditure of time. Facilities should be so constructed and maintained as to invite use and provide satisfaction in their use. To achieve this, warm, running water that is emitted via a (single faucet) mixing valve, soap in any usable form, and either disposable towels or warm-air dryers must be provided and constantly maintained.

A minimum of one lavatory per 25 school members is usually required. Lavatories should *not* be equipped with stoppers. In mass toilet rooms, a circular or semicirculatory gang wash fountain may be substituted for individual lavatories. Placement of both lavatory and toilet facilities in early elementary classrooms is highly desirable. Some youngsters come to school with no knowledge of how to use toilets or lavatories, toilet paper, or soap and towels. They need to be taught.

Toilets should be located convenient to classrooms on each floor, with separate units for boys and girls. They should be well lighted, clean, screened, and well ventilated in accordance with state and local codes. Only open-front toilet seats should be used. They are easier to keep clean than closed-front seats and are less likely to serve as a mode of transmission of pubic (crab) lice. Floors and walls should be easy to clean and impervious to water.

Minimal standards usually call for one toilet seat per fifty boys, one urinal per thirty boys, and one toilet seat per thirty girls.

All such facilities must be appropriate or adaptable to the sizes of those who use them. This recommendation should be interpreted in terms of ranges rather than averages. Selection of equipment should also be made with the needs of handicapped persons in mind. Persons confined to wheelchairs require low drinking fountains, as do small individuals. Every mass toilet room should have a wide entrance, exit doors, and at least one wide toilet stall that is equipped with handgrip bars.

Adequate and well-kept toilet and handwashing facilities must be provided in the locker rooms and health suite as well as in the locations previously mentioned. Special facilities must also be placed in locations that are convenient for the use of cafeteria workers, for whom frequent handwashing is a must. School administrators and other staff members generally insist on having their own private facilities. It can be argued, however, that facilities used by students would be better policed and better maintained by the custodial staff if they were also used by teachers and administrators.

Shower and swimming pool facilities. Showers are ordinarily found in schools in conjunction with athletic and physical education programs, and then usually in junior and senior high schools only. Although youngsters sweat before puberty, body odor problems do not occur as a result of sweating until after puberty. The reason is that unlike the always active eccrine sweat glands, the aprocrine glands, which only become active at puberty, produce sweat that contains organic matter. This material is then broken down by bacterial action to yield unpleasant odors. In view of the earlier ages at which puberty is now occurring, it appears desirable to introduce showering after physical activity as early as grade 5. At least a few showers should be included in every school plan for the benefit of adult members who use activity facilities and for youngsters from homes in which bathing facilities are inadequate.

Where showers are provided in connection with physical education and athletic facilities, the minimum number of shower heads provided should equal at least one fourth the number of individuals who will use them in any given period. There should be at least 10 to 12 square feet of floor space under each shower head. All gang shower heads should be served by mixing valves, preferably of the variety that automatically controls water temperature. Showers utilize considerable amounts of water and heat. They are likely to be overused and therefore wasteful. Teachers can be encouraged to skip showers when the class activity has been only mildly vigorous.

Showers, dressing room floors, and pool decks should be surfaced with nonslip ceramic tile. They should be washed daily with hot water and detergent. A disinfecting final wash with a standard household chlorine bleach solution (1 part of bleach to 8 of water) may be left and allowed to dry. Drying is facilitated by installation of mechanical dehumidification. A clean towel service provided by the school is much preferred over towels that are brought from home.

Ringworm infection (athlete's foot) and plantar warts (virus-caused warts on soles of feet) pose a nuisance and a public relations problem. Parents and students tend to blame such infections on unsanitary showers, locker rooms, and pool decks. There may be some justification for this belief in respect to plantar warts, but athlete's foot appears to be primarily a problem associated with individual susceptibility and foot hygiene. Some authorities recommend that students wear shower clogs. Individuals susceptible to athlete's foot can best

control it by drying the feet carefully with a clean towel, especially between the toes, and by daily use of a drying foot powder. So-called antiseptic foot baths and spray devices are worse than useless.

All pools should be designed, constructed, and operated to meet state and local board of health requirements. In general, these regulations require a recirculating system equipped for chlorination and filtration and prescribe acceptable ranges for chlorine and pH levels. Filtration will remove suspended particles of dirt. Chlorination and pH control are designed to control bacteria and algae growth. Paul* found that except for staphyloccoccal organisms bacterial levels are determined more by pH and free chlorine levels than by swim load. Staphylococcus levels rise with the number of swimmers present and are not significantly affected by either pH or chlorine levels. He concluded that it is not essential to test pools for bacterial content if recommended pH levels, chlorine content, and swim load are held to recommended levels. Paul's study was not so designed as to permit quantification of acceptable swim load levels. A pH range of 7.4 to 7.6 and an available chlorine level of 1.0 to 2.0 parts per million are generally recommended and are consistent with Paul's data.

Constant surveillance of the pool whenever swimmers are in the area is essential to safety. Someone other than the instructor should supervise the showers and locker rooms. Users should be required to shower before entering the pool. If suits are worn, they should be clean, which means that they should be supplied by the school, not the students. The generally accepted temperature ranges for comfort call for pool water temperatures between 72° F and 78° F, with air temperatures between 75° F and 82° F.

If the purpose of school swimming pools is to teach students to swim, then high pri-

---

*Paul, R. A.: An environmental model for swimming pool bacteriology, Am. J. Public Health **62:** 770-772, June 1972.

ority for swimming pool placement should be assigned to elementary schools. If their purpose is to provide facilities for athletic competition, then they belong in secondary schools, which is where most of them are now located.

A few school pools have been designed for year-round school-community use by equipping them with roofs that may be moved aside for summertime use or by encasing them in flexible enclosures that are supported by forced warm air during unseasonable weather.

Ionizing radiation and microwave ovens. *Ionizing radiation* should not ordinarily be a significant problem in most schools, since few schools are equipped with medical or scientific x-ray equipment. Where such equipment is used, it is essential that it meet current federal and state standards of construction, installation, and use. Surveillance of science laboratories and instructors should be maintained to insure that radioactive materials and equipment are not introduced into the school environment for instructional purposes. Some instructors may not be aware that *no* level of exposure to ionizing radiation is known to be safe and that fetuses and growing young people are particularly susceptible to its effects. In areas where uranium and other radioactive materials are mined or are present in significant amounts in nature, the sand or building material that is used in school construction should be monitored and cleared for use. Schools should not be located near such mines.

Microwave ovens are found increasingly in schools. Some are used for the rapid heating of school lunches. Others may be introduced for use in home economics instruction. They cook and heat food quickly and efficiently. Their known hazards include the possibility that accidental exposure of human beings to microwaves may result in cooked human flesh, eye damage, or malfunction of certain types of cardiac pacemakers. Preventive measures include the use of shielding devices, interlocking door and switch systems, and posting of warning

notices. A survey of industrial microwave ovens included one that was designed to heat school lunches, and which was found to be among the safest of all those tested in terms of leakage and potential for occupational exposure at eye level. The researchers noted that attendants require training in the safe use of microwave ovens.* Consumers Union tested models of counter-top microwave ovens that were designed for home use and found that all 15 met current standards of the Federal Bureau of Radiological Health. However, the report concluded that none could be deemed safe for home use because of the overloading and other misuse to be expected in the home.†

Illumination. The provision of good school lighting is a highly technical task, requiring the guidance of lighting specialists. The design of good lighting for a large, open classroom is much more difficult than that for a smaller, traditional classroom. Teachers and school health personnel, however, should understand what constitutes good school lighting so that they may use it efficiently and recognize defects that need correction. It is important to realize that a change in the color or glossiness of paint on room walls or the introduction of new furniture or furniture arrangements, for example, may change the quantity or quality of illumination for better or worse.

The quantity, quality, and distribution of lights are related to comfort and to the efficient performance of visual tasks. Most schoolrooms are lighted by a combination of natural and artificial light sources. *Natural* light consists of both direct sunlight and indirect light that is reflected from exterior surfaces such as snow or adjacent buildings. Such lights costs nothing, but its high intensity and the possibility that it may shine directly into human eyes and thus produce

---

*Eure, J. A., Nicolls, J. W., and Elder, R. W.: Radiation exposure from industrial microwave applications, Am. J. Public Health **62:**1573-1577, Dec. 1972.
†Microwave ovens: not recommended, Consumer Reports, April 1973, pp. 223-230.

discomfort and possible eye damage must be recognized. It is very difficult to control. *Artificial* light in schools is usually produced by electrical fluorescent or incandescent bulbs. Incandescent bulbs are inefficient; much energy is lost in the production of heat. They do, however, introduce a feeling of warmth and interest. Fluorescent bulbs are cooler and more efficient. The light produced by modern fluorescent bulbs is much like daylight in quality. Artificial light is relatively easier to control than natural light. Indirect lighting, in which light sources are hidden in wall recesses, provides lighting of high quality and high cost. Semidirect lighting, in which light sources are shielded from direct view, provides an economical and acceptable substitute.

The quantity of light *emitted* by any source is measured in terms of candle power. A standard one-candle power source is kept at the U.S. Bureau of Standards. The quantity of light *present* in any given space is measured in units called *footcandles*. One footcandle of light is the amount of light from one standard candle that reaches a surface 1 foot away. Some of the light that falls on a surface will be absorbed, and some will be reflected. The amount that is reflected from the surface is expressed in units called *footlamberts*. The number of footlamberts equals the number of footcandles that fall on the surface times the *reflectance* of the surface. For example, if 30 footcandles of light fall on a green chalkboard with a reflectance factor of 50%, 15 footlamberts of brightness are emitted from the chalkboard. The amount of light that reaches the eye is usually expressed in footlamberts.

A sufficient amount of light is essential to eye comfort and visual acuity. There is no evidence that insufficient lighting in classrooms presents a health hazard. Specific recommendations vary with the authority consulted, with the reflectance of environmental surfaces, and with the nature of the visual tasks to be performed. Recommended values vary from a low of around 10 footcandles in corridors, to 20 or 30 footcandles

in regular classrooms, to a high of 30 to 50 or more footcandles in areas where difficult visual tasks are performed, such as sewing white cloth with white thread. In general, gains in visual acuity and comfort are small with increases in intensity of over 20 footcandles.

Because of the difficulty in controlling natural light, authorities disagree as to whether or not windows should be provided at all in classrooms. If windows are provided, some form of shielding must be provided against sunlight, snow, and other outside sources of glare. Venetian blinds, shades, drapes, low-transmission glass, awnings, and shrubbery all provide shielding, and all have their advantages and disadvantages. Venetian blinds, for example, are easily adjustable to admit the amount of outside light and air desired. Their initial and maintenance costs are high, however.

Windowless classrooms do not entirely solve the glare problem. Glare is created by large *brightness differences* in light within a room, regardless of their source. Relatively bright light that is emitted directly into the eyes of an individual by either a light fixture or a light, glossy surface is glare. Windowless classrooms also tend to evoke a feeling of claustrophobia, but this may be relieved by installing dioramas, terrariums, or tanks of fish in wall recesses.

Regardless of whether windows are used, no brightness difference ratio within any individual's field of vision should exceed ten to one. Differences of less than five to one or even three to one are considered more desirable. At the same time, zero brightness differences throughout a room are to be avoided because monotony results; therefore, sharp contrasts between bright and dark surfaces are to be avoided. Such contrasts can be held to a minimum in several ways. Flat rather than glossy surfaces on walls, ceilings, floors, and chalkboards are desirable. Reflectances from ceilings should be 70% to 90%, from walls 40% to 60%, and from floors and furniture 30% to 50%. Chalkboards must be dark enough to allow chalk writing to be visible and nonglossy enough to make them insignificant as a source of glare. Reflectance should not exceed 20%. Green nonglare chalkboards and yellow chalk give good results. Desk or table tops should have a nonglossy finish. Flat pastel paints on walls produce reflectances in the optimal range. Light sources should either be shielded or so located that they are not in the direct line of vision of any room occupant. To avoid reflections from task surfaces, the lighting system should provide a minimum of downward light immediately over desks. Much of the light on a task surface should come from wider angles so that it is not reflected into the eyes as glare.

In the maintenance of satisfactory illumination, teachers and students can watch natural and artificial lighting to see that lights are turned on or off (or dimmed if the room is equipped with manually controlled dimmer switches) according to need. In some newer or relighted buildings, the intensity of artificial lighting is automatically adjusted to balance it with natural light. Shades can be adjusted as needed. Seating can be rearranged to provide optimal comfort for students, including those who may be left-handed or have eye difficulties. Chalkboards can be kept clean. Sources of glare within the room may be covered with nonglossy art work. Dirty fixtures or burned-out lights should be reported, repeatedly if necessary.

Acoustics and noise. Increasing attention is being given to noise control and sound-proofing in school buildings. Noise may be defined as unwanted sound. Noise within a school space is composed of unwanted sounds that are created by occupants and ambient or background noise admitted from the outside (such as traffic noise) and such inside noises as those created by mechanical equipment such as blowers. Noises have two measurable qualities, intensity and pitch. As human beings perceive sounds, loudness depends not only on intensity but also on pitch.

The following units of measurement are among several used to measure these qualities of sound:

decibel (dB). A ratio of the intensity of a sound to a physical base unit. The decibel scale is logarithmic. For each increase in intensity of 10 dB the actual sound pressure increases 10 times. Thus, 110 dB is 10 times more intense than 100 dB.

dBA. A decibel scale in which values are weighted to reflect the impact that sound makes on humans more closely than does the C scale, which is a measure of physical pressure.

Hertz (Hz). The unit now currently used to measure sound pitch. It is equal to the formerly used unit, cps, or cycles per second.

Human speech varies from about 500 Hz to 5,000 Hz. Below and above that level, greater intensity is required if the sound is to be heard readily.

Kryter* has proposed that an ambient noise level of 35 dBA represents a maximum tolerance (comfort) level for more or less continuous exposure to noise in schoolrooms. Ordinary conversation is conducted at levels of about 40 to 60 dB at a distance of about 3 feet. Goldsmith and Johnson† conclude that permanent hearing damage may occur with average occupational exposures of over 75 dBA, which is about the level of noise made by a home clothes washer or a passenger car traveling 60 mph at a distance of 25 feet. Federal occupational standards, however, allow 8 hours' exposure per day to 90 dBA of sound (the equivalent of that produced by a motorcycle at 25 feet) or ½-hour's exposure per day to 110 dBA (which is about the same level of intensity as that produced by a rock band or a riveting machine).

Breysse‡ surveyed twelve schools that were adjacent to a jet airport and three that were located next to a busy freeway. Maximum sound levels of 90 dBA or higher were observed in five of the airport schools

---

*Kryter, K. D.: Non-auditory effects of environmental noise, Am. J. Public Health **62:**389-398, March 1972.

†Goldsmith, J. R., and Johnson, E.: Health effects of community noise, Am. J. Public Health **63:**782-793, Sept. 1973.

‡Breysse, P. A.: School noise, School Health Review **3:**4, 16-18, July-Aug. 1972.

with open windows. The freeway schools averaged 60 to 70 dBA throughout the entire school day, with peaks ranging from 87 dBA to 91 dBA. It is difficult to believe that teaching and learning, which involves speaking and hearing, can occur at all under such conditions. That it can and does is evidence of human ability to tolerate the intolerable.

Measures to prevent exterior noise from entering school buildings include support of communitywide noise abatement programs, the placement of schools in low noise locations, and shielding. Shielding measures include the provision of air conditioning so that windows need not be opened and the use of shrubs, trees, and earthen mounds as noise barriers. Optimal shielding can be attained through underground construction.

Noise that arises inside the school is more likely to present an annoyance that interferes with teaching and learning than a hearing hazard. Noisy school areas such as shops, gyms, playgrounds, and music rooms should be located apart from such quiet areas as classrooms, the health suite, the library, and administrative offices. Separate ductwork should serve noisy and quiet areas.

Reverberations of speech and other sounds from surfaces that are not sound absorbent make perception difficult. Reverberations are most troublesome in large spaces such as auditoriums and gymnasiums. One or more of a variety of sound-absorbent materials, including acoustical ceiling tile, fabric draperies, and carpeting, may be utilized to control reverberations. Traditional classrooms should be so designed and finished that soft speech can be heard and understood in any part of the room.

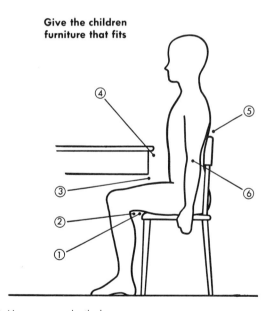

Give the children furniture that fits

1 No pressure under the knees

2 Free space back of inside angle of knee

3 Room above the thighs

4 Back edge of table overlaps front edge of chair

5 Low chair back, open at bottom; support for hollow of back only

6 Table top higher than elbow when arm is straight

Fig. 12-8. From the Yearbook, *American school buildings.* (Courtesy American Association of School Administrators.)

A physical barrier in the form of tall furniture in the central part of the room or overhanging ducts or beams that project down into the room from the ceiling may block or distort speech sounds. Conversely, a large, open classroom in which several activity groups function at once requires the placement of sound barriers between groups.

Teachers can help solve the noise problems by speaking softly and by keeping the volume of audio equipment turned low. When teachers speak loudly, students speak loudly in turn.

Seating. In school situations in which youngsters frequently move from one room or task to another and are not expected to sit or work in one place for very long, it may not be too important that seats and work surfaces be precisely fitted to the individual. It is part of the nature of children and young people to fidget and contort themselves into a variety of odd positions.

In situations in which long periods of sitting or performance of fine motor tasks such as writing or drawing are required, each individual should be provided with a seat and work surface that allow the practice of good sitting and writing posture (Fig. 12-8). The height of the work surface should be such that the individual may write without having to elevate one shoulder above the other.

Seating and work surfaces should be assigned by observing the individual seated and writing. A recent study showed that black youngsters have longer legs and arms and shorter trunks than whites and that boys have longer legs and arms and shorter trunks than girls. Thus, different seating may be required for individuals of the same height who vary in respect to sex or race.* A youngster may grow enough in the course of a few months to require a change of furniture.

Climate control. Modern methods of air conditioning make it possible to provide the kind of climate desired for classrooms, shops, gyms, and other areas of the school building. In contrast to the traditional little red schoolhouse, we now have many schools in which all air is conditioned. If our air were cleaner and schoolhouses smaller than they are, less complex systems would be required. Schools can be constructed or remodeled to utilize solar

*National Center for Health Statistics: *Body weight, stature, and sitting height: white and negro youths 12-17 years, United States,* DHEW Publication No. (HRA) 74-1608, Washington, D. C., 1973, U. S. Government Printing Office, pp. 10-13.

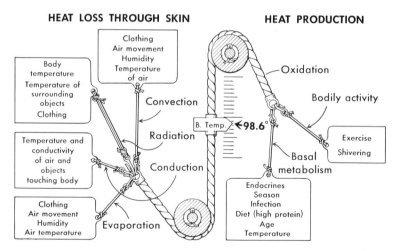

Fig. 12-9. Factors affecting heat production and heat loss. When heat production balances heat loss, normal body temperature is maintained.

energy not only for air heating and cooling but for water heating as well. Plans for a remodeled school in Atlanta are designed to obtain 60% of the school's energy needs from the sun.

Temperature and *air movement* assist the body in maintaining a balance between the heat produced in the tissues and the heat lost to the environment, if they are properly regulated. At ordinary indoor temperature ranges, *humidity* (air moisture) is of less significance to thermal comfort than are temperature and air movement, but high humidity does permit the lowering of room temperatures by a few degrees. The variables associated with body heat production and loss are illustrated in Fig. 12-9.

For adult males doing sedentary work, a dry bulb temperature range of 68° F to 72° F is generally recommended as optimal for comfort. Women, perhaps because of skimpier clothing and lower heat loss related to more ample subcutaneous fat deposits, are more comfortable at temperatures up to 75° F. School-age youngsters prefer lower temperatures because their metabolism rates exceed those of adults. Reduction of maximum cold weather classroom temperatures to 68° F (and possibly lower) as an energy conservation measure can readily be tolerated, especially if adult staff members compensate by wearing additional clothing and if a relative humidity between 30% and 70% is maintained. The presence of a source of radiant heat such as large window areas that are exposed to sunlight also makes it possible to lower air temperatures. Temperatures as low as 60° F in gymnasiums and 66° F in corridors may be tolerated as a result of exercise.

In summer, except when humidity levels of over 75% prevail, people readily adjust to temperature of 80° F or even 85° F. It is usually recommended that inside temperatures no lower than 15° F to 20° F below those prevailing outside be maintained. These standards imply that air cooling has been greatly overutilized.

Air movement velocities of around 25 to 50 feet per minute, or movement that is barely perceptible, are considered desirable in classrooms. In summer or in physical activity, higher velocities are desirable. The role of air movement in thermal comfort is to increase body-heat loss.

The air supply in a classroom should be exchanged for cleansed air at a rate of about 10 to 30 or more cubic feet per minute in order to remove body odors. The rate of exchange needed increases with crowding, higher room temperatures, and physical activity.

Large school buildings and auditoriums require the use of ventilation ducts and fans to maintain adequate air movement and exchange of air. In most large city schools and in other schools that are downwind from heavy industrial polluters, there is danger that polluted air and undesirable odors may enter the intake system. If inside-outside temperature differences are high, it pays to recirculate used air. In either case, the air should be cleansed. This can be accomplished by pulling the outside or used air through a sheet of water. This process removes particulates and soluble gaseous air pollutants. Excess water is removed from the air by eliminator plates before the air is cooled or heated and then distributed throughout the building.

Attempts have been made to disinfect school air supplies, but these efforts have not been proven to be either effective or safe.

Food and milk sanitation. The public school feeding program undoubtedly ranks among the largest food service operations in any given community. The potential for outbreaks of communicable disease caused by contaminated food and milk is high and can only be minimized through careful purchasing of milk and food and careful design and operation of food service facilities.

The design and equipment specifications for all school food, storage, preparation, and service facilities of a new or remodeled school should be carefully reviewed by a sanitary engineer or sanitarian and modified, if necessary, before they are accepted. Food and milk should never be purchased on the basis of low bid alone. The supplier's records of performance in delivery of sanitary products of high quality and in respect to sanitation violations should be of prime consideration. Preemployment medical examinations and tuberculosis screening of employees reveal nothing about their future health. They should, however, be continuously observed for signs of infection and excused from school with pay or assigned other work if these are noted. All food service employees should be trained in proper food handling and equipment operation procedures. They should be provided with clean garments, caps, and hairnets or headbands daily.

Once a food service is in operation, periodic inspection of the facilities, equipment, and performance of the staff by either a school or health department sanitarian is essential. Such inspections may include laboratory tests of milk and food samples and of the surfaces of supposedly clean dishes for bacterial contamination. The temperature and cleanliness of refrigerators, freezers, service units, and water in distributing units is checked. Recommended refrigerator temperatures vary from 32° F to 50° F, depending on the type of food stored. A temperature no higher than 0° F is required for freezers. Standards require that perishable food be kept for service at temperatures either below 40° F or above 140° F and that washed dishes be finally rinsed in a 180° F sanitizing spray. If dishes fail to dry without toweling, the final rinse is not hot enough.

Hand contact with food is to be avoided. Any foods of doubtful cleanliness or freshness must be discarded. If the facility is not equipped with garbage grinders, garbage must be stored in rodent- and flyproof containers near or at a service entrance and must be removed daily.

Solid waste disposal. It is possible to reduce the amount of garbage produced by school feeding programs, and thus reduce the size of the disposal problem, by serving preferred foods in their preferred forms. Students and staff can be surveyed to determine menu preferences, which are likely to vary with age and ethnicity. Discarded food can be monitored to determine items to be omitted from future menus. Student committees can be meaningfully involved in menu planning within the constraints imposed by nutritional guidelines and food costs. The palatability of school food, and thus its acceptance, can be improved by training cooks in methods utilized by successful restaurants. For example, the flavor of vegetables is greatly improved if they are cooked in small quantities, if they are somewhat undercooked, and if butter or margarine is added.

Schools also produce massive amounts of wastepaper. Schoolwide use of both sides of a piece of paper and acceptance of single-spaced typing can reduce waste. Used half-sheets for brief written material can be encouraged.

Recycling and reclamation of garbage, waste paper, and certain other wastes should be practiced if feasible. However, Kupchek* points out that the economic return from these procedures is limited and not always predictable. Not all trash is marketable at all times. Attempts by well-intentioned amateurs to poke through trash, sort it, and store it pose hazards of injury, infection, and infestation by rodents and other pests.

Probably the most valuable reuse of garbage is in hog feeding. For this purpose it must be properly stored and collected. Garbage can also be composted if there is a market, if a site is available well away from schools and residences, and if compost heaps are constantly maintained so as to control insect and rodent pests. There are well-designed incinerators that yield usable heat without seriously polluting the air, but they are costly to install and maintain, and they yield solid residues that require disposal.

There is no present method of community solid waste disposal that is inexpensive, feasible in all locations, or without some objection. Open dumps are the cheapest and

*Kupchek, G. J.: Recycling and reclamation, Am. J. Public Health **62:**1143-1147, Aug. 1972.

most obnoxious of the available methods. Use of grinders that feed garbage into the sewage system is feasible if the treatment system is adequate for the increased load. Sanitary landfill is satisfactory if appropriate sites are available and well maintained. Ocean dumping requires both careful site selection and some sorting of materials. As a responsible community agency, the school must exert its influence to ensure that its solid wastes are disposed of by the least objectionable method that is locally feasible.

SCHOOL AS A LABORATORY FOR ENVIRONMENTAL EDUCATION

The need for environmental education is illustrated by the results of a survey of middle- and working-class high school seniors from two school districts. Although 90% of them regarded the environmental situation as serious, fewer than half were willing to reduce their use of automobiles or electrical appliances by as much as a half, and only one third were willing to pay more taxes to clean up the environment.*

Mark Terry† has suggested a number of ways in which the classroom and the school can be used as a laboratory for environmental education. For example, materials and energy that are used can be traced to their sources. Various seating arrangements can be tried out and evaluated for their facilitation of communication. The use of certain resources, such as note paper, can be suspended for a time to learn whether or not they are essential. The impact of school waste on the community can be investigated.

In addition, the school environment could be evaluated in terms of some of the observable or measurable standards cited in this chapter. Students could then determine ways in which the school environment might be improved at the least cost in money, environmental resources, and pollution.

QUESTIONS FOR STUDY AND DISCUSSION

1. With what body does legal and moral responsibility lie for a safe and healthful school environment?
2. To what specific school officers may environmental responsibilities be delegated? How competent is each of these likely to be to assume this responsibility?
3. Who should be involved in the school plant planning process? What are the roles and responsibilities of the board, administrator, architect, and planning committee?
4. Ask any class member who has been involved in school plant planning to contrast the nature and extent of the involvement with that described in the text.
5. What are the implications of demographic data and available community resources for school plant planning? What examples of such implications can you cite from your own school experiences?
6. What are the implications of regular school placement of handicapped youngsters and of the ever changing nature of school programs for planning?
7. List the criteria for a desirable school site that are stated or implied in the text. In the consensus opinion of the class, what other desirable criteria should be added to the list? Evaluate an existing school site in terms of those criteria derived from the text or class discussion that are observable or measurable with instruments available to the class.
8. Follow the same process as that set forth in question 7 above to assess the adequacy of:
   a. The classroom in which you are meeting for health instruction in terms of illumination, acoustics and noise, seating, and climate control.
   b. A health service unit in a nearby public school, and the school's drinking fountains, handwashing and toilet facilities, food and milk service facilities including microwave ovens, and solid waste disposal.
9. Develop a similar list of nonobservable or nonmeasurable criteria for the school site and for each of the facilities listed in question 8. Translate these criteria into questions to be asked of knowledgeable persons in the school.
10. Determine the prevailing job qualifications and descriptions for building engineers and other maintenance staff members in your local school district.
11. How can the school environments investigated be improved at the least cost in resources and environmental pollution?

*Kilwein, J. H., St. Denis, G. C., and Hall, W. T.: The social class of young adults and their views on the environment: how much would you sacrifice? J. Sch. Health **44:**196-197, April 1974.
†Terry, M.: *Teaching for survival,* New York, 1971, Ballantine Books, Inc., pp. 49-106.

REFERENCES

Anderson, C. L.: *School health practice,* St. Louis, 1972, The C. V. Mosby Co.
Joint Study Committee of the American School Health Association and the National Society for the Prevention of Blindness: *Teaching about vision,* New York, 1972, The Society.

National Committee on School Health Policies of the National Education Association and the American Medical Association: *Suggested school health policies,* Chicago, 1966, AMA and NEA.

National Council on Schoolhouse Construction: *Guide for planning school plants,* East Lansing, Mich., 1967, The Council.

Nemir, A., and Schaller, W. E.: *The school health program,* ed. 4, Philadelphia, 1975, W. B. Saunders Co.

Sartwell, P. E., editor: *Maxcy-Rosenau preventive medicine and public health,* ed. 10, New York, 1973, Appleton-Century-Crofts.

Terry, M.: *Teaching for survival,* New York, 1971, Ballantine Books, Inc.

Wilner, D. M., Walkley, R. P., and Goerke, L. S.: *Introduction to public health,* New York, 1973, Macmillan, Inc.

school health policies, Chicago, 1966, AMA.

PART SIX

Health promotion and health problems

CHAPTER 13

🌿 Growth and development: related problems and school functions

An understanding of the growth and development of children and young people of school age is important to school professionals for several reasons. Youngsters are interested in what is happening to them as they mature, and some may need reassurance that the differences that they observe between themselves and their peers are indeed normal and healthy. There is need to differentiate healthy behavior and appearance from that which indicates possible health problems at any given stage. School health and health education program design appropriately varies to some extent with developmental stages, and healthy growth and development may be facilitated to some extent by appropriate school programs.

Throughout this chapter some terms that are used repeatedly require definition:

Growth. Increase in the size and weight of the body or its parts.
Development. Progress in or refinement of function of body parts or of psychosocial behavior or processes.
Maturation. The concepts of growth, development, and aging.
Puberty or **pubescence.** The time period during which the reproductive system becomes active. Dramatically marked in girls by the onset of menstruation; by the appearance of pubic hair in boys. Ushers in the longer period of adolescence during which general body and psychosexual growth continues to occur.

SOME BASIC CONCEPTS

A child is not a small adult. Children differ from adults not only in size but also in terms of body proportions and physiological and psychosocial functioning.

Children's heads are larger and their limbs longer in proportion to total height than are those of adults. By about age 10, their eyes and brains have acquired full adult size. Lymphoid tissues (tonsils, adenoids, lymph nodes, and thymus gland) are considerably larger in relation to the total body weight at around age 12 than they will ever be again. Genital tissues grow little until puberty and rapidly thereafter. Most other body tissues do not attain full adult size until the late teens. Children require more food and oxygen for their weight than adults do. They need relatively more protein for tissue growth. Their hearts beat faster because of their relatively small size, and children who are fit have relatively less stamina than do fit adults. Children are more susceptible to infections than adults because they are still in the process of acquiring their immunities.

Children have an amazing ability to learn, but they have not yet accumulated adult-sized stores of knowledge. Their behavior is child-like; they have not yet learned to control the ways in which they display or cope with their feelings. Their capacity for work develops during the elementary school years. Their capacity for love develops during adolescence and young adulthood.

Growth and development is an orderly process. Each stage of growth and development follows the previous stage in undeviating sequence: prenatal period, infancy, childhood, adolescence, and adulthood. Failure to achieve growth and development goals fully at any given stage decreases the likelihood of future achievement.

Erik Erikson* in his theory of psycho-

*Erikson, E. H.: *Childhood and society,* ed. 2, New York, 1963, W. W. Norton, & Co., Inc.

social development, which is perhaps the most useful for school professionals, postulates eight stages of human development. Two of these stages span the public school years. Healthy children enter school having achieved (1) a sense of *basic trust,* which results from having experienced affection and need gratification in early infancy, (2) a sense of *autonomy,* which means that they have come to view themselves as adequate persons, and (3) a sense of *initiative,* which means that they exercise their imaginations, test reality, and imitate adults. Children who have failed to achieve these stages may enter school jealous, inhibited, and distrustful of both others and themselves.

During the elementary school years healthy children achieve *industry.* They work hard, develop skills, discern the dif-

ference between fantasy and reality, and come to welcome competition. In Junior and senior high school they attain *ego identity* by experimenting with roles. They become certain that they are boys or girls, leaders or followers, and all that these terms imply. They emerge from school ready to love and work in the adult sense. Those who fail are sure of their inferiority, confused about their roles in life, and likely to become loners or sexually promiscuous.

Physically, middle childhood (from school entrance until puberty) is a period of slow, steady growth in height and weight. The adolescent *growth spurt* begins at about age 10½ for girls and age 12 for boys. It ends at about age 13 for girls (when significant numbers of them begin to get pregnant) and at about age 14¾ for boys. On the average, girls become taller than boys be-

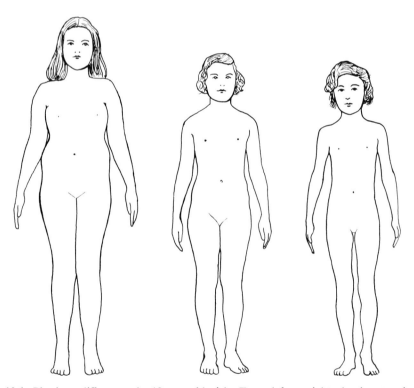

Fig. 13-1. Physique differences in 10-year-old girls. From left to right, dominant endomorph (6-3-3), dominant mesomorph (4-5-2), and dominant ectomorph (2-2-6). (Courtesy Dr. Stanley M. Garn, Yellow Springs, Ohio.)

tween the ages of 9 and 10, and boys become taller than girls between the ages of 13 and 14.*

Individual differences. Well children vary greatly from each other. Certainly there are some general signs of health versus illness, but healthy children are not as alike as new automobiles of the same make and model. Red cheeks that are normal for Jim may signify a fever for Henry. Differences in the nature of their skins account for the difference in their skin coloring and complexion. Normal variations in features or facial expressions may suggest a degree of fatigue or cheerfulness that does not exist.

Sharp differences exist in youngsters' emotional reactions. One may be excitable, another phlegmatic. Of another pair of healthy youngsters, one may be extroverted and the other introverted. One may possess high vitality and endurance, another may not.

These and other individual differences result from interactions between one's genetic potential and environmental influences. Techniques of genetic engineering are being developed that may be useful in overcoming problems of heredity, but the ethical propriety of their use is questioned by scientists as well as nonscientists. The environment can be modified, but the impact of the school environment is less than that of society as a whole.

Among the specific variables that influence growth and development are body type, endocrine gland production, nutrition, family socioeconomic characteristics, race, psychosocial influences, physical activity, and illness, which will be discussed briefly below. Although climate and geography are associated with differences in growth and development, we have no reason to believe that there is any significant cause-and-effect relationship. Rather, the supposed geographical and climate differences seem to be the result

of differences in genetic and environmental influences, which vary from place to place.

Body type. Differences in body type are apparent throughout life. Some persons are stocky with heavy bones, others are thin with fine bones, while others exhibit gradations between the two extremes. One way of describing differences in body build was proposed by Sheldon* in 1940. He used as the basis for his terminology the three primary layers of the embryonic germ cell layers (endoderm, mesoderm, and ectoderm), each of which seemed to have furnished the characteristics for a single, distinguishable type of body build. An *endomorph* is one whose massive digestive organs dominate the body economy and whose musculature is soft and thin. A *mesomorph* is a solidly built person with large, firm, strong muscles. An *ectomorph* is commonly referred to as a string bean, whose body is slender with small muscles, long arms, legs, and trunk. Sheldon recognized that many individuals cannot be readily categorized as belonging to one of three types and developed a rating scheme to indicate the relative dominance of each type as observed in an individual. An extreme ectomorph would be classified as a 1-1-7 (for endorphy 1, mesomorphy 1, and ectomorphy 7). An individual whose body build was at the midpoint in respect to each of the three groupings would be classified as 4-4-4. Examples of the three dominant types are presented in Fig. 13-1.

School professionals have many more useful things to do than to somatotype children, but the concept produced several implications of practical importance. First, we should not expect a healthy person to always conform to height-weight averages. A heavily muscled athlete who can in no way be accurately described as fat will be overweight according to height-weight charts or even, in some cases, according to

---

*National Health Survey: *Height and weight of youths 12-17 years, United States,* DHEW Publication No. (HSM) 73-1606, Washington, D.C., Jan. 1973, U.S. Government Printing Office.

*Sheldon, W. H., Stevens, S. S., and Tucker, W. B.: *The varieties of human physique,* New York, 1940, Harper & Row, Publishers.

charts that purport to set standards of weight by both height and body build. Second, neither we nor our students should allow ourselves to be pressured into extreme and strenuous dietary or exercise programs that are designed to change our natural body builds to conform with current fashionable notions of male or female attractiveness. It is futile, dangerous, and senseless to attempt to overcome body-build limitations imposed by healthy genes. Third, both dominant mesomorphs and endomorphs tend to accrue excess fat unless they adhere to sensible patterns of diet and engage in at least moderate amounts of physical activities. Although ectomorphs are unlikely to become fat, they benefit in other ways from sensible dietary and exercise behavior.

Endocrine gland production. All hormones can be said to influence growth and development in some way, if for no other reason than through their complex interactions. Human growth hormone (HGH), which is produced by the pituitary gland, appears to regulate directly a variety of metabolic reactions in concert with insulin. A deficiency of either hormone can produce dwarfism, which if detected early enough, is treatable by hormone injections. In rare cases, an oversupply of HGH produces giantism, or acromegaly, which can be effectively treated early by surgery or radiation of the pituitary gland. Thyroxine can be administered to children whose thyroid glands are insufficiently productive to stimulate normal growth. Androgens are male hormones that are produced by the adrenal glands in both boys and girls during puberty. They initiate the adolescent growth spurt and, in collaboration with other hormones, stimulate the hardening of the epiphyses (growing end of the long bones), which brings the growth spurt to an end.

One point of this brief and incomplete recital is that if *extreme* cases are identified early and then medically evaluated, *some* of them may be helped by a qualified medical specialist in endocrinology. Such treatment, however, does not appear to be successful in overcoming limits that have been genetically imposed.

Nutrition. The importance of nutrition in growth and development is sometimes obvious to the casual observer and sometimes not. Extremely undernourished youngsters, including some in the United States, may suffer from kwashiorkor (protein deficiency disease), or marasmus (calorie deficiency), while others may simply be undersized. Those who are extremely overnourished in terms of calories are too fat. In between are some youngsters who exhibit signs of mineral or vitamin deficiencies, whose hair and eyes are dull, whose skin is not elastic, or whose posture is poor but who fall within average height and weight limits. Still others show no outward signs of poor nutrition but may reveal some evidence of it as measured by laboratory tests or by food intake studies.

Sufficient calories and proteins appear to be the nutrients of greatest importance to growth. Calories are now believed to be essential to cell multiplication, while proteins are essential to cell enlargement. Altogether some 45 different nutrients have been identified as contributing to healthy growth. Most of these nutrients are provided qualitatively by the four basic food groups: (1) meat, poultry, fish, and eggs, (2) vegetables and fruit, including both dark green vegetables, citrus fruits, and tomatoes (vitamin C sources), and yellow vegetables (vitamin A sources), (3) enriched or whole-grain breads and cereals, and (4) milk and milk products (Fig. 13-2). A diet based on the basic four pattern may be deficient in iron and some other nutrients, however. Table 13-1 shows recommended quantitative protein and calorie allowances for most healthy children, youths, and young adults of average size and activity in the United States. Note that adults require fewer calories than do young people of junior or senior high school age.

Children whose growth is impaired by malnutrition have exhibited considerable ability to catch up on diets that are high in calories and adequate in proteins. Prolonged and severe nutritional deprivation, however, may cause some permanent deficiencies in growth and in brain development. It is difficult to determine whether the mental retardation noted by a number of researchers results from undernutrition or from the poor social environments in which nutritionally deprived children are usually raised.

It is believed that improvements in nutrition over time are responsible for the worldwide trends toward increased height, weight, and earlier sexual maturation that have been observed. These trends now appear to be leveling off.

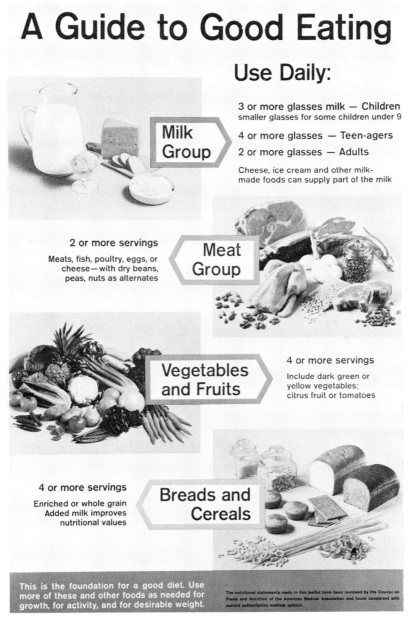

Fig. 13-2. Basic four food groups. (Courtesy National Dairy Council.)

Table 13-1. Recommended daily U.S. protein-calorie allowances by age and sex and for pregnancy and lactation

Sex	Age and size (pounds and inches)	Kilocalories	Protein (grams)
Children	4 to 6 (44, 44)	1,800	30
Children	7 to 10 (66, 54)	2,400	36
Males	11 to 14 (97, 63)	2,800	44
Females	11 to 14 (97, 62)	2,400	44
Males	15 to 18 (134, 69)	3,000	54
Females	15 to 18 (119, 65)	2,100	48
Males	23 to 50 (154, 69)	2,700	56
Females	23 to 50 (128, 65)	2,000	46
Pregnancy	Add	300	30
Lactating	Add	500	20

Adapted from Food and Nutrition Board: *Recommended dietary allowance,* ed. 8, Washington, D.C., 1974, National Academy of Sciences, National Research Council.

Socioeconomic characteristics and race. It is almost a truism that socioeconomic status is significantly associated with everything else. Although individual differences exist, middle- and upper-class children are significantly bigger, grow more rapidly, mature earlier, and score higher on all kinds of intelligence tests than do lower-class children. Socioeconomic status is usually measured in terms of parental education, income, and occupation. The poor and the less educated are less able than the affluent and better educated in the United States to provide adequate nutrition, decent housing, and medical care for their youngsters. In the United States, black youngsters are more likely than white youngsters to come from homes of low socioeconomic status and, as has been noted, belong to a culture that is different from that of whites. It is therefore difficult to distinguish genetic racial differences from socioeconomic and cultural differences, but it is important to the health and welfare of black youngsters to try to do so.

For example, comparisons of intelligence test results have consistently shown black youngsters to score lower than white ones, on the average. Recent studies of national samples of children showed, however, that while whites outperformed blacks on subtests of the Wechsler Intelligence Scale for Children, which were developed using only white children, black and white scores were essentially equal when controlled for family income and measured by a modification of the Goodenough-Harris (draw-a-person) test.* Another National Health Survey study of hematocrit levels, a test for anemia, revealed that black teenagers have lower levels than white. Careful and complex data analysis provided no grounds for concluding whether this difference was caused by racial and genetic, socioeconomic, cultural differences, or some combination of these factors.† A number of studies have revealed that black youngsters exceed whites in agility and general athletic performance, a fact that may be related to genetic differences.

Psychosocial influences. There is clear and convincing evidence that emotional deprivation retards both physical and intellectual growth. Very small babies need to be cuddled, and premature infants who are not fondled but who receive otherwise good quality care are retarded in growth compared with those who are thus stimulated.

*Health Services and Mental Health Administration: *Intellectual development of children,* DHEW Publication No. (HSM) 72-1012, Washington, D.C., 1971, U.S. Government Printing Office; and *Intellectual maturity of children,* DHEW Publication No. (HSM) 72-1095, Washington, D.C., 1972, U.S. Government Printing Office.
†Health Resources Administration: *Hematocrit values of youths 12-17 years,* DHEW Publication No. (HRA) 75-1628, Washington, D.C., 1970, U.S. Government Printing Office.

Older children whose parents give them toys, books, and love do far better in school than those whose parents neglect or abuse them. Although the psychophysical mechanisms by which the ill effects of deprivation occur are not understood, the presence of good parents in socioeconomically deprived homes may very well account, at least in part, for the many slum youngsters who achieve well in school and later life, physically, intellectually, and emotionally.

Physical activity. There is no evidence that physical activity or the lack of it has any significant influence on height. Those who are physically active tend to weigh less than those who are inactive, because active people store and maintain less fat. Activity yields not more muscle fibers but larger, heavier, and stronger ones. Activity improves respiratory and cardiac function and bone strength.

Physical activity, however, is not without its hazards to growth and development. Growing long bones such as those in the legs and arms are soft at the ends (epiphyses) where growth occurs. Jolts and jars incidental to activity can damage the epiphyses and halt or retard growth. Jolts and jars to the head can cause brain damage. Damage to joints as a result of either overexertion (as in baseball pitchers) or injury (as in football) is more likely to occur in growing individuals than in mature ones.

Illness. Illnesses tend to retard growth in relation to their severity. With slight illnesses the retardation is slight and tends to be overcome after recovery. Severe illnesses may result in more or less permanent decreases in stature. Rheumatic fever results in significant heart damage in some cases.

MEASUREMENT AND EVALUATION OF GROWTH AND DEVELOPMENT

The height, weight, intellectual achievement, and physical fitness of students in most schools in the United States are measured periodically to provide a basis for assessment of growth and development. Measurement of psychosocial development is rare, probably because of the fear of parental protests and the recognition that available instruments are not as valid, reliable, or as easy to interpret as measurements of physical and intellectual growth seem to be. Much of the difficulty lies in interpretation. We tend to evaluate the growth and development of individuals against *group* standards, which often are derived from study populations that are not representative of the whole population, and we assume that every youngster ought to equal or exceed the group average, which is a statistical impossibility.

The question of first importance to be answered in assessing growth and development is: Is this individual growing and developing? To answer it, we need only compare present measurements with previous ones. It is also useful to determine how much an individual deviates from the norms or averages of the age, and the sex and racial or ethnic group to which he or she belongs, but this troublesome question then arises: How much variation indicates that a problem probably exists? To this question, we have no firm answers.

Height and weight. Heights and weights are inaccurately measured in most schools, but if interest is delimited to whether or not a youngster has gained in height and weight over a year's time, some errors can be tolerated. Height is measured by means of a fixed standard, usually attached to the beam scale on which weights are measured. A movable crossarm attached at right angles to the standard is lowered through the hair until it just touches the crown of the scalp. Height is read directly from the standard. A T square should be used to test the angle because the instrument may become bent with use. Reasonably accurate measurement requires that the measurement be taken with shoes off and with the shoulders, buttocks, and heels pressed firmly against the upright. Accuracy of measurement can be increased by routinely scheduling measurements for the same time of day. Individuals are somewhat taller in the morning than they are in the afternoon.

Beam scales are much more accurate than spring scales, but they should be checked occasionally by use of standard weights. Ideally, subjects should be weighed naked, or nearly so. In practice, a reasonable compromise is to conduct weighing with shoes off. Weights should be taken at the same time of day and with the bladder empty.

Individual heights and weights, together with the dates taken and the birthdate, usually become a part of the health record and may be reviewed to determine whether or not growth is occurring.

Table 13-2. Weight range of boys and girls 6-17 years of age by single year of age and height*

Height in inches	6 years	7 years	8 years	9 years	10 years	11 years	12 years	13 years	14 years	15 years	16 years	17 years
Girls												
						Interquartile range of weight in pounds†						
Under 41.3	35-39											
41.3-43.2	40-45											
43.3-45.2	43-49	40-44										
45.3-47.2	48-54	43-49	43-52									
47.3-49.1	52-62	48-55	46-54	49-56								
49.2-51.1		52-63	52-62	53-62	52-58							
51.2-53.1		56-65	58-67	57-66	57-65	60-69						
53.2-55.1			64-77	64-77	62-77	64-78	58-71					
55.2-57.0			75-93	71-89	71-81	69-82	73-91	67-88				
57.1-59.0				73-102	78-94	76-94	78-94	84-97	80-105	93-116	99-120	88-101
59.1-61.0					82-99	84-106	86-104	86-104	94-118	98-116	101-119	98-118
61.1-63.0						94-122	95-119	97-119	102-123	102-122	107-124	107-127
63.1-65.0						102-134	104-126	105-126	107-132	111-133	114-135	111-127
65.1-66.9							111-132	115-136	115-136	122-145	118-148	122-144
67.0-68.9							112-181	107-144	124-155	126-158	128-147	122-145
69.0-70.9									127-142	119-156	136-178	132-166
71.0-72.8												
72.9-74.8												
74.9-76.8												
Boys												
41.3-43.2	37-41	—	—	—	—							
43.3-45.2	40-45	41-46	—	—	—							
45.3-47.2	44-50	44-50	43-49	—	—							
47.3-49.1	48-55	48-54	49-54	49-54	—							
49.2-51.1	53-60	53-60	53-60	53-61	—							
51.2-53.1	—	57-66	59-67	58-65	55-61	61-71						
53.2-55.1	—	63-71	64-76	63-74	58-66	65-75	67-76	64-77				
55.2-57.0	—	—	69-77	70-83	64-74	71-82	70-80	71-86				
57.1-59.0	—	—	—	71-103	70-80	77-91	79-90	80-91	87-93			
59.1-61.0	—	—	—	—	77-92	83-101	84-101	84-100	86-106	94-101		
61.1-63.0	—	—	—	—	81-95	94-120	92-111	92-113	92-113	103-125	98-120	106-127
63.1-65.0							99-123	103-128	105-124	103-124	106-128	116-136
65.1-66.9							108-132	109-131	114-137	117-135	116-141	124-148
67.0-68.9							132-146	118-148	121-145	125-148	127-148	131-158
69.0-70.9								132-155	129-154	132-153	134-160	136-162
71.0-72.8									144-170	142-173	142-169	144-173
72.9-74.8										139-186	154-199	155-178
74.9-76.8										153-227		150-199

From National Center for Health Statistics: *Facts of life and death,* DHEW Publication No. (HRA) 74-1222, Rockville, Md., 1974, Public Health Service, Health Resources Administration.
*Height in inches without shoes; weight in pounds, partially clothed. Values shown represent range of weight within which 50 percent of children of given height and age would fall. Approximately 25 percent would weigh less and 25 percent more than these values.
†The middle 50 percent of the weight range: $P_{75} - P_{25}$.

Much staff time can be saved by training and utilizing older students or adult volunteers to measure and record heights and weights. Such involvement probably has some educational value if it is preceded by instruction in the purposes as well as the techniques of measurement and recording.

Measurements can be compared with tables that give average height and weight-age-sex values (Table 13-2). The danger of this procedure is that unjustified concern may be aroused when an individual varies from group norms. Such tables are often out of date and do not take into account differences in body build or ethnicity. The use of such tables is therefore not recommended as a sole criterion for evaluating underweight or fatness.

More elaborate methods of measurement and recording are used in some schools. For example, calipers may be purchased to measure pelvic and chest widths in addition to height and weight and thus permit comparison of individuals with group norms that take body builds into account. Height and weight measurements may also be recorded on sex specific charts like those shown in Fig. 13-3. However, such procedures are time-consuming.

A relatively new technique for measuring body fat is available. This involves the measurement of skinfold thicknesses by use of special calipers and comparison of these measurements with recently computed sex-age-race norms and percentile ranks. The technique will be described and discussed in a later chapter.

Intellectual achievement. Numerous studies have led us to believe that middle-class learning ability, or ability to achieve high scores on intelligence or achievement tests, does not change significantly with maturation. Compared with others of one's sex, age, and ethnic group, one's percentile rank tends to remain about the same. It has been demonstrated that intellectual achievement is adversely affected by such environmental factors as early malnutrition, illness, lack of sensory stimulation, cultural differences

not taken into account in test construction, and the absence of hope that one can succeed. However, individuals exist who have overcome such deficits and whose IQ scores have increased dramatically.

As in the case of physical growth, we therefore expect healthy youngsters to learn as they mature, but neither to forge ahead of nor lag behind others in their group in intellectual achievement. When lags do occur, health appraisal devices should be used to determine if a health problem such as hearing loss or brain damage has occurred. An examination of the home-school environment may reveal the presence of such defects as a psychotic or abusive parent or teacher. Late bloomers exist who occasionally forge ahead of their last performance, but these, like those who lag behind, are rather rare.

One other use of intelligence or achievement testing is to identify students who may qualify for admission to special programs for gifted or retarded learners. Placement on the basis of test scores alone is not desirable, because they do not assess social abilities, which may enable rapid or slow learners to function acceptably in average classrooms.

Physical fitness. There are tests for the measurement of physical fitness in terms of either task performance or physiological functioning. Those now used in schools are usually of the task performance variety. For example, the testing program developed in the late 1960's by the President's Commission on Physical Fitness may be used to assess strength, flexibility, and agility by the ability of the individuals to perform such tasks as situps, pullups, and squat thrusts. Physiological tests such as the measurement of oxygen consumption during the performance of some standard exercise are usually used only in research work.

The President's Commission recommended that a progressive exercise program follow testing to increase fitness to a level appropriate to the developmental level of each child.

CHARACTERISTICS AND NEEDS OF CHILDREN AT DIFFERENT STAGES OF MATURATION

It is by first-hand observation of individual youngsters that we determine their stage of development, health, and educational needs. Observation is facilitated, however, by a knowledge of the general characteristics of typical children and young people at various stages in the course of their school years. There are appreciable changes in any 3-year period, and in any class some individuals will have grown or developed more than others. Also, age in years or grade in school are only rough measures of stages of development, but it is not feasible to assess the developmental age of each student more accurately by such available means as taking hand-wrist x-rays for comparison with national norms for ossification of epiphyses. For these reasons, it seems suitable to present the characteristics and needs of school-age youngsters by 3-year age and sex groups.

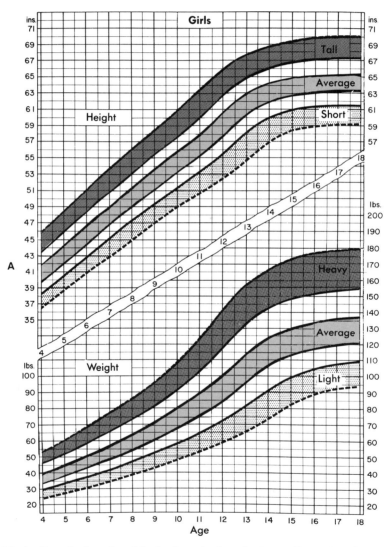

Fig. 13-3. A, Growth chart for girls. **B,** Growth chart for boys. Charts **A** and **B** are available from the American Medical Association and the National Education Association. (Courtesy Joint Committee on Health Problems in Education.)

Children 6 to 8 years of age
(grades 1 to 3)
Physical traits

Physical growth is slow and steady.

Front teeth are liable to be missing during this period.

Deciduous teeth are being replaced, and interest in teeth is increasing.

Eyes are still developing.

Many 6-year-olds are still farsighted, and muscles of accommodation fatigue easily.

Brain reaches approximately its full weight by the end of this period.

The youngster tires easily and recovers quickly.

Breathing begins to be less diaphragmatic and more costal.

Sleep requirements gradually decline.

Posture is likely to be poor, especially in tall children.

Movement tends to involve the whole body.

Children are clumsy with their hands but enjoy cutting, pasting, painting, drawing, and handling simple tools.

At age 6, childhood diseases and infections are prevalent, but they gradually become less common.

The eustachian tubes are short, wide, and straight, and middle-ear infections occur.

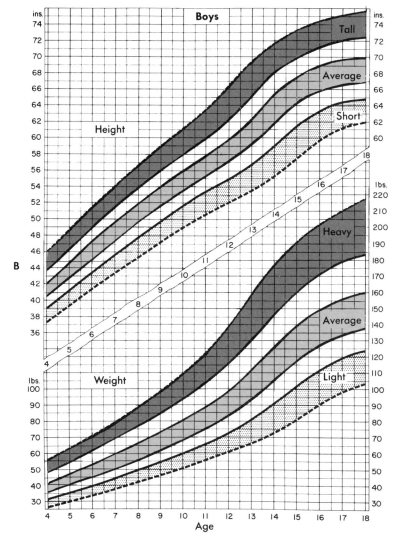

Fig. 13-3, cont'd. For legend see opposite page.

ntal traits

iildren like riddles and slapstick jokes.

ey are interested in specific information but not in generalizations.

They enjoy simple tasks within their capacities.

They like repetition.

Attention span is short.

Memory is strengthening.

Questions about sex differences are asked.

Dramatic play and make-believe comic books and animal stories are enjoyed.

Imagination is active.

Children love pets.

They like to produce well-made objects.

This is sometimes called the eraser age.

Social and emotional traits

Children are more self-centered than group-centered.

Being fair is very important. They are tolerant of others.

Children want to feel that they have done right, and wrongdoing leaves them unhappy and worried.

They are boisterous, energetic, and daring.

Praise is important to them.

Interest in competition awakens.

Their sense of responsibilities is growing.

Gradually these children begin to accept blame and to apologize.

Children are interested in growing.

Cleanliness is not important to them.

Boys and girls are interested in the same things.

They imitate their parents and teachers.

Health needs and desirable developmental experiences

Children need activities for the large muscles and practice in improving posture.

Vigorous games and outdoor play with running, chasing, hunting, throwing, catching, and climbing are desirable, as are singing games and rhythms.

Boys and girls play together.

Daytime rest is helpful.

Children profit by dramatic play and opportunity for creativity, such as fingerpainting or clay modeling.

Habits of cleanliness may need improvement.

Work periods should be short and ample time given for any task.

There is need for opportunity to develop leadership through various social situations.

Opportunities to agree or disagree in a desirable manner are needed.

Children need safety protection and instruction.

These children need expanding opportunities for oral self-expression.

Good eating habits should be encouraged.

Some children may need to learn to like new food.

Understanding and friendship on the part of the teacher are of great importance.

There is a need to begin education about sex and family life.

Children 9 to 11 years of age
(grades 4 to 6)
Physical traits

Children tend to be physically active, working and playing to the peak of capacity.

Slouching posture is frequent.

Blood vessels increase in size, but heart remains small.

Replacement of primary teeth continues.

Growing bones are easily injured.

Proficiency in physical skill is increasing.

Girls begin to grow more rapidly than boys.

Motor coordination and eye-hand coordination are increasing.

Different parts of the body may begin to show uneven growth.

Functions of the eye are becoming well established, and the eye adjusts for both near and far vision more readily.

Brain has stopped increasing in size.

Girls begin to reach menarche.

Mental traits

Attention is given to subjects of interest for longer periods of time.

There is increased interest in constructive projects.

Interest in books about adventure, science, nature, and home life is increasing.

Interest is increasing in exploring, experimenting, and in how things are made and how they work (including the human body).

Memory is high.

Ability to budget time is increasing.

Ability to plan and work with a group in improved.

Social and emotional traits

Children are still self-assertive and apparently selfish, but tendency to cooperate in games appears.

Children are interested in the group, team spirit, and peer approval.

They enjoy competing and matching skills with others.

They desire status in the gang or club and are willing to assume more responsibility.

Some antagonisms toward the opposite sex appear.

Emotions are becoming more stable.

Special friends are likely to be chosen among the child's own sex.

The sexes have different recreational interests.

Increased independence appears when away from the family group.

Hero worship appears.

Children are anxious to be chosen and to do well.

Sex modesty is characteristic.

Health needs and desirable developmental experiences

A balanced program of big-muscle activities and quiet activities is needed.

Children need more formal games of great physical activity involving chasing, hunting, and throwing; these are such games as prisoner's base, three-deep and tag games, which call for individual speed and skill but not great endurance.

Opportunities to practice good health habits should be supplied.

Boys and girls should have separate play areas.

Activities should involve cooperative or team play and should give individual satisfaction.

Time periods to complete group projects should be sufficiently long.

Opportunities for creative expression should be given.

There is a need for guidance in setting personal goals and evaluating achievements.

Opportunities to discuss social and personal problems, to make decisions, and to be independent are needed.

Learning for life-long memory should be provided.

Safety precautions are necessary.

Children need opportunities to learn and use social skills.

Acceptance by the group is important.

Access to a wealth of biographical and other reading materials should be made available.

Children should be protected against the danger of becoming overfatigued.

They need guidance in problem-solving and critical thinking.

The emotional climate should be conducive to the discussion of personal problems.

Children need opportunities for success and achievement.

They need opportunities to collect, identify, and classify objects.

Attention to body mechanics is necessary.

The need for dental care is universal.

Children need checks of vision and hearing.

Sex education should be provided regarding developmental changes.

Youth 12 to 14 years of age (grades 7 to 9)

Physical traits

This is the age of puberty, characterized by rapid acceleration of bodily growth.

Heart and lungs are developing rapidly.

Appetites are often enormous and dietary excesses are common.

Difficulties with elimination may appear.

At age 12 the eyes reach maximum growth and acuity.

Arms and legs are out of proportion to the trunk. Awkwardness occurs.

Skin problems are common.

Tooth decay is common.

Bones and ligaments are not yet strong enough to withstand heavy pressure.

Girls are maturing more rapidly and are bigger than boys.

Postural defects are more obvious.

Endurance is small, and children are easily fatigued.

Girls are more precise in their movements than boys.

Reproductive organs are growing, and secondary sex characteristics are appearing.

Mental traits

Pupils enjoy working on concrete problems.

Ability to apply scientific problem-solving approaches is increasing.

Wider variations in abilities and capacities appear.

Attention span continues to increase.

Charts, maps, and diagrams are increasingly useful.

Reading rates approach the adult level.

Desire for creative expression is growing.

Interest in problems of human relationships is increasing.

Social and emotional traits

Daydreaming is common.

Emotions are somewhat unstable.

Confusion and timidity may appear in social situations.

There may be rapid changes in mood.

Frustration may grow out of conflict with parents or peers.

Hostility to adults may appear.

Interest in team play and competitive games is increasing.

Positive reactions to ideals are strong if properly presented.

Fears and anger are common.

The approval of the peer group is becoming more important and that of adults less important.

There is a desire to conform in language, dress, and manner to peer culture.

Hero worship is general.

Friends are mostly of the same sex.

Interest in personal appearance is increasing.

Interest in the opposite sex is beginning. Some pregnancies occur.

There is increased interest in team play and competitive games.

Health needs and desirable developmental experiences

Competitive games involving quickness and skill and only moderate fatigue or emotional stress are desirable, such as relay races, swimming, rowing, bicycling, touch football, softball, field hockey, tennis, and volleyball.

Group sports need supervision.

Eyes, ears, and teeth may require attention.

Much rest is necessary.

Privacy and independence are needed.

Sound group guidance is important.

Practice is needed in selecting an adequate diet, in leading and following, and in improving body mechanics.

Youth need reassurance that they are normal and to understand growth and development.

They need to express, examine, and learn to control emotions.

Specific education regarding VD, sex, and drugs is essential.

Youth 15 to 17 years of age (grades 10 to 12)

Physical traits

Physical coordination becomes adequate.

Heart is becoming larger.

Growth is nearing completion.
Trunk increases in proportion to length of legs.
Skeletal growth is complete at ages 15 to 17 for girls and at ages 17 to 19 for boys.
Endurance and strength increase rapidly.
Graceful and controlled movement is possible.
Posture is improving for most students.
Acne is a common emotional problem.
Appetites are hearty, but fad dieting is common.

Mental traits

There is expanding interest in the exact and behavioral sciences.
Students possess increased capacity in organizing their own activities.

Social and emotional development

Emotional problems increase.
These students tend to be idealistic, inconsistent, sensitive, and insecure.
They resent restraint and orders.
They need approval.
Interest in the opposite sex and in grooming is increased.
The peer group is a dominant force.
Accident rate is very high.
They feel a growing independence from parental rule.
They often have a critical attitude toward parents and teachers.
Pregnancy, VD, too early marriage, and drug and alcohol use are common problems.

Health needs and desirable developmental experiences

Regular and vigorous physical exercise is necessary.
Competitive sports including baseball, soccer, football, basketball, tennis, golf, volleyball, swimming, softball, and field and track are desirable.
Individual guidance and approval are required.
Help is needed in developing self-discipline, orderliness, self-reliance, self-esteem, self-confidence, adaptability, and a sound philosophy of life.
Fine coeducational activities such as social dancing, volleyball, tennis, and badminton provide wholesome recreation.
Hiking and camping are desirable.
Safety education including driver education is needed.
Education for family life is essential.

SIGNS OF HEALTH AND ILLNESS

Children who conform to the growth and development characteristics listed above are likely to be healthy. Children who deviate from these patterns may either be ill or early or late developers. In addition, a healthy youngster exhibits vitality, good skin and muscle tone, and whatever skin color is normal when he or she is healthy.

On the other hand, chronic fatigue and listlessness, and abnormal skin tone and color denote probable illness. In the following chapters specific physical defects and illnesses are considered in some detail. The conditions and actions listed below are some of the danger signals that teachers commonly observe and report in working with supposedly well children:

Eyes
Blinks frequently
Rubs eyes
Eyes water
Holds books too close or too far
Squints to see book or chalkboard
Crossed eyes
Inflamed eyes or crusted lids

Ears
Picks at ears
Discharge from ears
Frequent earaches
Fails to hear questions

Nose and mouth
Mouth breathing
Chronic signs of a cold
Sore throat

Behavior
Restlessness or hyperactivity that is inappropriate to stage of development
Listlessness
Social or intellectual behavior that is inappropriate to stage of development
Poor food habits
Shy, withdrawn behavior
Stuttering or other speech defects
Emotional disturbances
Antisocial behavior
Behavior that is too good

General conditions
Failure to learn
Tires easily for age
Poor posture for age
Skin rashes
Extremely fat or thin
Poor coordination for age

Teacher observations provide information that will be helpful to the school nurse, school physician, or parent in the absence of school health service professionals. They are not diagnoses; they do not prove that something is wrong, only that it might be. However, early detection of illnesses, followed by diagnosis and treatment if indicated, may prevent disruptions in growth and development that might otherwise result.

FACILITATING GROWTH AND DEVELOPMENT

Two school programs, food service and physical activity, facilitate growth and development directly to some extent if properly conducted. It is not to be expected that these programs will fully compensate for genetic, home, or community deficiencies. Their positive effects are not always readily apparent after short periods of participation in them. Their goal is to help establish patterns of dietary and exercise behavior that will promote not only growth and development but also positive health in adult life.

Food services. Through participation in the U.S. Department of Agriculture's federal-state programs, or independently of them, schools may provide breakfast or milk, which may be accompanied by fruit or crackers, as a midmorning or midafternoon snack in addition to the traditional noon lunch. Some schools offer all three services, others serve one or two of them, and still others serve no food at all. The present purpose of these programs is to provide both nutrition and education—education in nutrition, etiquette, and the importance of relaxed eating and cleanliness. Again, these purposes are achieved in some schools but not in others. Some effort is required to integrate school nutrition education with feeding programs, but it has been and can be done.*

Integration requires the provision of opportunity for students and staff to study menus and to participate in menu planning within Department of Agriculture guidelines. It requires their involvement in making and keeping the eating place physically clean and socially pleasant, whether it be cafeteria or classroom. It means providing opportunity for students to taste and learn about the values of new foods and hope-

fully to enjoy them. Early elementary children enjoy preparing and eating samples of new foods. Upper elementary children are ready to learn why a new food is nutritionally desirable. Junior and senior high school students are ready to learn relationships between specific nutrients and health.

In one controlled study, the nutritional status of children in two school districts was assessed in the fall and again in the spring. Those in the district that served both breakfast and lunch improved much more in nutritional status than did those in the district that served lunch and midmorning milk.* In another study the investigator was unable to show any significant difference in height, weight, or hematocrit levels between students who participated in the school lunch program and those who did not. He noted, however, that the results may have been affected by absenteeism.†

A study of breakfast practices among senior high school students in El Paso revealed that half the students came to school with either no breakfast or a poor one and that a majority of the breakfasts that were eaten lacked a vitamin C source and/or milk. Too late, not hungry, and didn't like the food served were reasons commonly given for no breakfast or a light one. A majority said that they were hungry before 11 AM.‡ A Massachusetts survey that included grades 1 to 12 revealed that breakfasts that were classed as good were eaten by only 5% of the elementary children and 3% of those in senior high school. Those eating no breakfast at all increased from 4% in the early elementary grades to 29% in senior high school.§ The Iowa Breakfast

---

*Sinacore, J. S., and Harrison, G.: The place of nutrition in the health curriculum, Am. J. Public Health **61:**2282-2289, Nov. 1971.

*Emmons, L., Hayes, M., and Call, D. L.: A study of school feeding programs, II: effects on children with different economic and nutritional needs, J. Am. Diet. Assoc. **61:**268, Sept. 1972.
†Paige, D. M.: The school feeding program: an underachiever? J. Sch. Health **42:**392-395, Sept. 1972.
‡Harris, W. H.: A survey of breakfast eaten by high school students, J. Sch. Health **40:**323-325, June 1970.
§Callahan, D. L.: Focus on nutrition: you can't teach a hungry child, School Food Journal, Sept. 1971, p. 25.

Studies produced evidence that an adequate breakfast resulted in better attitudes and better school performance.* In another study, representatives of schools participating in the USDA breakfast program reported that the breakfasts served at school resulted in decreased numbers of students who showed physical signs of hunger (headaches, stomach pains), improved classroom performance and behavior, and decreased absenteeism and tardiness.†

Thus, the preponderance of the evidence is on the side of a school feeding program that includes breakfast as well as lunch. None of the studies cited attempted to demonstrate the value of midmorning or afternoon snacks. However, the milk snack may well have real educational values, and it may serve to prevent the pangs of hunger that interfere with schoolwork and send many students to the health service. It may also add to the comfort of those students who are subjected to long bus rides to and from school.

In addition to its use as a snack food, milk may also be served to supplement lunches that are brought from home. The one problem associated with milk as either a snack or as a part of the breakfast or lunch program is that significant numbers of students, most of them black, are deficient in lactase, a body enzyme essential to the digestion of milk sugar. When these youngsters drink milk, they suffer from gas, bloating, and diarrhea. They can, however, tolerate fermented milk products (cheese or yogurt), which supply essentially the same nutrients as milk.‡

Program requirements. The basic USDA

school breakfast program regulations require that schools*:

A. Operate the breakfast program on a nonprofit basis for all children regardless of race, color or national origin.
B. Serve breakfasts that . . . include: milk, fruit, full strength fruit or vegetable juice, bread or cereal. Schools are encouraged to serve a meat or meat alternate as often as possible.
C. Provide breakfasts free or at a reduced price to children whom local school authorities find are unable to pay the full price. Children getting free or reduced-price breakfasts must not be identified or discriminated against in any way.

National school lunch program regulations require that lunches also be provided free or at reduced rates to the poor and that if lunch is offered by the school, it be offered to all students. In addition, lunches must conform to the Type A pattern; that is, they must include milk; meat or a meat substitute; vegetables, fruits, or both; and bread and butter or margarine. On the average, lunches are expected to meet one third of the recommended dietary allowances established by the National Research Council of the National Academy of Sciences.

Innovations. Many schools, especially those in older buildings, have no facilities for food preparation and service. Innovations designed to make food service possible in such schools include central kitchens and satellite feeding, and the use of frozen or canned entrees. In satellite or central feeding, lunches are prepared in a central kitchen, which may or may not be located in a school. The lunches are then either delivered hot or reheated in microwave ovens or by other means in satellite schools and are thus served in much the same manner as meals served on commercial airline flights. Frozen or canned entrees are also heated by whatever means available and served with fruit, milk, or other items. The

---

*Cereal Institute: *A complete summary of the Iowa breakfast studies,* Chicago, 1962, The Institute, pp. 57-59.
†The Food Research and Action Center: *If we had ham, we could have ham and eggs . . . if we had eggs,* New York, 1972, The Center.
‡Paige, D. M., Bayless, T. M., and Graham, G. C.: Milk programs: helpful or harmful to Negro children? Am. J. Public Health **62:**1486-1488, Nov. 1972, Paige, D. M., and Graham, G. C.: School milk programs and Negro children, J. Sch. Health **44:**8-10, Jan. 1974.

---

*Food and Nutrition Service: Handbook for volunteers: child nutrition programs, U.S. Department of Agriculture Publication No. FNS 10, Washington, D.C., 1970, U.S. Government Printing Office.

equivalent of a Type A lunch is thus provided.

Another problem has been that of trying to get nutritious food past finicky taste buds and down reluctant throats. One response has been the development of "engineered foods." For example, a cream-filled cake was developed and approved by the USDA, which together with milk meets the same nutritional requirements of the breakfast program.

The advantage of such innovations must be weighed against their disadvantages. The preparation of foods elsewhere than in the individual building is efficient, economical, and permits food service in buildings that lack facilities. On the other hand, opportunities for student involvement in the program and ability to offer foods acceptable to cultural or ethnic groups are limited. Engineered foods and the nutrients that they contain are eaten, but their use is likely to

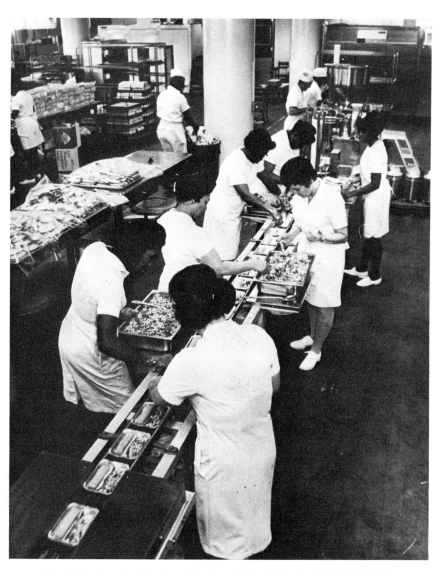

Fig. 13-4. A central kitchen. (Courtesy School District of Philadelphia.)

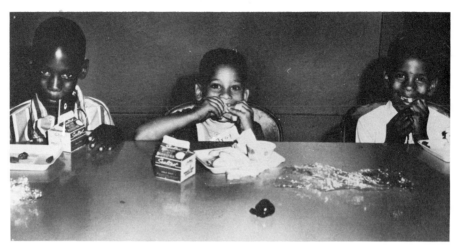

Fig. 13-5. Satellite feeding of students. (Courtesy School District of Philadelphia.)

teach students that a piece of cake and a glass of milk constitute a nutritious breakfast, which, of course, they do not.

Unmet needs. Hiemstra* has noted that it is possible to serve a lunch that meets Type A standards but fails to provide sufficient iron or other nutrients. Bowden† points out that although American male adolescents eat diets that are better balanced nutritionally than those of their female peers, athletic training tables promote food habits that foster obesity and possibly heart disease in later life, because of their over-emphasis on meat and eggs. When fad dieting, especially vegetarianism, is practiced without knowledge of how to achieve balance in such a diet, the life and health of those (primarily females) who are prone to such fads are endangered. Both males and females tend to substitute nonnutritious snacks for meals.

Bowden goes on to suggest that high schools improve nutrition education by making it less repetitive, by making it coeducational, and by emphasizing the interrelationship between food and physical activity.

*Hiemstra, S. J.: Nutritional standards in school food service, J. Sch. Health **42:**317-319, June 1972.
†Bowden, N. J.: Food patterns and food needs of adolescents, J. Sch. Health **34:**165-168, March 1973.

In addition, nutritious snacks can be substituted for empty-calorie snacks in school vending machines. The rights of vegetarians to adhere to their beliefs must be respected, but guidance can be given in how to achieve balance by the addition of eggs and milk or by using an appropriate variety of vegetable protein sources.

Hopefully, the movement toward certification of athletic coaches in the United States will eventually result in improved nutrition for athletes. In the meantime, schools should recognize that many if not most coaches only think they know something about nutrition, and they should insist that nutritional advice to athletes and training table menus be made the responsibility of a home economist or dietitian rather than the coach.

Activity programs. School-centered physical activity programs include supervised or unsupervised play periods before and after school and at recesses, formal physical education programs, and competitive intramural and interscholastic athletics. In addition, school facilities and personnel may be utilized in the conduct of community recreation and athletic programs. If properly planned and conducted, these programs provide not only the physical exercise youngsters need for healthy growth and development and good posture but also develop skills and activity practices that can contribute to health protection and promotion throughout life. Poorly planned and conducted programs increase the likelihood of physical injury and may encourage the development of the warped value systems evident in the atrocious behavior of many adult spectators at athletic events.

Unorganized activities before and during the school day provide opportunity for youngsters to work off some of their need for movement and undoubtedly result in improved classroom conduct. For safety's sake, supervision by trained adults should be provided. It is desirable that younger and older students be segregated and that space and equipment suitable to each age group be provided. The probable benefits are well worth the cost if the danger of expensive lawsuits arising from accidental injuries is considered.

Physical education programs. The primary purposes of physical education are to develop movement skills and to introduce students to a variety of activities from which each individual may select those that he or she finds most appealing. Physical education classes alone cannot provide all the activity that youngsters need.

At the early elementary grade levels (through grade 3) big muscles are developing. Short spurts of vigorous activity need to be provided in view of the lack of stamina and the short attention spans characteristic of youngsters at this age. These youngsters need to learn and practice running, climbing, throwing, catching, and jumping. They are not yet ready for complex, highly organized, competitive games. Most enjoy fundamental rhythm activities such as skipping, games that combine songs and movement, and very simple dances. These boys and girls share all activity interests, are the same size, and will play together without difficulty.

Upper elementary youngsters are generally ready to increase skill levels, to tolerate longer periods of vigorous activity, and to become interested in competitive games. Boys and girls tend to segregate themselves,

however, and at about the fifth or sixth grade levels girls begin to be noticeably larger than boys. It is possible to bring boys and girls together for some activities while permitting them to pursue their sex-specific interests on other occasions. In junior and senior high school, major emphasis should be placed on learning lifetime activities such as swimming, social dancing, bowling, skating, golf, and tennis. At these higher grades, interest in developing heterosexual relationships can serve to motivate physical education class participation if coeducational classes are conducted.

Many youngsters present medical excuses from physical education activities in the form of notes from their personal physicians. The real reasons behind many of these notes include overprotectiveness on the part of the parents and the failure of physical educators to provide a wide variety of activities suitable to the needs and interests of every child. Given a suitable range of activities that encompasses quiet games, more vigorous activities suitable for individuals who are temporarily or permanently handicapped in any way, and activities suitable for individuals with a wide range of skill levels, there is no reason why such excuses need to be accepted at all. Adaptive physical education programs of this kind require adequate staff and facilities and interpretation of the program to health care professionals and parents. The message to be delivered is: We *do not* accept medical excuses from physical activity classes. We *do* accept medical advice about the kinds of activities suitable for individual students, and we will provide such activities.

Athletics. Unfortunately, many if not most schools and school systems pour funds, staff time, facilities, and equipment into a few interscholastic sports in which only the talented few can participate. Instead, emphasis should first be placed on a wide variety of intramural and interscholastic sports in which resources are utilized for the benefit of all children and young people. Desirable program guidelines have been formulated for competitive athletic programs for children of elementary school age, most if not all of which are appropriate for secondary school programs also.* Included among these guidelines are:

1. Proper physical conditioning of participants
2. Competent teaching and supervision of the sport
3. Modification of the sport, equipment, and facilities to the maturity level of the participants
4. Suitable and properly fitted protective equipment
5. Matching of participants by size, skill, and physical maturation
6. Safe, well-kept facilities
7. Periodic medical appraisal of participants
8. Presence or ready availability of medical care during practice sessions as well as games
9. Established policies and procedures for the care of injuries
10. Limitation of participation to those in the upper elementary grades or above
11. Parental permission for participation
12. Avoidance of excessive publicity, promotion, participation in play-offs, inappropriate spectator behavior, and similar pressure-producing activities

Most authorities agree that boxing has no place in any school program at any level. The objective of boxing is to injure one's opponent, and the injuries frequently include brain concussions. Many authorities hold that sports that include high risk of collision, such as football, hockey, and soccer, are best restricted to well-matured senior high school students to minimize the risk of epiphysial injury. Peewee baseball poses risks to the immature throwing arm joints of young pitchers, and epiphysial injuries may result from sliding into base. For

young players, touch or flag football, played on a shortened field and with time periods reduced in number and duration, represents a reasonable substitute for the conventional game. If the use of any one pitcher is limited to two innings per game and sliding into bases is eliminated, then baseball can be suitably modified for young players. As it is now conducted in the United States, Little League baseball must be condemned for its win-at-all-costs attitude as well as its attendant risk of injury.

QUESTIONS FOR STUDY AND DISCUSSION

1. Define the concepts: growth, development, maturation, pubescence, and adolescence.
2. What are some of the ways in which children differ from adults?
3. What are some of the ways in which healthy children of the same age and sex differ?
4. Equate Erikson's two stages of psychosocial development that occur during the school years to the approximate grade levels during which they occur. What are the implications of these two stages for school health and health education?
5. State the approximate age parameters of the adolescent growth spurt for boys and girls. What are the implications of growth spurt differences for school health and health education?
6. List the factors that affect growth and development and describe the nature and effects of each factor.
7. Describe methods cited of measuring growth and development, and evaluate the usefulness of each in school programs. If possible, demonstrate correct ways of measuring height and weight.
8. Describe the characteristics and needs of typical boys and girls at each 3-year school-age group.
9. What common observable signs indicate possible problems of the eyes, ears, nose and mouth, behavior, or other conditions? What is the significance of teacher observation of such signs to growth and development?
10. Describe the nature and purposes of each of the present U. S. Department of Agriculture school feeding programs. What are the effects of these programs? What federal program requirements exist?
11. Describe and evaluate recent innovations in school feeding programs.
12. Evaluate a school feeding program that you have experienced against the guidelines stated or implied in the text. How would you change the program to improve it in terms of the nutritional and educational needs of students and staff?

*American Association for Health, Physical Education, and Recreation: *Desirable athletic competition for children of elementary school age,* Washington, D.C., 1968, The Association, pp. iii-viii.

13. List desirable features of school physical activity programs cited in the text. Add to these lists other desirable features that you consider likely to facilitate growth and development and lifetime activity. Use the list to evaluate a school program known to you.

REFERENCES

American Association for Health, Physical Education, and Recreation: *Desirable athletic competition for children of elementary school age,* Washington, D.C., 1968, The Association.

Andrews, G., Saurborn, J., and Schneider, E.: *Physical education for today's boys and girls,* Boston; 1960, Allyn & Bacon, Inc.

Bucher, C. A.: *Foundations of physical education,* ed. 6, St. Louis, 1972, The C. V. Mosby Co.

Eisner, V., and Callan, L. B.: *Dimensions of school health,* Springfield, Ill., 1974, Charles C Thomas, Publisher.

Erikson, E. H.: *Childhood and society,* ed. 2, New York, 1963, Norton, W. W. & Co., Inc.

Krogman, W. M.: *Child growth,* Ann Arbor, 1972, The University of Michigan Press.

National Committee on School Health Policies: *Suggested school health policies,* Chicago, 1966, American Medical Association.

Nemir, A., and Schaller, W. E.: *The school health program,* ed. 4, Philadelphia, 1975, W. B. Saunders Co.

U.S. Clinical Research Centers Branch: *How children grow,* DHEW Publication No. (NIH) 73-166, Washington, D.C., 1972, U.S. Government Printing Office.

Wallace, H. M., Gold, E. M., and Lis, E. F.: *Maternal and child health practices: problems, resources, and methods of delivery,* Springfield, Ill., 1973, Charles C Thomas, Publisher.

Wheatley, G. M., and Hallock, G. T.: *Health observation of school children,* ed. 3, New York, 1965, McGraw-Hill, Inc.

CHAPTER 14

❧ Eyes, ears, and learning disabilities

Some children and young people have difficulty learning because they do not see, hear, or speak well; others have difficulty because they have a variety of other problems characterized as learning disabilities. Styes, conjunctivitis, and earaches cause discomfort. Defective color vision may be vocationally handicapping. This chapter deals with the nature of these kinds of problems and with the helpful things that can be done about them through school health and health education.

EYE PROBLEMS

Eye problems encountered among school-age children and youth include not only refractive errors such as near-sightedness and astigmatism but also crossed eyes, a variety of inflammations, and eye injuries. Each of these problem categories are considered in this section.

Problems of visual acuity. Recent National Health Survey vision tests revealed that about three fourths of the 6- through 11-year-olds in the United States have normal (20/20) or better distance vision and that a similar proportion has normal or better near vision. About 70% of the 12- to 17-year-olds have normal or better distance vision, and 84% of them have normal or better near vision. About 15% of the children and 12% of the youth have moderate to severe eye-muscle imbalance, that is, their eyes do not track properly.* Some of

*U.S. Health Service and Mental Health Administration: *Binocular visual acuity of children,* DHEW Publication No. (HSM) 72-1031, Washington, D.C., 1972, U.S. Government Printing Office; U.S. Health Service and Mental Health Administration: *Visual acuity of youths 12-17 years, United States,* DHEW Publication No. (HSM) 73-1609, Washington, D.C., 1973, U.S. Government Printing Office.

those with less than normal vision will function adequately whether they are treated or not, but many will benefit from the use of glasses or other forms of treatment.

The most common specific problems of this type encountered among school-age children and youth are hyperopia, myopia, astigmatism, strabismus resulting in dim vision, and color vision deficiency.

Hyperopia usually results from the eyeball being too short from lens to retina. The focused image falls behind the retina instead of on it, and the perceived image is blurred (Fig. 14-1). Most infants are born hyperopic, and most outgrow the problem as the eyeball becomes rounder with age. This developmental trend is consistent with the improvement observed in near vision acuity from childhood to youth in the National Health Survey data previously cited. Many individuals remain hyperopic throughout life, however. Individuals who are hyperopic attempt to accommodate to their problem by using the ciliary muscles to adjust the crystalline lens of the eyes (Fig. 14-2). Such accommodation is easier in childhood when the mucles are stronger and the lens more elastic than in later life. Some succeed; but the greater the hyperopia, the greater the effort required to accommodate, and the greater the fatigue that results from attempts to read books or perform other near vision tasks. In addition to lens accommodation, hyperopic persons tend to adjust to visual tasks by holding the book or other near work at a greater than usual distance from their eyes. Thus, students with hyperopia tend to complain of blurred vision and of tired eyes after reading or performing other close work a short time, and they hold

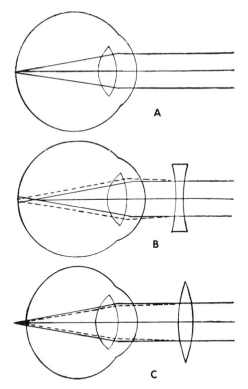

Fig. 14-1. A, The normal, or emmetropic, eye is of the proper depth, and the image forms upon the retina. **B,** The nearsighted, or myopic, eyeball is too long, and a concave lens is needed to make the image fall on the retina. **C,** The farsighted, or hyperopic, eyeball is too short, and a convex lens is needed to make the image fall on the retina.

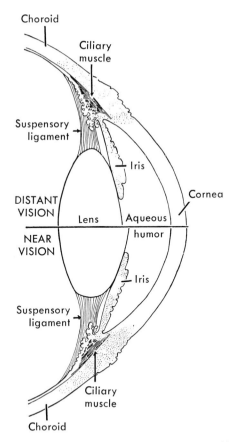

Fig. 14-2. Diagram illustrating the changes taking place during accommodation in the eye. (From Turner, C. E.: *Personal and community health,* St. Louis, 1967, The C. V. Mosby Co.)

visual tasks at a greater than usual distance from the eyes. Extreme hyperopia sometimes results in crossing of the eyes. Those with hyperopia do not necessarily see better than others at a distance, but hyperopic individuals see better at far distances (120 feet or more) than they do at close range.

Not all hyperopic youngsters require corrective lenses, but many are relieved of fatigue, crossed eyes, and discomfort by use of convex (plus sphere) lenses that are prescribed by an eye specialist. Whether the corrective lenses need to be worn at all times or only when reading depends on the extent and nature of the problem. Youngsters with uncorrected hyperopia are not helped by placing them near the blackboard. They are helped, however, by the large type characteristic of books designed for children of early elementary age. It is not uncommon for a child who enters school with hyperopia to outgrow the condition, acquire normal or better (emmetropic) vision, and then proceed to myopia at some time during the elementary school years.

Myopia is the opposite of hyperopia in many ways. Instead of the eyeball being too short from lens to retina, it is too long, and the focal point of the light rays falls in the front of the retina, thus producing blurred vision when viewing distant objects. Myopic individuals hold their books close to their eyes, choose to sit near chalkboards and television sets, and may squint in an effort to see distant objects. Reading and other close work is not uncomfortable for them;

they tend to prefer reading to playing ball. Myopia tends to appear during the school years and to get worse instead of better with age. Corrective lenses are concave (Fig. 14-1) and appear thick. Corrective lenses do not make the basic myopia either better or worse, but they do wonders for the distant vision of myopic youngsters. Many myopic youngsters choose to wear their lenses only for distant viewing and to take them off when reading or drawing, while others prefer to wear them all the time. This practice does no harm. The purpose of the lenses is to improve visual comfort and efficiency.

Astigmatism is usually caused by an unequal curvature in the cornea, the rather tough outer window of the eye (Fig. 14-2), and sometimes of the lens. With this inequality one cannot see vertical and horizontal lines clearly at the same time, even by using the ciliary muscles to accommodate.

There are three types of astigmatism. In *hyperopic astigmatism* the focal points of the vertical and horizontal planes are behind the retina, but one is closer to the retina than the other. In *myopic astigmatism* both points are in front of the retina, again at unequal distances from it. In *mixed astigmatism* the focal point of one plane is in front and the other behind the retina. The strain of attempted accommodation by use of the ciliary muscles leads to the same symptoms of fatigue associated with reading as are experienced by those with hyperopia.

Most persons have some degree of astigmatism, but most do not require correction. When the astigmatism is severe enough to require correction, the condition may cause youngsters to dislike reading and to develop dimness of vision. It is therefore important to identify and refer those most likely to require correction before or during grades 1 to 3. Eye specialists prescribe a combination of lens types to correct the problem.

Strabismus, sometimes referred to as crossed eyes or squint, is caused by an imbalance in the strength of one or more of the opposing muscle pairs that turn or posi-

tion the eyes. Imbalance may cause the eyes to turn inward (esophoria) or outward (exophoria). Strabismus is important not only because it interferes with binocular vision but, more important, because it leads, in some cases, to a condition called amblyopia ex anopsia, or lazy eye blindness, if it is not detected and corrected early in life. This dimness of vision in one eye results from suppression of perception of images emanating from it in the brain in an effort to adjust to poor binocular vision.

Amblyopia ex anopsia can be prevented by early and adequate treatment of strabismus, preferably beginning before the child enters school or shortly thereafter. If left until later, treatment may fail either to prevent or correct amblyopia and may have only cosmetic value. One treatment method involves patching the eye in which vision is better in order to force use of the eye in which vision is poor. The stronger muscle of the imbalanced opposing pair may be surgically weakened to correct the imbalance. Glasses may be prescribed for some children to correct any refractive error in the unpatched eye. Eye exercises may be prescribed in some cases. The choice of the treatment methods to be used in a particular case should be dictated by the professional judgment of the eye specialist rather than by parental or child preference. The most commonly used method is a combination of glasses and patching.

Color vision deficiencies are sex-linked hereditary traits. National Health Survey data reveal a prevalence of red-green deficiency of 7% to 7.5% among boys and less than 1% among girls in the United States. Less than 1% have blue-yellow deficiencies. Racial differences are insignificant.* Such deficiencies are not treatable;

*U.S. Health Service and Mental Health Administration: *Color vision deficiencies in children, United States,* DHEW Publications No. (HSM) 73-1600, Washington, D.C., 1972, U.S. Government Printing Office; U.S. Health Service and Mental Health Administration, *Color vision deficiencies in youths 12-17 years of age, United States,* DHEW Publications No. (HRA) 74-1616, Washington, D.C., 1970, U.S. Government Printing Office.

the victims and their teachers must learn to live with them, but they do limit vocational choices. Lampe and his associates* have found no significant difference in the academic achievement of pupils who are color deficient and those who are not.

Detection of visual acuity problems

Observations. Evidence of possible problems of visual acuity that may be observed by teachers, nurses, or parents include:

Holding a book too near or too far when reading.

Not seeing distant objects, such as material on the chalkboard, clearly.

Crossing eyes.

Squinting or frowning in attempting to see.

Rubbing the eyes excessively.

Complaining of blurring or double vision in seeing or eye tiredness.

Shutting or covering one eye when reading.

Tilting the head to see better.

Blinking excessively when doing close work.

The Joint Committee of the American School Health Asssociation and the National Society for the Prevention of Blindness† recommends that those exhibiting signs or complaints that may indicate eye problems be referred for a professional eye examination even though screening test results are within normal limits. However, Eisner and Callan‡ note that two evaluative studies of school screening methods show that overreferrals based on teacher observation alone exceed 60%, while underreferrals based on observation were 52% to 58%. The school nurse should

evaluate those students who were reported by the teachers to show signs of symptoms of vision problems prior to making a referral. The nurse can reobserve student behavior, ask pertinent questions, perform an individual screening test, and utilize professional judgment, keeping in mind that some youngsters who pass any screening test do need a professional eye examination.

Snellen chart. The familiar Snellen chart, which is available in either letter or illiterate E form (Fig. 14-3), is utilized either alone or in conjunction with other tests in all school vision screening programs conducted in the United States. When it is used alone, its overreferral rate is 33% to 35%; underreferral has been found to be 16% in one study and 51% in another,* which may reflect the use of different standards or techniques. The advantages of using the standard Snellen wall test chart are that it is inexpensive and easy to administer and interpret, and that it detects significant myopia, some types of astigmatism, and amblyopic conditions. Disadvantages are that any bright youngster can memorize the chart if it is open to view before testing, that it requires 22 feet of clear floor space to administer, that it is difficult to maintain standard conditions of lighting, and that it fails to detect pure hyperopia and some cases of astigmatism and muscle imbalance. The chart can be used or adapted for use at a distance of 10 feet, however.

Readings are expressed in fractions; the numerator indicates the distance at which the test is administered (usually 20 feet), and the denominator indicates the smallest line of type correctly read (three out of four symbols) at that distance. The referral point should be determined locally in consultation with ophthalmologists and optometrists; the level usually selected is 20/40 or worse in either eye.

Because the Snellen wall chart eye test is so commonly used and because teachers

*Lampe, J. M., Doster, M. E., and Beal, B. B.: Summary of a three-year study of academic and school achievement between color deficient and normal primary age pupils: phase two, J. Sch. Health **43**:309-311, May 1973.

†Joint study committee of the American School Health Association and the National Society for the Prevention of Blindness, Inc.: *Teaching about vision,* New York, 1972, National Society, p. 18.

‡Eisner, V., and Callan, L. B.: *Dimensions of school health,* Springfield, Ill., 1974, Charles C Thomas, Publisher, p. 60.

*Eisner, V., and Callan, L. B.: *Dimensions of school health.*

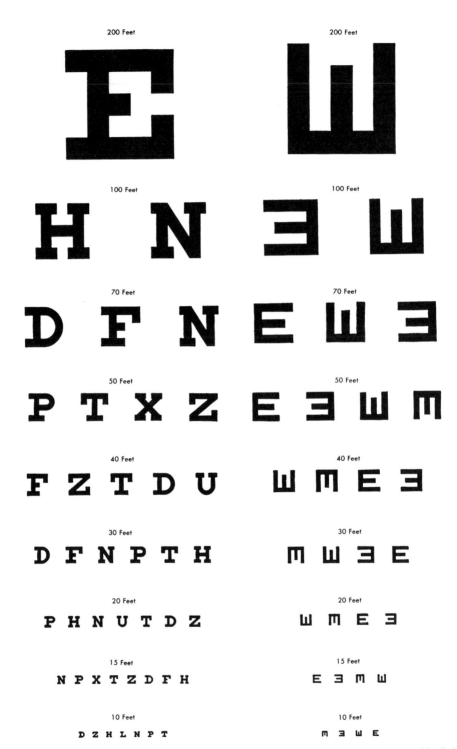

Fig. 14-3. Snellen charts are used for testing visual acuity. The E chart is used with little children and illiterate persons. (Courtesy National Association for the Prevention of Blindness.)

as well as nurses are often called upon to administer it, instructions for the preparation and conduct of testing are provided below.

PREPARATION FOR ADMINISTERING THE SNELLEN TEST.* The Snellen chart must meet standard specifications concerning the size and spacing of letters or symbols. Checking these standards is a technical task that can be avoided by purchasing charts from reliable sources.† Two types of charts are commonly used, one with letters and the other with the symbol E in various positions. The latter may be used with children from about 3 years of age and up, the former with children old enough to read letters easily.

Two pieces of cardboard are needed for covering the parts of the chart that are not being used. One 9 × 11½ inches is used to cover the upper half of the chart, leaving the 50-, 40-, 30-, and 20-foot lines exposed. A smaller card, 9 × 3¼ inches, can be clipped on the chart to cover the section below the 20-foot line. One window card, 11 × 14 inches, with a centered square hole of 1¾ × 1¾ inches should be used to show a single letter through the hole as the test proceeds. The center hole permits this to be done for the 20/20- to 20/70-foot lines. The card should be held vertically for the 70-foot line; horizontally for the others. Results are more reliable when the child sees only one letter at a time.

When the symbol E chart is used with small children, the teacher or other tester should have two large E's mounted on either side of the cardboard. These are used to familiarize children with the various positions of the E and make it possible for the tester to check to see exactly how the child sees the symbol.

Once the equipment is ready, attention should be given to other arrangements. Illumination on the chart should be 10 to 30 footcandles, evenly diffused over the chart, and with no glare. The amount of illumination may be checked through use of a light meter.* General illumination should be not less than one fifth of the chart illumination, and there should be no bright light in the child's field of vision. In order to gain the child's complete confidence and cooperation, the test must be given in a quiet room and with a reasonable degree of privacy. The tester should be friendly and patient.

The chart should be hung at average eye height and a line marked 20 feet away. Children may stand or sit when being tested. If they are standing, their heels should touch the 20-foot line; if they are seated, the back legs of the chair should touch the line.

TESTING PROCEDURE. For valid results children must be at ease and should be encouraged to do the best they can. Children who are being tested for the first time with the E chart need to be taught how to indicate the direction of the shafts of this symbol in its different positions.

Both eyes should be open during the test. The eye that is not being tested should be covered with a small card or folded paper that rests obliquely across the nose. For reasons of sanitation and aesthetics, each child should have his or her own individual card or paper.

A standardized routine avoids confusion and facilitates recording. The following procedures are recommended:

1. If a child wears glasses, test him or her with the glasses.
2. Test the right eye first, then the left.
3. Begin with the 30-foot line and follow with the 20-foot line. (Some testers prefer to begin with the 40-foot line.) It is not necessary to test below the 20-foot line.

*The following two sections are from National Education Association and American Medical Association: *School health services*, Washington, D.C., and Chicago, 1964, NEA and AMA.
†Equipment may be obtained from the National Society for the Prevention of Blindness or the American Medical Association. A Snellen chart with built-in illumination may be obtained from Goodlite Co., 7426 Madison St., Forest Park, Ill.

*A light meter may be purchased. Frequently, one may be obtained from the local health department or light company.

4. Keep unused parts of the chart covered, using the window card to expose single letters. This improves concentration and prevents memorization.

5. Move promptly and rhythmically from one symbol to another at a speed with which the child can keep pace.

6. Consider that a child sees a line satisfactorily if he or she reads correctly three out of four symbols.

During the test, note if the child strains to see. Evidence of this includes tilting the head, watering of the eyes, excessive blinking, thrusting the head forward, frowning or scowling, squinting, or closing one or both eyes. Observations of this nature should be recorded and the child referred for examination.

With the test completed and results recorded, the next step is the selection of pupils for whom an eye examinataion is to be recommended. Children failing the screening test should be retested before recommendations are made for referral.

Other tests. A simple test may be added to the use of the Snellen wall chart as previously described to increase its sensitivity and thus reduce the percent of underreferrals. This test should not be used with students who fail the Snellen test. Its use, however, is also likely to result in increased overreferrals. The test involves the use of plus sphere lenses to attempt to read only the 20-foot line on the Snellen chart. The plus sphere glasses (usually ground to +2.25 diopters for use with students below the fourth grade or to +1.75 diopters for use above) are placed on those who pass the Snellen test. Because the glasses correct for hyperopia, those who can read the 20-foot line with them on are suspected of having hyperopia and are referred for a professional examination.

The Snellen test, together with the plus lens test and a test for muscle imbalance (cover or Maddox rod), has been incorporated in a number of vision-testing machines, which are frequently used in schools. These machines are constantly being improved, and recent evaluative data are not available.

Data collected some years ago showed performance roughly comparable to that obtained by use of the Snellen chart alone. The machines are expensive, but they are also convenient; they maintain standard lighting conditions, and the tests are not subject to memorizations. Their use is not generally recommended in schools where follow-up of vision referrals is less than 85% to 90% successful. Adoption should be preceded by local or state committee consideration.

The school vision-testing program with the best reported overreferral (6%) and underreferral (2%) record is the Modfiied Clinical Technique.* The technique resembles that used by eye specialists for diagnosis. It includes instrument examination of the eye and is therefore performed by professional eye specialists. For this reason it is considered by many to be unsuitable for routine use in schools. It can be argued that the role of the school should be limited to screening out and referring those who appear to require a professional examination and should not encompass providing such examinations. Furthermore, jealousy and antagonism may be aroused among eye specialists in the community who are not involved in the program and on whom the ultimate success of the school vision program is dependent.

Defective color vision is best detected by use of color plates that are designed for the purpose, such as the Ishihara and HRR plates, or the Farnsworth F-2 single color plate test. Tests can be administered reliably as early as the first grade, but there is no need to do so that early.

While color vision testing need be administered only once to each pupil, use of the Snellen or other tests selected should be repeated according to a locally developed plan. The plan should include testing of preschoolers (4- and 5-year-olds) with the

---

*Blum, H., and others: *Vision screening for elementary schools: the Orinda study,* Berkeley, Calif., 1959, University of California Press.

Snellen illiterate E chart (or some special form of it) alone. Preschool testing is vitally important to the early detection and treatment of amblyopia ex anopsia due to strabismus. The same test can be repeated at kindergarten or first grade. Repeat vision testing, utilizing both the Snellen and other tests, is often scheduled at approximately grades 2, 5, 8, 10 and 11, and prior to driver education. In addition, testing is recommended of new students who come into the system at any grade, all teacher or parent observations, self-referrals, and all students who exhibit evidence of learning disability or behavior change. All students who wear glasses or contact lenses should be retested on schedule. Testing should also be offered to all school staff members who wish to participate. Those past 40 tend to develop *presbyopia,* a loss of elasticity of the crystalline lens, which makes near vision difficult and which is correctable by use of bifocal or trifocal lenses.

Referral and follow-up of visual acuity problems. Except for vocational counseling, no referral is indicated for those with color vision deficiencies, because the problem cannot be corrected. Such students, their parents, and their teachers should be informed, however, to enable them to be aware of the problem and to cope with it. For other suspected problems of visual acuity, referral should be made for a professional eye examination. Parents and students need to understand that failure to pass a school vision screening means that a professional eye examination is needed. It does *not* mean that the individual necessarily requires corrective lenses or any other form of treatment. Some may need referral to whatever resources the school and community provide for financial assistance or free examinations and treatment.

The final decision as to whether an optometrist or an ophthalmologist should be consulted is the business of the parents and students, not the school. The child's usual source of medical care may provide referral. The school can and should provide basic, factual information on which a decision can

be made. Such information includes these definitions:

ophthalmologist or **oculist.** A physician who specializes in the diagnosis and treatment of diseases of the eye and who is prepared to treat such diseases medically, surgically, or through the prescription of corrective lenses.
optometrist. A licensed nonphysician practitioner who is prepared to diagnose, measure, and treat refractive errors and eye muscle disturbances through the prescription of corrective lenses and exercises, but not by means of surgery. Optometrists in some states are now permitted to use or prescribe appropriate drugs.
optician. A technician who grinds corrective lenses and fits glasses as prescribed by an ophthalmologist or optometrist.

In most communities, optometrists charge less for their services and are able to schedule appointments sooner than ophthalmologists. Ophthalmologists are, however, prepared and legally permitted to prescribe medication and perform surgery when such services are needed.

In the interim between the time when students are referred for professional eye care and when diagnosis and treatment, if any, have been provided, common sense adjustments in classroom procedures may be helpful. Referred students should be permitted to position themselves in the classroom wherever they can see best. Some may have to stand directly in front of the chalkboard to see what is on it; others may be helped by seating themselves in a place where lighting is of high intensity and quality. Teachers should make allowances for difficulties in respect to visual task assignments and expectations. When professional diagnosis has been completed and following treatment or in the course of it, the source of eye care may make recommendations regarding school management. This practice should be encouraged by the school by providing a form that the eye specialist may use to report back to the school.

Some parents and students resist the use of corrective lenses on the mistaken grounds that they weaken the eyes and that eye exercises are the appropriate means of correcting any eye problem. Eye exercises are a useful means of treating strabismus when combined with another mode of treatment, but lenses provide better and more comfortable vision in the presence of other problems, and the person becomes accustomed to them. There is no credible evidence that properly prescribed and fitted lenses weaken the eyes in any case. Cosmetic objections may be overcome by selecting either fashionable frames or contact lenses.

Contact lenses are often chosen by athletes who engage in collision sports and by those with severe myopia as an alternative to the thick glasses prescribed for that condition. Disadvantages of contact lenses include their high cost, the difficulty of caring for them properly, the initial discomfort experienced by many who use them, and the discomfort that may result from wearing them for too long a period in a day.

Those who opt for glasses may choose between dress safety, industrial safety, and plastic resin glasses. Industrial safety glasses are the heaviest but offer the greatest degree of protection against injury. Resin plastic glasses are the lightest but are easily scratched and offer moderate safety protection. Dress safety glasses are moderately light and afford considerable safety protection. When broken, they do not shatter but crumble into small particles. Once fitted by an optician, glasses should be rechecked by the eye specialist who prescribed them.

Students and parents can benefit from the above and other relevant consumer information that can be provided by the school. It is clear that in choosing a source of eye care or a type of corrective lens there is no one right answer for everyone, but a poor choice can be costly or detrimental.

School management of visual disabilities. Most students have normal or better vision either without or with corrective lenses and need no special consideration. Fewer than 1% of noninstitutionalized U.S. children and youth are blind or partially sighted with the best correction obtainable. These youngsters are both educationally and vocationally handicapped and therefore require special services.

Partially sighted persons are commonly defined as those whose vision in the better eye is between 20/70 and 20/200 with a correcting lens. *Blind* persons are defined as either those whose vision in the better eye is 20/200 or poorer with a corrective lens or whose visual field in the better eye is 20° or less. (Most of us have a visual field of 180°; we can see our hands when our arms are stretched straight out at right angles to our bodies and our eyes are focused straight ahead.) Relatively few "blind" persons are completely without sight.

In-school guidance should first seek to help blind and partially sighted individuals to set realistic goals for themselves, bearing in mind that those with visual disabilities have proved their ability to learn to move about in the same physical and social worlds as fully sighted individuals with minimal assistance and that the presence and nature of other disabilities must be considered. Overprotection is more often a problem than the selection of goals that exceed the capability of the visually handicapped person.

The federal-state vocational rehabilitation agency will provide expert vocational guidance, beginning at about age 16 or 17, as well as financial and other assistance in achieving goals.

Appropriate school placement of blind and partially sighted students is often within a regular classroom in a regular school, but they may require the assistance of an itinerant special education teacher who provides special materials and equipment as well as information and advice to the regular classroom teacher. Some schools house a special education resource room in which handicapped youngsters spend part of each day with a special education teacher and helpful supplies and equipment. Some who are unable at first to cope with regular placement may benefit from temporary placement in a special classroom or special school situation. Residential schools for the blind provide excellent special teaching and resources but impose undesirable social segregation. The appropriate choice among these alternatives depends on the nature of the individual as well as the range of resources available.

Regardless of placement, blind and partially sighted persons require training in orientation and mobility. Orientation involves the use of cues provided by sounds, the way surfaces feel, and a knowledge of the environment to determine where one is. Blind students also often require the helpful assistance of others in establishing their orientation, especially in schools that are new to them. As they learn the school environment, their need for such assistance decreases.

Mobility (skill in moving about) also improves with experience. It may be aided by a trained dog, sighted guide, or cane. A sighted guide is most helpful when the unsighted person holds the guide's arm rather than the other way around and when the guide walks a bit ahead of the blind person so that turns and steps can be anticipated.

Blind students will generally be aided in scholastic tasks by learning braille, by using tape recordings, and by using paid or volunteer readers. Partially sighted students can often read conventional materials by use of high light intensities focused on the task and with the aid of magnifying lenses.

Eye inflammations. Red, inflamed, or sore eyes are observed rather frequently. Some cases are caused by infections that may spread from person to person. Most cases may benefit from definitive diagnosis and treatment by a physician. Cases are best identified by observation by teachers and nurses and by attention to student complaints.

Blepharitis is a chronic inflammation of the eyelid margins. White scales or yellow crusts at the base of the eyelashes, loss of eyelashes, and redness and swelling of the eyelids are often obsesrved. Victims may complain of soreness or itching or that light is painful. This condition is not regarded as communicable, but it should be seen by a physician. Treatment is difficult.

Styes are infections that are localized around hair follicles in the margin of the eyelid. They are small cones, filled with pus,

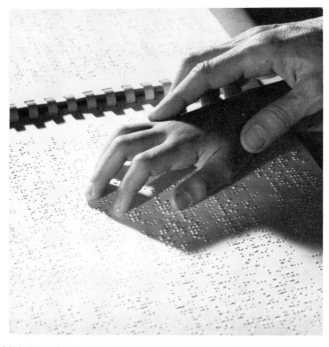

Fig. 14-4. Learning braille. (Courtesy Frank Gordon from A. Devaney, N.Y.)

that cause a sensation of "something in the eye" if they touch the eyeball. They usually burst and drain by themselves. If styes appear one after the other, or if one is particularly painful or persistent, the services of a physician may be helpful.

Conjunctivitis (commonly known or referred to as pink eye) is a catch-all term that means inflammation of the conjunctiva (the mucous membrane that lines the inner surface of the eyelids and the exposed surface of the eyeball). Conjunctivitis is marked by redness, tears, and itching, smarting, or burning of the eyelids. There may be a discharge of pus. Some cases result from allergic reactions, which of course, are not communicable. Others are caused by either bacterial or viral infections, which may spread throughout the group by those whose fingers touch papers or other objects contaminated by victims and who then touch their own eyes. Except for the case of an individual who has a history of allergic conjunctivitis and whose inflammation coincides with probable exposure to an implicated allergen, it is difficult to distinguish between the allergic and communicable forms. Therefore, all students with conjunctivitis should be excluded from school and referred to a physician for treatment except for those known to have an allergic basis.

Prevention and care of eye injuries. At the elementary level, eye injuries tend to occur during play as a result of carelessness in carrying or using sharp objects or by contact of a moving individual with some object in the environment. Preventive measures include adult supervision of play and enforcement of common sense rules of safe behavior, such as carrying sharp objects at a walk and with the points held down, and the identification and protection or removal of environmental objects that might injure a child's eyes. Although fights between children are to be expected, it may be helpful to explore alternative ways of settling arguments both in class and in disciplinary conferences with those guilty of fighting.

In secondary schools, shop and laboratory activities pose hazards to eye safety. Some states have followed the example of Ohio where, in 1963, a law was enacted requiring all students and teachers engaged in specified shop and laboratory activities to wear industrial quality eye protective devices and permitting boards of education either to furnish such equipment free or to provide it at cost. Standards for industrial quality safety eye and face protective equipment are published and revised from time to time by the American National Standards Safety Institute.

Eye injuries are not only painful but also frightening because of the potential loss of vision. They occur frequently enough that every school professional should know appropriate school and home first-aid procedures:

1. A particle on, but not embedded in, the white of the eye or the inner surface of the eyelid is best removed by allowing tears to wash it out. Tears constitute the safest, most effective eyewash available. If the particle is under the upper lid of the eye, tear washing is facilitated by drawing the upper lid over the lower one. If tearing fails to remove the object, flushing the eye with tap water may help. Often an object can also be removed by rolling the eyelid back over a clean applicator stick and touching the object with a bit of clean, moistened cotton or gauze. If this fails, medical attention is indicated.

2. Particles on the surface of the cornea (the transparent covering over the iris and pupil) or that are embedded should be removed by a physician only.

3. Any penetrating wound of the eye requires the immediate services of an ophthalmologist. In any of these cases, pain may be relieved to some extent by *loosely* covering both eyes with a sterile bandage. *Never* exert pressure on an injured eye. If the eye or eyelid is bleeding, let it bleed.

4. Chemical burns of the eye should be

flushed with water from a tap or poured from a clean container for 15 minutes before transporting the victim to an ophthalmologist or to a hospital accident ward for further treatment. *Never* try to neutralize the chemical with another. *Never* use an eyecup; they are always inadequate in volume and almost always dirty from disuse.

5. Blows to the eye are too often dismissed as unimportant. Some authorities believe that all "black eyes" should receive medical attention. There is no question that medical care is required whenever a blow to the eye is followed by a complaint of blurred or double vision or of seeing a shadow or curtain in the eye, the appearance of blood under the cornea, and unequal pupil size. The possibility of the fracture of bone around the eyes is another indication for referral. The immediate application of cold wet cloths reduces the swelling associated with a black eye.

Eye health education. Kindergarteners and first graders can be taught to appreciate the sight they take for granted by trying to identify familiar objects in the dark or with blindfolds on and then by looking at the same objects. Other blindfold games can contribute to the appreciation of sight. Students can learn how to cooperate in vision-screening tests by pointing in the direction that the "legs of the table" (the illiterate Snellen E) point. They can learn to carry sharp-pointed objects with the points down. Later in the early elementary grades they may learn how the crystalline lens focuses light on the back of the eye so that objects can be seen and that some persons wear glasses to overcome focusing problems. They can experiment with lenses to discover that they bend light. They can develop their own rules for protecting eyes at play. Use of proper lighting and the trick of resting eyes by looking away from one's work occasionally to reduce fatigue can be demonstrated and learned. The importance

of a good (basic four) diet to healthy eyesight can be stresssed.

At the upper elementary or middle school and secondary levels pupils may be ready to learn that adequate amounts of vitamin A foods (such as dark green and yellow vegetables, liver, and whole milk) prevent an eye disease, xerophthalmia, which can lead to blindness, but that excessive vitamin A intake (100,000 IU or more daily) as practiced by some faddists can lead to perceptual ocular disturbances. Adequate intake of the B complex vitamins is also essential to eye health. Study of the nature and management of common vision problems, of relevant consumer information, of eye safety in school, shops, and labs, and of first aid for eye injuries is also appropriate for older students.

Each time that a solar eclipse is about to occur, all students need to be warned that *any* form of direct viewing, including the use of darkened glass, is hazardous. Indirect viewing such as via television is safe.

EAR PROBLEMS

The early recognition of hearing loss is extremely important not only because it may interfere with school achievement but also because the development of clear speech and social skills is facilitated by good hearing. Estimates of prevalence vary with the methods and standards used to assess the disability. Audiometric tests of a sample of noninstitutionalized U.S. youth, 12 to 17 years of age, indicate that about 1% have losses that interfere only with the ability to understand faint speech, while about 0.2% have frequent difficulties with normal speech.* These estimates probably understate the extent of the problem because those in institutions were not included and because pure-tone audiometry does not detect some cases of failure to perceive

---

*U.S. Health Resources Administration: *Hearing levels of youths 12-17 years, United States,* DHEW Publications No. (HRA) 75-1627, Washington, D.C., Jan. 1975, U.S. Government Printing Office.

speech correctly. Other estimates run as high as 3% to 6%.

Types of hearing impairment. Hearing impairment may be either congenital or acquired after birth. There are two main types of hearing loss, conductive and sensorineural. *Conductive loss* is localized in the area of the external auditory canal, eardrum, and middle cavity of the ear (Fig. 14-5). Causes include impacted ear wax and small objects such as bits of eraser or beans that children stuff in their ears, broken or scarred eardrums resulting from trauma or infections, untreated middle ear infections, and otosclerosis (fusion of the conductive small bones in the middle ear or overgrowth of spongy bone in the inner ear, uncommon in children, which blocks the oval membrane to which the stapes communicates sound impulses). Many cases of conductive loss can be successfully treated by medical or surgical intervention. *Sensorineural losses* include defects of the structures of the inner ear through which sound pressure impulses are received by nerve endings, damage to the nerves through which sound sensations are transmitted to the brain, and damage to brain centers where sensations are perceived and in-terpreted. Known causes of sensorineural loss include prolonged exposure to loud noises that damage structures in the cochlea (an occupational hazard of rock musicians).

The occurrence of German measles (rubella) in pregnant women frequently results in sensorineural loss in their offspring. The occurrence of meningitis or scarlet fever in childhood or youth may also result in hearing loss unless it is discovered and effectively treated early. Sensorineural losses from any of these causes are rarely if ever successfully treated, and hearing aids are helpful only in selected cases. The best that can be reasonably expected is to maintain residual hearing abilities and to utilize such rehabilitative measures as lip-reading instruction and speech therapy.

Prevention of hearing impairment. Those who hear well tend to take their ability for granted. Thus, the first step in the prevention of hearing loss, as in the prevention of blindness, is to develop an appreciation of the sense of hearing. One approach is to attempt to carry on classroom interactions for a period of time without use of speech or hearing; communication forms are limited to writing or to gesturing and other nonverbal modes. Children need to be

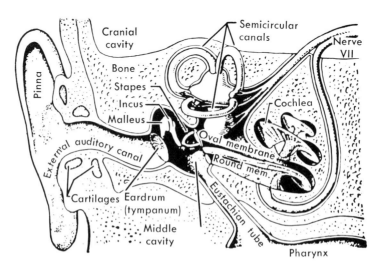

Fig. 14-5. Diagram of the ear. (From Storer and Unger: *General zoology,* ed. 4, New York, 1965, McGraw-Hill, Inc. Used by permission.)

taught that the insertion of any object small enough to penetrate the external auditory canal may block the passage or damage the eardrum and that accumulated or impacted ear wax should be removed by a medically qualified person only.

Both parents and children need to be taught that undiagnosed or inadequately treated infections can result in hearing loss. Upper respiratory tract infections can travel from the pharynx up the eustachian tube and into the middle ear cavity. Thus, the first step in their prevention is early detection and medical treatment of sore throats and similar infections. The first sign of a middle ear infection (otitis media) may be an earache, a feeling of fullness in the ear, or a noticeable reduction in hearing acuity. The infection results in an accumulation of fluid in the middle ear. As the fluid pressure increases, earache develops. If the infection continues untreated, the pressure may result in rupture of the eardrum and visible signs of drainage through the canal. (For example, a wad of cotton in a child's ear is often a sign of drainage.) Unless the perforation is large, it usually heals itself. However, rupture and healing can produce a scarred eardrum that lacks some of the resilience necessary to conduct sounds to the small bones (malleus, incus, stapes). Eardrums may also be ruptured as a result of deep diving or of blows to the ear. The eustachian tube, the function of which is to equalize ambient and middle ear pressure, may become chronically blocked as a result of either repeated infections or excessive growth of the tonsils or adenoids. Such chronic otitis media imposes the risk of accumulation of thick gluey matter in the middle ear, which may result in hearing loss. All of these conditions may be alleviated by medical or surgical treatment to prevent or alleviate resultant hearing loss. Acute upper respiratory tract infections such as colds commonly produce a measureable but temporary hearing loss.

Detection of hearing defects

Observations. The observable signs of hearing loss are subject to misinterpretation, because any of them may result from other causes. They include:

1. Inattentiveness.
2. Asking to have questions repeated.
3. Watching the face of a speaker closely.
4. Directing one ear toward the speaker.
5. Difficulty in copying dictation.
6. Irrelevant responses to or difficulty in answering easy spoken questions.
7. Mistakes in pronunciation of words.
8. Speaking too loudly or too softly in relation to ambient noise levels.
9. Scholastic achievement below the student's level of ability.
10. Failure to respond to speech or other sound stimulus the source of which is to one side or behind the student.

Those who present any of the manifestations listed above should be tested or at least observed independently by the school nurse or other health service professional prior to referral. In addition, all who have signs or symptoms of ear infections should be referred for immediate medical attention. This group includes those who complain of earache that lasts more than an hour or so, those who show signs of a draining ear, or those who have frequent respiratory tract infections or earaches.

Audiometry. The cornerstone of the detection program in most U.S. schools today is pure-tone audiometric testing. Audiometric procedures have replaced the *whisper* and the *watch tick* tests. These older tests present sounds of unknown intensity and pitch. The pure-tone audiometer, on the other hand, presents sounds of intensity and pitch that are selected by the tester. *Group pure-tone audiometric testing,* in which a whole classroom of students, each of whom receives sounds through earphones rigged to a single audiometer, is tested at once, has also largely been abandoned. A study by Yankauer and his associates[*]

---

[*]Yankauer, A., and others: Comparative evaluation of three screening methods of detection of hearing loss in school children, Am. J. Public Health **44:**77-82, Jan. 1954.

showed that group testing failed to identify as many children with true hearing loss as individual tests and that individual tests required only a little more time than group tests.

Individual pure-tone audiometry encompasses the use of several different types of tests. *Sweep check testing* is often utilized as an initial screening device because it is easy to administer and requires relatively little time. All sounds are presented at a single predetermined level of intensity (number of decibels) over a predetermined range of frequencies (measured in Hertz units or cycles per second). The subject either hears or fails to hear each sound presented. The intensity level selected increases with the ambient noise level of the testing location. Pitch levels often are selected to encompass the approximate speech range (500, 1,000, and 2,000 Hz) or may extend somewhat above and below this range. Overreferrals, however, tend to occur at low frequencies in the presence of high ambient noise levels. Each ear is tested separately, with the person tested seated so that the movements of the dials by the audiometrist are hidden. When students receive orientation to the testing procedure as part of their educational preparation for it, they can be tested at a rate of one every 3 or 4 minutes.

Threshold testing requires more time than the sweep check but produces data used to construct an audiogram or line graph that shows the extent of hearing loss at any pitch tested for each of the two ears. At each frequency tested the audiometrist presents the tone at various levels of intensity until the lowest number of decibels at which the subject hears the sound is identified. The additional information obtained by threshold testing provides not only an indication of the severity of a loss but also nondiagnostic clues as to its nature. Although a conductive loss may involve either one ear

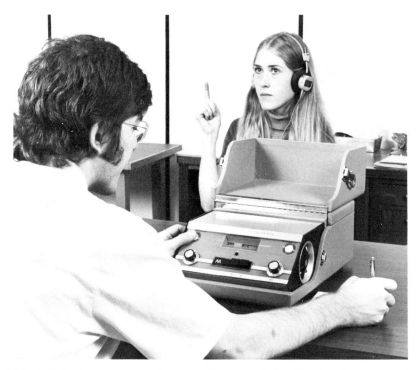

Fig. 14-6. Individual pure-tone audiometry. (Courtesy Maico Hearing Instruments, Inc., of Minneapolis.)

or both, and sensorineural loss may be either partial or complete, conductive loss is *never* complete because the bone that surrounds the ear is capable of conducting sound to the inner ear structure. Conductive losses tend to occur predominantly at low frequencies, while sensorineural losses tend to occur at high and middle frequencies. Threshold testing may be used to rescreen those first selected by means of sweep check testing, or it may be used both as an initial screening procedure and as a retest.

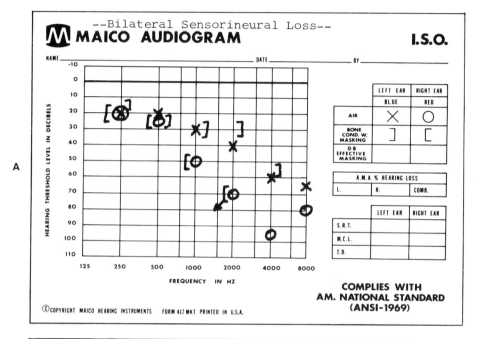

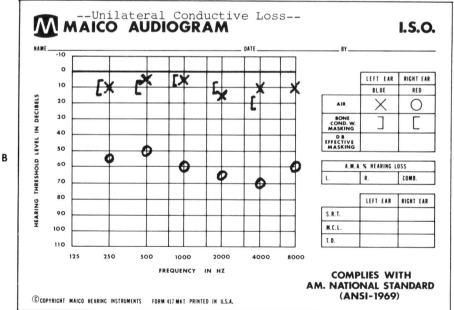

Fig. 14-7. A, Audiogram typical of bilateral sensorineural loss. **B,** Audiogram typical of unilateral conductive loss. (Courtesy Maico Hearing Instruments, Inc., of Minneapolis.)

In any case, both initial testing and re-testing should *always* precede referral. The initial testing and the retest should be separated in time by at least 1 week to reduce the number of overreferrals caused by colds or other transient infections. If school audiometers are recalibrated frequently, as they should be, the possibility of instrument error is reduced.

In some programs those whose sweep check and/or threshold test so indicates are referred for professional evaluation without further in-school investigation. In other programs additional tests may be provided or an examination by an otologist (physician ear specialist) offered before referral. Some state health departments provide acoustically treated vans or trailers equipped for diagnostic testing and the services of a professional audiologist for use in local school-community programs. These services are especially valuable in outlying areas where community speech and hearing centers are nonexistent and where there are few or no otologists in practice.

One of the special diagnostic tests that may be made available is the *bone conduction test*. In a standard sweep check or threshold test, sound impulses are transmitted to the external auditory canal by air from an earphone head set. In a bone conduction test, sound impulses are transmitted by way of vibrators placed on a bony prominence next to the ear. The sound impulses thus bypass the outer and middle ear segments and are picked up directly by the sensory organs of the inner ear. If losses in the bone conduction audiogram closely match those revealed by threshold testing, a sensorineural loss is indicated. If the bone conduction audiogram shows significantly better hearing than the threshold test, a conductive loss is indicated, and the probability that a properly fitted hearing aid will be useful is high (Fig. 14-7).

Another special test is called the *speech perception test*. This requires a special audiometer operated by a person with advanced training in audiology. Standard lists of words are presented at selected intensi-ties to determine not only the threshold at which spoken words are correctly identified but also whether the person tested is able to perceive spoken words correctly.

Prereferral examinations. A prereferral otological examination complemented by diagnostic testing capability serves several useful functions. If excessive wax or foreign objects are blocking the ear canal, the obstruction can readily be removed by the otologist. A repeat threshold test conducted on the spot often reveals the obstruction to be the sole cause of the loss, in which case no referral is needed. In other cases, the working diagnosis made by the otologist is helpful in determining which students should be referred to their personal physicians and which to otologists or to speech and hearing clinics. The otologist may also make helpful recommendations for school management. If the examination culminates in a brief conference between the otologist, the student, a parent, and the school nurse, the likelihood that the case will be appropriately and successfully followed up is greatly enhanced.

Scheduling and conduct of testing. Hearing defects in children and youth tend to occur most often at younger ages, and both the extent of the loss and its resulting defects in social and speech development tend to worsen with age and lack of treatment. A desirable school-community hearing screening program therefore begins with the testing of preschoolers. Preschool, kindergarten, and retarded children, however, are often unable to cooperate in standard audiometric testing. Play audiometry, a technique in which the child responds to audiometric tone by dropping an object in a box, may be used. Routine screening is much more productive when conducted at elementary grade levels than later. Thus, mass screening is usually scheduled more frequently during the elementary years than later. From two to four tests may be scheduled during the elementary grades, perhaps one at the middle or junior high school levels and one or none during senior high school. Testing should be provided for all new entrants and for all parent, teacher, or self-referrals at any level, and each year or two for any youngster previously found to have a hearing loss. It should also be offered to any school staff member who wishes to be tested.

Persons who administer hearing tests require training not only in audiometric techniques but also in the art of eliciting and interpreting responses of young or retarded children. Some states require certification as an *audiometrist,* which may be obtained by the successful completion of college courses in audiometry. In others, volunteers or school nurses may receive informal in-service training to administer sweep checks and threshold tests. Diagnostic testing and the interpretation of audiograms require more advanced training, such as that received by certified *audiologists,* who may be employed by larger local school districts or by state health departments.

Referral and follow-up procedures. Standards and procedures for referral should be developed at the local or state level in consultation with otologists and other hearing and speech specialists. Since various decibel loss scales that vary in number value equivalence are used in the United States, it would be inappropriate and confusing to state standards here. A troublesome question is whether initial referral should be made to the child's usual source of health care or whether the child and the parent should be presented with a list of qualified medical otologists and/or speech and hearing clinics from which to select their own specialized source of help. It is something of a breach of ethics to bypass a personal physician, but there is a risk that the personal physician may not make a specialist referral when indicated. One possible compromise is to suggest that the parent request a specialist referral from the child's personal physician. In any case, the earlier indicated medical treatment is begun, the greater the probability that the condition will be improved or alleviated.

Pending definitive diagnosis and treatment, those students with a mild or moderate hearing loss may be placed in a location within the classroom near the teacher. Those with profound losses as well as those with mild or moderate losses are helped if the teacher or other speaker faces them. Speakers who enunciate words clearly are better understood, but excessively loud speech is not necessarily helpful.

Speech (lip) reading instruction is helpful in many cases. Those whose loss results in speech deterioration benefit from speech therapy provided either in the school or at a nearby speech clinic. As in the case of defects of visual acuity, the goal is to keep those with hearing losses in the educational mainstream if at all possible. Some, especially those with other handicaps in addition to hearing loss, may benefit from special class or special school placement. The options are similar to those provided for blind or partially sighted students.

Some parents of children who are hearing handicapped tend to rush out and purchase a hearing aid. This is usually a costly mistake and one that is preventable by adequate referrals and counseling procedures. Hearing aid salesmen abound who pose as qualified experts and who are all too willing to sell an aid to anyone with the cash and desire to buy one. The recommendation to buy an aid should come only from the otologist or clinic that provides definitive diagnosis and care. Aids are needed and helpful only in relatively few cases.

Application of the preventive measures stated earlier in this section to those with losses is of vital importance. Prevention of ear injury and the early detection and treatment of ear infections serve to help preserve residual hearing ability.

SPEECH IMPAIRMENTS

Speech disorders are more common among young children and males than among older children and females. That many of them reflect the individual's stage of development is apparent from the observable improvement in children's speech that occurs at about the third grade. Some speech impairments are related to such identifiable health problems as hearing loss, missing or misaligned teeth, cleft palate, and certain central nervous system impairments. Others are described as functional; that is, they have no detectable cause. Some are mildly annoying; others make effective communication nearly impossible. Estimates of prevalence vary widely, depending on the standards used to classify speech as normal or abnormal.

Systems of classification of speech disorders also vary. For example, they may be classified by cause (defective breathing or resonance, for example) or by the properties of the speech produced. What we observe are problems of articulation (pronunciation), voice production (intensity, pitch, accent), and fluency (stuttering, inappropriate pauses).

Speech defects are first identified by teacher observation in many schools and referred by the teacher to a speech correctionist for evaluation. In some elementary schools the speech correctionist screens all children in one or more of the early grades. Clearly, hearing testing and other health appraisal testing techniques should be utilized to identify and refer for evaluation and care those with possible basic organic health problems. The speech correctionist may refer some cases to a speech pathologist (Ph.D. specialist) for evaluation. Many of those with either organic or functional problems are benefitted by the services of a speech correctionist who may provide instruction on either an individual or group basis. If speech correction services are not available in the school, they may be available elsewhere in the community.

LEARNING DISABILITIES

Many youngsters fail to learn well despite average or better intelligence and despite little greater prevalence among them of visual, hearing, or demonstrable organic neurological lesions than might be found in a population of "normal" youngsters. Their behavior is often obnoxious and always frustrating to their parents, teachers, peers, and themselves. A long list of labels has been applied to them, among which are learning disability, minimal brain dysfunction, dyslexia, hyperkinesis, and minimal brain damage. They are typically disorganized, impulsive, anxious, and often antisocial. They

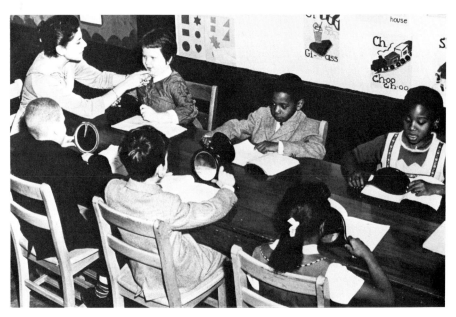

Fig. 14-8. Group speech correction. (Courtesy School District of Philadelphia.)

cannot stick to a useful task, but often perseverate (that is, repeat the same words or actions over and over again when it is pointless to do so). Coordination tends to be poor. Most are overactive, some are underactive. They vary wildly in mood. Estimates of prevalence range from 5% to 25% or higher.*

Miller points out that the labels explain little and that they may only be consequences of societal insistence on conformity in social and cognitive behavior, but he suggests that the concept is at least useful in calling attention to the needs of these children for special health and education services. He suggests that they, like others, will benefit from individualized expert attention and from attempts to understand the nature of their individual problems and to provide for their individual needs by conjoint medical, educational, and psychological diagnosis and planning. This requires community programs for preschool screening, the careful study of all those who exhibit learning problems in school, the provision of individualized school programs with accompanying special education service, and a variety of community services to assist not only the children with learning disabilities but also their parents.

In-school programs might include readiness testing upon kindergarten entrance, developmentally based kindergarten and early elementary programs, nongraded classes, provision for instruction of children and youth by their preferred modes (auditory or visual), and the further development of learning centers or laboratories.

Controversy surrounds the use of drugs in the management of these youngsters. Stimulant drugs are usually used, with the paradoxical result that many of them are calmed down to the point where their behavior is easier to tolerate and learning

may improve. But the condition (or conditions) and the mechanisms of drug action are unclear. It may be argued that their use does nothing to alleviate basic causation and that it further encourages the popularity of psychoactive pill popping. The use of such drugs should certainly not be routine, and any possible undesirable side effects noted in school or at home should be reported promptly to the practitioner by whom they were prescribed.

Useful educational modalities include physical activities designed to improve coordination, arts and crafts, psychological counseling if an emotional problem exists, remedial education, language therapy, and perceptual-motor training. For some, isolation in an environment devoid of distracting stimuli and the presentation of a single learning task at one time have proved helpful. Rewards for successful task completion, discipline that is firm but sympathetic, and assistance in task organization are useful approaches both in school and at home.*

Some states, notably California, have pioneered in special education services for children wtih learning disabilities, but there is a national shortage of prepared special educationists. Needed services vary in quality and availability from place to place. The Association for Children with Learning Disabilities and its state-affiliated parent groups can provide helpful information.†

QUESTIONS FOR STUDY AND DISCUSSION

1. What is the physical nature, importance, and usual means of correction of each of the problems of visual acuity, including color vision deficiency, cited in the text?
2. What are the advantages and disadvantages of each of the types of vision-screening tests cited in the text? Approximately when or how often should vision testing be conducted?
3. Describe appropriate referral and follow-up of defects of visual acuity. What are some of the problems faced by youngsters with

*Miller, C. A.: Minimal brain dysfunction. In Wallace, H. M., Gold, E. M., and Lis, E. F.: *Maternal and child health practices, problems, resources and methods of delivery,* Springfield, Ill., 1973, Charles C Thomas, Publisher, pp. 1,149-1,165.

The child with minimal brain dysfunction, Rockville, Md., 1974, American Occupational Therapy Foundation, Inc.
†2200 Brownsville Road, Pittsburgh, Pa. 15201.

defects and by their parents, and how can the school help in solving these problems?
4. What is the nature of and appropriate school response to each of the eye inflammations described in the text?
5. How may eye injuries be prevented, and how should each type of eye injury be cared for?
6. What important objectives for eye health education are suggested in the text? What other important objectives can you add?
7. Why are hearing impairments important?
8. Distinguish between conductive and sensorineural hearing loss in terms of causation, anatomical location, nature of loss, and prognosis for cure.
9. What measures are helpful in the prevention of hearing loss?
10. Prepare a list of health education objectives for hearing conservation education. Suggest an appropriate teaching method and grade level placement for each objective.
11. Distinguish between each of the methods of hearing defect detection used in schools in terms of nature, purpose, and usefulness. What schedule for screening testing is recommended, and why?
12. What are the advantages and disadvantages of the prereferral otological examination?
13. What referral and follow-up procedures are recommended for youngsters with suspected hearing defects?
14. Assign one class member the role of school nurse and another the role of an uninformed or misinformed parent of a child with strabismus or profound hearing loss. Give the role players time to prepare; then stage a counseling session in which the nurse tries to inform and guide the parent to appropriate action.

15. Describe the general nature and appropriate school management of (a) speech impairment, and (b) learning disabilities.
16. In small group discussions try to reach consensus about how you would like to be treated by your peers and school professionals if you were a student who was: (a) partially sighted or blind, (b) profoundly deaf, (c) severely speech handicapped, or (d) a victim of learning disabilities. (Assign one handicap to a group.)

REFERENCES

Bryan, D.: *School nursing in transition,* St. Louis, 1973, The C. V. Mosby Co.

Eisner, V., Callan, L. B.: *Dimensions of school health,* Springfield, Ill., 1974, Charles C Thomas, Publisher.

Henderson, J.: *Emergency medical guide,* ed. 3, New York, 1973, McGraw-Hill, Inc.

Joint Study Committee of the American School Health Association and the National Society for the Prevention of Blindness, Inc.: *Teaching about vision,* New York, 1972, The Society.

Nemir, A., and Schaller, W. E.: *The School health program,* Philadelphia, 1975, W. B. Saunders Co.

Wallace, H. M., Gold, E. M., and Lis, E. F.: *Maternal and child health practices, problems, resources and methods of delivery,* Springfield, Ill., 1973, Charles C Thomas, Publisher.

Weiner, F.: *Help for the handicapped child,* New York, 1973, McGraw-Hill, Inc.

Wheatley, G. M., and Hallock, G. T.: *Health observation of school children,* ed. 3, New York, 1965, McGraw-Hill, Inc.

CHAPTER 15 ❧ VD, the common cold, and other plagues

We have seen that the infectious diseases are relatively insignificant as causes of death in the United States today. Among U.S. youngsters who were 5 to 14 years of age in 1970, only one group of communicable diseases (influenza and pneumonia) ranked among the ten leading causes of death, causing fewer than two deaths per 100,000 persons.* National Health Survey household interview data,† however, indicate that in the survey year 1972-1973 respiratory tract conditions, including colds and influenza resulted in an average of about 270 days of school absence per 100 youngsters of 6 to 16 years of age, or more than half of all school absences due to illness. Digestive disorders cost about 24 days of absence per 100 students, while other infective and parasitic diseases resulted in about 73 lost school days per 100 students. Most communicable disease occurrences produce no lasting ill effects, but some do. For example, about one in four infants born to mothers who suffer rubella (3-day measles) during the first trimester of pregnancy are born with severe defects.

SCHOOL AND COMMUNITY RESPONSIBILITY

Primary responsibility for the control of communicable diseases in the United States is vested by law in state and local health departments. Specific statewide requirements are set forth either in statutory laws

---

*National Center for Health Statistics: *Facts of life and death,* DHEW Publication No. (HRA) 74-1222, Rockville, Md., 1974, Public Health Service, Health Resources Administration.
†National Center for Health Statistics: *Current estimates from the health interview survey,* DHEW Publication No. (HRA) 74-1512, Rockville, Md., 1973, Public Health Service, Health Resources Administration.

enacted by state legislatures or in rules and regulations (administrative laws) promulgated by the state boards of health. For example, state statutes or regulations may require certain immunizations as a prerequisite to school admission or that those with certain diseases be excluded from school attendance until the illness is rendered noncommunicable by time or treatment. Local departments of health may establish similar regulations that are more restrictive than those established by the state but may not relax state requirements.

School health service personnel are required to follow state communicable disease control laws and regulations regardless of whether they are employed by the local health department or the school district. School districts have been required by the courts to comply with emergency orders issued by local health officers in epidemic situations, but in the absence of an epidemic or other similar situation, they may or may not be bound to do so, depending on the extent to which powers have been delegated to local health departments. Nevertheless, any truly effective program of communicable disease control is much more dependent on joint planning and action by school and health department staff members and community providers of health care than on legislative requirements.

BASIC CONTROL PROCEDURES

From the viewpoint of school health and health education, four basic procedures are useful in the control of communicable diseases. Not all of these procedures are useful in the control of every communicable disease, nor are all of them equally effective. These procedures are: (1) health education, (2) immunization, (3) early detection of cases combined with definitive treatment and/or temporary exclusion from school, and (4) environmental control measures. In addition, the issues of closing schools during epidemics and of school practices in respect to the convalescent student are discussed in this section.

Health education. There are a number of simple personal health practices that provide at least a moderate degree of protection against a variety of communicable infectious diseases and that can be promoted through health education. Health education can also be utilized to enlist cooperation in disease prevention through the communal procedures of immunization, early detection, treatment or isolation, and environmental controls.

Personal health practices that may be helpful in reducing the spread of infectious diseases include thorough handwashing after going to the toilet and before eating. Covering coughs and sneezes may also be of some value. An adequate, well-balanced diet is believed to increase individual resistance to infection. Although it is generally regarded as polite to share things, those children who share caps and combs are also likely to share scalp ringworm (a fungus infection) and head lice, while individuals who share sex partners are also likely to share syphilis and gonorrhea.

Health education with respect to immunizations is important for at least two reasons. First, it encourages maintenance of desirably high levels of immunization by informing parents and students of legal requirements, the importance of immunizations, and when, where, and how they may be obtained. Second, it can reduce concerns

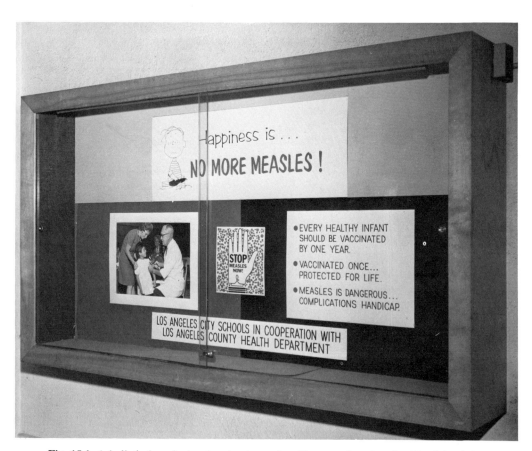

Fig. 15-1. A bulletin board educates about measles. (Courtesy Los Angeles City Schools.)

about discomfort associated with procedures by demonstrating or showing pictures of them in advance. Most youngsters today have already experienced hypodermic injections and have learned that they do not hurt very much. The compressed air injectors used in many mass immunization programs are formidable in appearance, and it helps if children can observe one and learn how it works. One unnecessarily frightened, crying child in an immunization line can make the whole experience a harrowing one for everyone involved.

There is some danger in attempting to teach children and young people the signs and symptoms of communicable diseases. They may imagine that they have certain diseases whether they do or not, and they may attempt unjudicious self-medication. On the other hand, self-observation of indications of syphilis and gonorrhea is essential to the control of these particular diseases.

Student, teacher, and parent involvement in planning and assistance with the conduct of in-school immunization programs may make preparatory education more meaningful and effective than would otherwise be

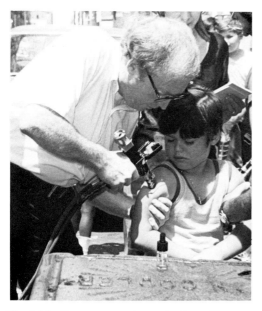

Fig. 15-2. Street corner immunization. (Courtesy Philadelphia Department of Public Health.)

the case. Most persons are willing to learn about procedures in which they are to be actively involved; fewer are willing to acquire information if they perceive it as irrelevant to their own actions. This principle also applies to education with respect to environmental sanitation.

Immunization. An effective school-community program of immunization against a specific disease depends first of all on the availability of an effective vaccine against that disease. Theoretically, no vaccine is 100% effective, but some of them approach that level. Smallpox vaccine, for example, must be credited with the absence of cases in the United States since 1949, as a result of which this vaccine is now used only to protect those who might be exposed.

The vaccines used to prevent diseases in presumably well and unexposed populations are primarily *active* vaccines. Active vaccines are made up of either killed disease-producing organisms or of live ones that are so weakened or modified (attenuated) that they do not cause disease. As a result of administration of an active vaccine, most individuals produce antibodies that assist natural body defenses in destroying the same organism should it invade the body in the future. During the time that antibodies are being produced by the body, active vaccines afford little or no protection. They are therefore usually of little or no value to a person who has already been exposed to a disease; that is, they are slow to act. Once antibodies have been formed, however, the body cells that produce them retain the ability to produce them again, in some cases for 1 or more years, in other cases apparently for life. Active vaccination may therefore be described as long lasting. Active vaccination can occur naturally; any person who has once had measles, for example, is unlikely ever to have it again.

A *passive* vaccine is composed of antibodies against a disease-producing organism or toxin that have already been manufactured by the body cells of another human or other animal. Once injected, these antibodies are immediately ready to attack the organism or toxin that stimulated their production in the first place. Passive vaccines, therefore, are quick acting. The individual who receives a passive vaccine, however, is unable to replicate the antibodies it contains. Thus, passive vaccines are short lived. Like active vaccines, passive ones vary in effectiveness. Antibodies produced by a nursing mother may be passed along to her infant in her milk, thereby providing some degree of temporary natural protection against certain infections. In general, artificial passive vaccines are reserved for use in persons who have been exposed to a disease.

The effectiveness of immunization programs also depends on the administration of vaccines to nearly all members of the population who are at risk of exposure to those diseases against which the selected vaccines provide protection. An effective school-community immunization program, therefore, is one in which:

1. Diseases are identified to which the local population is at risk and for which effective vaccines are available.
2. An outreach program is planned and conducted to bring the susceptible population in for immunization. This includes those who require booster doses as well as initial vaccinations.
3. The selected immunizations are offered at no charge and at times and places convenient to all.
4. The immunization status of individuals in the population is periodically assessed, and those in need of immunization are notified.

Thus, effective programs are preplanned and continuously operated. They aim to reach infants and preschoolers as well as those in school. Crash programs should rarely, if ever, be required.

It is not essential that 100% of the population be immunized against a disease. If 95% are immunized with a vaccine that is 95% effective, then only ten individuals in a hundred will be unprotected. The proportion of immune individuals required to achieve an acceptable degree of group im-

munity varies not only with the effectiveness of the vaccine, but also with the means by which the disease is transmitted and other complex factors. The point to be remembered is that it is usually quite safe to allow conscientious objectors (or the merely obstinate) to go unimmunized. If the immunization is legally required, court action to enforce the requirement is rarely worth the cost in effort and negative public relations.

Immunization time schedules are revised from time to time as new and improved vaccines are developed and as knowledge is accumulated with respect to the need for revaccination for specific diseases. In general, it is recommended that U.S. children receive their first immunizations for diphtheria, whooping cough (pertussis), tetanus, and polio during infancy (the first year of life). After the first birthday, protection against measles, German measles (rubella), and mumps is recommended. It is especially important that girls receive rubella vaccine before adolescence, when they risk pregnancy. Readministrations of the diphtheria, tetanus, pertussis, and polio vaccines are recommended at intervals during the preschool years. These should be repeated (with the exception of pertussis) at about the time of kindergarten entry. Tetanus and diphtheria vaccinations should be repeated at about age 15.*

Influenza vaccine is sometimes recommended for infants and aged persons and for teachers and others whose jobs place them in high risk of exposure. Influenza vaccine is about 70% effective, and to be effective it must be administered annually. Teachers, especially young men, who are not known to have had mumps, should receive mumps vaccine. Mumps in adolescents and adults carries with it the risk of orchitis, an inflammation of the testes (which is especially painful) and ovaries. In general, childhood viral respiratory tract

---

*Recommendations of the Committee on Infectious Diseases, American Academy of Pedriatics, 1971.

Table 15-1. Reported cases and registered deaths for 1963-70, United States from selected communicable diseases

Diseases	1963	1964	1965	1966	1967	1968	1969	1970
Diphtheria								
Cases	314	293	164	209	219	260	241	435
Deaths	45	42	18	20	32	30	25	30
Measles								
Cases (thousands)	385	458	262	204	62	22	26	47
Deaths	364	421	276	261	81	24	41	89
Poliomyelitis								
Paralytic cases	396	106	61	106	40	53	18	31
Deaths	41	17	16	9	16	24	13	7
Whooping cough								
Cases (thousands)	17	13	7	8	10	5	3	4
Deaths	115	93	55	49	37	36	13	12
Gonorrhea								
Cases (thousands)	278	301	325	352	405	465	535	600
Deaths	23	13	9	18	11	1	3	9
Syphilis								
Cases (thousands)	124	114	113	105	103	96	92	91
Deaths (thousands)	3	3	2	2	2	0.6	0.5	0.5
Tuberculosis (all forms)								
Cases (thousands)	54	51	49	48	46	43	39	37
Deaths (thousands)	9	8	8	8	7	6	6	5

Source: National Center for Health Statistics.

diseases are much more serious when they occur in adulthood than in childhood.

Of the diseases for which reported cases and registered deaths are shown in Table 15-1, diphtheria, measles, poliomyelitis, and whooping cough are all preventable through immunization and have been so for each of the years shown. The record is not as impressive for them as it should and could be, because effective immunization programs have not been conducted in many communities. A recent Federal Court decision (Reyes versus Wyeth Laboratories) culminated in a ruling, the burden of which was to require that the recipients of vaccines administered in mass immunization programs must be informed by the manufacturer of the risks as well as the benefits involved. Curran* suggests that this principle could apply to any prescription drug distributed in clinics. This further com-

plicates the task of organizing and conducting immunization programs.

Early identification of cases. Early identification of cases of communicable disease together with their subsequent isolation or exclusion from school is both difficult and relatively ineffective as a control measure for most of the diseases that are commonly found in schools. There are diseases (such as syphilis and gonorrhea) for which exclusion from school is useless and inappropriate. There are other diseases (such as impetigo) in which isolation and exclusion from school are effective in preventing spread. Diseases spread by the respiratory tract route are typically communicated from one person to another well before any signs or symptoms of illness appear, and to complicate matters further, respiratory tract diseases pass through a prodromal period (in which the victim feels ill but the disease is not diagnosable) during which signs and symptoms are indistinguishable from those of a common cold.

*Curran, W. J.: Public health warnings of the risk of oral polio vaccine, Am. J. Public Health **65**:501-502, May 1975.

If identification is followed by treatment that is of benefit to the victim (again, as in the case of syphilis, gonorrhea, or impetigo), then early detection is worthwhile. Our record for gonorrhea (Table 15-1) indicates that this disease is out of control. Although effective treatment is available for it, we have no very reliable method of early detection. Blood tests for detection and effective treatment are available for syphilis, and the downward trends indicate progress. There is, however, no effective cure for the common cold or other diseases of viral origin; the best that can be done is to alleviate the symptoms to some extent.

Early identification of cases of a few serious diseases followed by notification of parents in time for them to take some useful preventive action is worthwhile. For example, parents should be notified of the occurrence of meningococcal meningitis in a classroom and advised to consult the child's usual source of medical care for preventive treatment. It is also important that pregnant girls in contact with unimmunized school children exposed to rubella be notified and urged to seek medical advice.

Primary responsibility for the early detection of cases of communicable diseases in American schools rests with the teacher. Teachers who know their students are better able than anyone else to determine when a youngster seems to be acutely ill. Also, definite signs of illness often develop in the afternoon in a child who appeared perfectly well in the morning. It is neither desirable nor necessary for the teacher to diagnose the illness. If signs of illness appear, the youngster is usually better off at home if someone is there, or resting in the cot room if adult care is not available at home.

Signs and symptoms that should cause teachers to suspect the presence of a communicable disease and (in accordance with local policy) to refer a student to the nurse, to isolate a student at school, or to send him or her home include:

Fever
Unusually flushed face
Unusual pallor
A rash or spots on the skin
Swelling of neck glands
Persistent coughing or sneezing
Red or sore throat
Stiff or rigid neck
Headaches
Nausea or vomiting
Red or watery eyes
Dizziness or headache
Chills or fever
Disinclination to play or work
Pains in chest, limbs, or back of neck
Diarrhea

Readmission standards and procedures should be developed locally or at the state level by school and health officials jointly. It is essential that these be revised frequently in light of changing medical knowledge.

In addition to teacher observation, two types of screening tests are now commonly used in schools to detect communicable diseases. One is a skin test to detect tuberculosis contacts and cases, and the other is the use of a Wood's (ultraviolet) light to detect scalp ringworm infections. Little, if any, in-school screening use has been made of blood tests that are available for syphilis or certain other diseases.

Environmental sanitation. School environmental procedures and standards that help to prevent the transmission of certain diseases have been presented in Chapter 12. These measures are primarily useful in the control of those diseases spread through the ingestion of contaminated food, milk, and water. Attempts to control the spread of respiratory tract diseases in schools by sanitizing air have not proved useful.

Epidemics and school closing. School closing as a means of breaking a threatened or real epidemic is mentioned here only to make the point that it does not work. By the time school closing is considered, the disease is already well spread not only within the school but also within the community. Students will continue to associate with their friends whether school is closed or open. It is useless to keep schools open, of course, where so many students and teachers are absent that no significant teaching or learning is taking place.

Convalescence and the school. Most students who have been ill return to school during the period of convalescence rather than waiting until they have fully recovered. It is generally recommended that physical exertion be held to a minimum during this period on the grounds that resistance to other infections is low. Full participation in physical education activities should be avoided. Children should be observed carefully during convalescence for signs of possible complications such as earaches. Influenza convalescence does not always progress smoothly, and intermittent attendance following recovery from this and other debilitating infections is to be expected.

SOME SPECIFIC DISEASES
OF SCHOOL IMPORTANCE

There are certain communicable diseases that occur frequently enough among the school population or that are important enough in other respects that school professionals should be acquainted with them. Some of them are discussed in Appendix A. Others are discussed below.

Venereal diseases and the school. Gonorrhea and syphilis are the common venereal diseases of concern in the United States at this time. Nearly all the cases that occur among school-age children (even those in the elementary grades) and youth are spread by intimate sexual contacts, that is, through sexual intercourse and oral-genital or genital-anal contacts, whether heterosexual or homosexual. Incidence data are unreliable; we know as a result of surveys that many cases that are diagnosed and treated are not reported by physicians even though reporting is required by law. The nationally reported cases (Table 15-1) suggest that there is continuing upward trend in gonorrhea occurrence, but that syphilis occurrence may be decreasing.

There is no vaccine against either disease available at this time. No natural immunity develops as a result of gonorrhea infection; frequent repeated infections are common. With repeated attacks of the same strain of syphilis some degree of resistance does appear to develop against syphilis, but the degree of protection thus obtained is not high. Health education and the early detection and antibiotic treatment of cases and contacts are thus the only potentially effective means of control available at this time.

Health educators cannot dictate the behavior of individuals. They can only present choices and permit discussions, which hopefully will lead young people to choose protective behaviors that the young people regard as sensible and feasible for them. Also, teachers can only go as far as school administrators and the community will allow them to go. Encouragement of open, frank, and comprehensive classroom discussion of the venereal diseases and methods of controlling them is the natural result of increasing adult recognition of the VD problem.

Traditionalist opinion in our society holds that sexual intercourse should be delayed until marriage, or at least until engagement. Many youngsters accept and are guided by this viewpoint, but the sex urge is basic and strong. Given the information that masturbation is a useful and risk-free way of relieving sexual tension, some will use it as a substitute for sexual outlets that entail risk of venereal infection. Young people, however, do fall in love and wish to express that love in physical ways. Some will be content with kissing and petting for a while, particularly if petting includes mutual manual genital stimulation to orgasm. Although this practice carries with it some risk of venereal infection, the risk is small. Syphilis can be transmitted from the genitalia of one partner to the bloodstream of the other through cut or scratched skin. Gonorrhea, on the other hand, requires the warm, moist, dark environment provided by mucous membranes. Sooner or later most of us are satisfied by nothing less than genital-genital, genital-oral, or genital-anal intercourse, preferably with a loved partner. This carries no risk of venereal infection if a monogamous relationship is developed and maintained, but relatively few humans confine their sexual relationships to a single partner, as mallard ducks and many other animals do. Even so, risk of infection can be substantially reduced by the use of condoms during intercourse and/or thorough soap and water washing of the genitalia afterwards. A few schools have provided condoms to students. Many young people are too embarrassed to ask for them at the prescription counters of drugstores, but many if not most druggists treat such requests in a neutral way, knowing their importance not only in the prevention of disease but of unwanted pregnancy also.

Early detection of venereal infections among school-age children and youth depends almost entirely on recognition by the individual of signs and symptoms. Occasionally a case will be identified when a student is named as a sex contact by another victim in the course of a health department investigation, and premarital or prenatal blood tests for syphilis may bring other cases to light.

In males, the first sign of gonorrhea infection is a thick, yellowish discharge from the penis, which first appears 3 to 9 days after exposure. This is usually accompanied by itching and burning of the urethra and pain upon attempted urination. Some strains of the causative organism, *Neisseria gonorrhoeae,* cause relatively asymptomatic infections, however. Females are not so fortunate. In them, a certain amount of vaginal discharge is normal, and early gonorrhea infection may either be unaccompanied by discomfort or may produce relatively minor itching and burning. (In cases acquired through oral or anal exposure, discomfort, inflammations, and discharge are associated with those areas.) Later in the course of the genitally acquired disease, the infection may spread further into the genitals and urinary systems. From there it may enter the bloodstream, and as a result sterility, arthritis, and heart damage may occur.

Syphilis, which is caused by infection with the spirochete *Treponema pallidum,*

first manifests itself by the appearance of a sore (chancre) at the point of infection about 3 weeks after contact. The sore (which in some cases fails to appear at all) heals by itself in 4 to 6 weeks. Disappearance of the chancre is followed by the secondary stage, which is usually characterized by an infectious rash of the skin and mucous membranes. Within several weeks to a year the secondary signs disappear, to be followed by a latent period that may last anywhere from a few weeks to several years. Tertiary syphilis, when it finally appears, may result in cardiovascular or central nervous system damage. In the primary stage, females are often at a disadvantage in that the initial chancre, which is painless, may be hidden in the vagina.

The use of scare tactics in venereal disease education, based on the unfortunate late effects of syphilis and gonorrhea, has been tried in the armed services with no discernible useful results. Such tactics have no place whatever in school health education, but young people must recognize that VD is difficult to detect in its early stages and that the consequences of failure to prevent or detect and treat it are serious.

Detection is worthless unless it leads to treatment. Fortunately, a number of state legislatures have recognized this fact and have enacted laws that permit physicians and clinics to diagnose and treat venereal diseases in minors without informing parents or obtaining their consent. This means that health educators can inform students of these rights and of the existence of community clinics that they can attend if they suspect that they have VD. Health service workers can also refer individual students to such clinics and assure them that their parents need not be informed. Thus, students can be relieved of the fear of parental wrath and reprisal that have kept many of them from seeking treatment in the past. Specific information about clinic hours, policies, and assurance (if this can be given honestly) that clinic patients will be treated humanely and that their identity will be kept in confidence also promote student utilization of diagnostic and treatment services. For example, some clinics no longer interview young people about their sex contacts, in part because the process discourages prospective patients and in part because staff time for follow-up of contacts is simply not available. Instead, patients may be asked to address envelopes for follow-up by mail. Treatment of contacts of suspected cases is not always preceded by diagnosis, because many persons come in for diagnosis but fail to return for treatment. In general, the better acquainted students are with local resources, the more likely they are to use them.

Neither physical environmental controls nor exclusion of infected persons from school is of practical value in VD control.

Common cold and other respiratory tract diseases. On the average, each person in the U.S. has between two and three or more *colds* a year. The incidence is highest in young children and decreases somewhat with age. Colds develop 12 to 72 hours after exposure to either the coughs and sneezes of another cold victim or to papers or other articles that are contaminated by nose or throat discharge. The causative organism may be any one of a large number of different viruses. Vaccines that are intended to provide immunity have proved ineffective. As in the case with other viral diseases, the only known cures occur with the passage of time. Cold victims are often said to recover in 7 days with treatment and in a week without it. Large doses of vitamin C have not been shown unequivocally to either prevent colds or abort them. Medical consultation is a waste of the physician's time and the patient's money. Neither environmental control measures nor isolation of cold victims can be said to have any significant effect in prevention.

Nasal stuffiness can be relieved by hot showers, water vaporizers, or by use of phenylephrine hydrochloride nose drops or sprays (.025% for children, .05% for adults) no more than two or three times a day. General discomfort may be reduced by aspirin that is taken in accordance with package directions. These measures are suggested for home, not school, use.

The main concern of the school is whether what appears to be a cold is, in fact, a cold and not the prodrome of some other disease. If a temperature of 101° F (rectal) or higher is present, or if a rash develops, then it is only reasonable to assume that the "cold" is, in fact, a case of some such disease as measles, rubella, chickenpox, or scarlet fever, all of which are communicable diseases of public health importance.

Influenza is caused by one of several types of influenza viruses. An annual injection of influenza vaccine is moderately effective in preventing the disease; this is usually recommended for teachers, but only for those students who are not in good health. The symptoms are like those of a cold plus chills, fever, general misery, and headache. The mode of spread, the short incubation period, and the resistance of the disease to drugs and antibiotics are other characteristics shared with the common cold. Influenza patients, however, belong at home in bed until recovery, which usually occurs in a week or less. Aspirin to reduce fever accompanied by high fluid intake helps make the course of influenza a little more bearable. Returning convalescents need a few days of reduced activity to recover fully.

Measles and rubella are other respiratory tract diseases of viral origin. For these diseases, the available attenuated live virus vaccines are highly effective. Both diseases begin with cold symptoms and produce a rash, but with measles typical small white spots (Koplik spots) also appear in the mouth. Both diseases are more severe in adults than in children. Exposed persons who are not well enough to tolerate these diseases may be protected by prompt injection of a passive vaccine (immune serum globulin, or ISG). All those with measles or rubella belong at home, not in school, but the disease is well seeded in the school before the first case is discovered. The itching associated with measles may be relieved by calamine lotion, and fever is reduced by aspirin.

Chickenpox, like measles and rubella, is characterized by a rash and is more severe in adulthood. It is highly contagious, and the rash resembles blisters. Calamine lotion relieves itching. This is important because scratching the eruptions is likely to leave scars.

Infectious mononucleosis is a common disease among adolescents that is believed to be viral in origin. There is no known means of preventing, controlling, or curing the disease. Onset typically occurs with fever, headaches, and general body discomfort. The lymph nodes are enlarged, and a sore throat is common. In some cases jaundice develops; thus, mononucleosis may be mistaken for hepatitis. Recovery occurs usually in about 2 to 3 weeks, but convalescence may be prolonged and is accompanied by lack of stamina and ability to concentrate on school or other tasks.

Meningococcal meningitis, or inflammation of the membranes that cover the brain and spinal cord, is a frightening disease because of the delirium (and sometimes coma) and muscle rigidity that accompany it. The meningococcus bacterium is one of several organisms that cause meningitis, and thanks to present methods of prevention and treatment, fatalities are nowhere near as common as they once were. The disease is not nearly as communicable as it generally is believed to be. Dull and Dowdle* estimate that only about one in a thousand individuals who harbor the organism in their throats develop the disease. Nevertheless, outbreaks occur occasionally in schools. The disease is spread (like other respiratory tract infections) through close person-to-person contact and begins to appear 2 to 10 days after exposure. When it does occur in schools, parents and students should be notified with the suggestion that they consult their personal physicians for possible preventive treatments. Preventive mea-

sures include drug prophylaxis and the possible use of an active vaccine now available for one form of the disease. Reporting of cases to public health authorities is mandatory.

Scarlet fever and strep throat are each caused by certain streptococcal bacteria. Scarlet fever is the same disease as streptococcal sore throat except that in scarlet fever a red skin rash is present. These diseases are usually spread in the same manner as the common cold or by contaminated food. There is no effective vaccine against them, but streptococcal infections are readily curable by antibiotic therapy. Anyone with a high fever accompanied by a red, swollen sore throat, flushed face, and swollen lymph nodes in the neck should be suspected of having a streptococcal infection. Exclusion from school and referral to the individual's source of medical care for diagnosis and treatment are appropriate procedures, together with readmission upon the recommendation of the physician.

Streptococcal infections are sometimes followed by a serious, long-term illness called rheumatic fever, which is treated primarily by an extended period of bed rest. Repeated streptococcal infections, especially among rheumatic fever patients, increases the possibility that rheumatic heart damage may follow rheumatic fever. Young rheumatic fever patients therefore receive penicillin prophylaxis for several years to prevent reinfection.

Tuberculosis (TB) is a bacterial infection that usually spreads from person to person in the same manner as the common cold. It usually involves the lung tissues, but it may also invade other body structures. The steady downward trend in cases and deaths in the United States (see Table 15-1) is largely a result of effective early detection and treatment programs. Case-finding techniques are skin tests and chest x-rays. Modern antituberculosis drugs have sharply reduced the cost and time of treatment. Although a vaccine (BCG) is available, it has been used in the United States only among health care professionals and in

---

*Dull, H. B., and Dowdle, W. R., In Sartwell, P. E., editor: *Maxcy-Rosenau preventive medicine and public health,* New York, 1973, Appleton-Century-Crofts, p. 149.

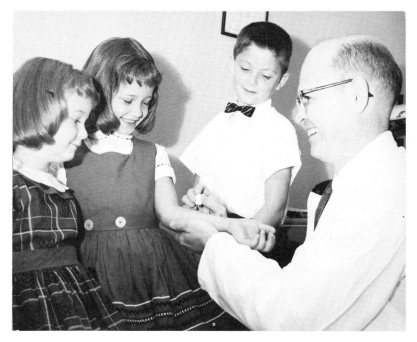

Fig. 15-3. Tuberculosis skin testing. (Courtesy Lederle Laboratories.)

certain poverty areas where the prevalence of the disease has remained high. There are two reasons why BCG vaccine has not been more widely used. One is the belief that recipients become and remain positive to the skin test, and therefore this case-finding technique would no longer be useful. The other reason is that the effectiveness of the vaccine is moderate or low at best. From a recent study of its effectiveness among children and youth in Puerto Rico, Comstock and his co-workers* concluded that its effectiveness among those not previously positive to the skin test was only 29%.

Most states and local school districts either mandate or offer skin tests and chest x-rays to both students and adult staff members. Required programs have frequently grown out of unfortunate incidents in which an infected school staff member has spread tuberculosis to students. Generally, the skin test is used as the primary screening device,

and positive reactors are then x-rayed. This procedure minimizes both the cost of the program and the exposure of individuals to radiation.

The success of a school-community TB case-finding program depends, first, on a well-planned and conducted program of health education before the testing. Second, success depends on the availability of professionals to follow up both those screened positive and the human contacts who may have exposed them to tuberculosis in the first place.

Health education must be directed to the students and staff members who are to be tested and to the parents of students to be tested. The basic objectives must include:

1. Encouragement of willing participation in the program.
2. Alleviation of the fears that naturally result from a positive skin test or chest x-ray.

Participation is encouraged by the existence of a legal requirement, and the nature of the requirement, if any, should be explained. Willingness to participate is en-

---

*Comstock, G. W., Livesey, V. T., and Woolpert, S. R.: Evaluation of BCG vaccination among Puerto Rican children, Am. J. Public Health **64:** 283-291, March 1974.

couraged by explaining that the purpose of the program is to discover cases of TB at an early stage so that they can be effectively treated with drugs to protect both the patient and those who come in contact with the patient. Willingness is also encouraged by explanation of the simple and relatively painless nature of the skin test. Recipients should understand that the test is *not* a vaccination, although the procedure is similar to vaccination.

A positive tuberculin skin test produces an observable reaction. Most reactors, therefore, have good reason to believe that they are positive before the reaction is evaluated by a nurse or physician. The resulting anxiety can be alleviated in advance by explaining that a positive skin test is produced by prior *exposure* to the disease and is not necessarily proof that one has active tuberculosis. Likewise, a single positive chest x-ray does not necessarily mean active TB; other tests are required to establish a diagnosis of active TB. In the event that tuberculosis is present, modern treatment halts the disease process and protects others without seriously interfering with the activities of the patient.

The recommended procedure is to provide related education to students and parents both before and at the time that parental consent slips are distributed. It is wise to word the consent slip in such a way that permission for both follow-up x-rays and the initial skin test is obtained at the same time. Because of the anxiety aroused by tuberculosis, all students and their parents should be notified of negative as well as positive results. Immediate follow-up of family and other close contacts of positive reactors (which involves further skin tests and x-rays) is important.

Diphtheria and poliomyelitis are diseases that rarely occur except in communities where immunization programs are inadequate or neglected. Both begin with cold-like symptoms. Diphtheria progresses to high fever, sore throat, and prostration. The diphtheria bacillus sometimes causes the development of white or gray patches on membranes in the throat or on the tonsils. The bacillus also produces a toxin (poison) that may cause neuritis or heart damage. The disease, however, is medically curable. Polio, without paralysis, is difficult to recognize; aching muscles and a stiff neck are common symptoms, which are shared with many other diseases. Polio is caused by a virus; thus, no curative treatment is available. Supportive treatment during the acute phase of paralytic polio helps to maintain life. Physical therapy helps restore functions of body parts disabled by paralysis. The suspected occurrence of either disease should be reported to the health department. Diagnosis should provide impetus for improvement and extension of the community-school immunization program.

Skin infections and infestations. The diseases discussed in this section are often referred to as nuisance diseases, perhaps because they are more annoying than debilitating. Some of them are communicated from objects or other persons to their victims. Others are not regarded as communicable but instead result from ecological imbalance in which the resistance of the individuals is lowered for some reason and an infective agent that normally coexists in relative peace with its human host multiplies and causes trouble.

Lice and *scabies* are two such diseases that are classified as communicable and that are caused by small multicelled animals rather than by viruses, fungi, or bacteria. For this reason, they are more properly referred to as infestations than as infections.

Lice may infest the hair of the head, the clothes and torso, or the pubic hair (crab lice). Three different kinds of lice are involved. Such infestations are sometimes referred to as pediculosis, a more elegant term than lousiness. Lice feed on blood, which they obtain by biting, which in turn results in itching and scratching. These are the most obvious signs of infestation. They lay their eggs (called nits) on hair or clothing to which they are quite firmly glued. Nits appear as small white objects,

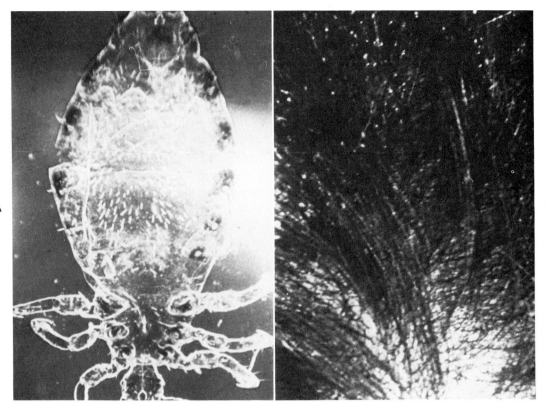

Fig. 15-4. A, Head louse. **B,** Louse nits. (Courtesy Reed & Carnrick.)

not unlike bits of dandruff, and are observable on close inspection, but other bits of material are sometimes mistaken for nits. Lice themselves may be observed, but they are quite small, about an eighth of an inch long.

Lice may be transmitted from one person to another by close contact, including sexual intercourse, or by using clothing or personal articles such as combs that belong to another. They may also be picked up from toilet seats, gym mats, upholstered furniture, and similar objects.

A variety of effective pesticides are available in a variety of convenient forms such as shampoos and ointments for the treatment of louse infestations. The new pesticides, which have largely replaced DDT, effectively eradicate both lice and nits. Clothing, of course, should be laundered or dry cleaned concurrently with treatment of the person. Some of the new preparations are classified as prescription items and others are not. All include instructions for use.

Scabies (the 7-year itch) is caused by a small mite that burrows under the skin, laying its eggs as it proceeds along a line. The itching is more severe at night and during exercise than at other times. Scratching and itching (usually localized in the finger webs, the fronts of the wrists, under the arms, at the belt line, or in the general area of the buttocks and external genitalia) characterize the disease. More than one student in a classroom or more than one member of a family is likely to be infested.

Some of the same preparations (those containing benzyl benzoate) that are effective against lice are also effective against scabies.

Since both lice and scabies can and do spread through a classroom, most schools exclude infested youngsters during the day or two required for treatment and concurrent laundry of clothes.

Fungus infections seem to require individual susceptibility as a necessary condition for their occurrence. Fungi form spores that are resistant to treatment and that are generally present in the environment, waiting for a susceptible person to appear. The most common fungi infections in the U.S. schools are athlete's foot (tinea pedis), scalp ringworm (tinea capitas), and jockstrap itch (tinea cruris). Like lousiness and scabies, they are often referred to as nuisance diseases. Fungi thrive in warm, dark, moist environments, and preventive environmental measures therefore are directed to keeping showers and locker rooms especially clean, light, dry and well ventilated. Health education can promote personal cleanliness, including emphasis on drying well with a clean towel after bathing.

Athlete's foot and *jockstrap itch* are best controlled by the environmental and health education procedures noted above. A clean towel service for physical education students is helpful in preventing both of these types of infections. Use of clean undergarments daily, including clean athletic supporters for boys, is also recommended for the prevention of jockstrap itch. Careful drying of the feet with a clean towel after showering, use of clean socks daily (absorbent socks made of cotton or wool help), use of a nonmedicated drying foot powder (talcum), and ventilated shoes are also useful control measures for athlete's foot. So-called sanitizing foot baths or sprays are useless and a waste of school funds.

Exclusion of students with jockstrap itch or athlete's foot from showers or swimming probably does little if anything to control the spread of these infections. Those with severe athlete's foot in which open sores are present may be excluded from shower or swimming to protect them against secondary bacterial infections. These students may also benefit from medical treatment prescribed by their personal general physician, a dermatologist, or a podiatrist. Other victims (or all students) may be instructed

to wear shower clogs, or disposable paper slippers may be provided. Such footwear at least has some public relations value and may afford some degree of protection.

Scalp ringworm rarely occurs after puberty. This fungus infection is spread from one person to another or from a pet to a person. It may be spread by direct contact, by common use of such items as caps, combs, and barber tools, or by contact with contaminated bus or theatre seats or other furniture. It appears as round, patchy areas of near baldness on the scalp. The skin is reddened and may itch to some extent. When a case is discovered in a classroom, the usual procedure is to inspect all the pupils by shining a special ultraviolet lamp called Wood's light on their scalps. A green-yellow phosphorescence indicates the presence of infection. Infected persons need not be excluded from school. They do, however, require treatment. Treatment includes both daily shampoos and the use of prescription medications for a number of weeks under the supervision of a physician.

Warts are probably mildly communicable, but there is no need to treat them as such because one is either susceptible or not and because the virus that causes them is widespread anyway. Their appearance on unclothed parts of the body is disconcerting to both victims and others. When they occur on the soles of the feet they are called plantar warts, and the pressure of walking presses the wart inward and is often painful. They can be removed by physicians or podiatrists, but they frequently return. Left untreated or treated by prayer, charms, and incantations, they also disappear (but perhaps less quickly than under medical intervention), and they also return in time. Eventually, many wart victims appear to develop some sort of resistance to them, and they disappear forever.

Cold sores (or herpes simplex) are also caused by a virus. Apparently, almost all of us acquire the virus at some point in our lives. It lies dormant and appears under infection or such stress as is caused by an impending wedding, final examination, or sunburn. They eventually dry up and disappear by themselves, with or without treatment.

Cold sores are sometimes confused with a bacterial skin infection called *impetigo contagiosa*. This highly contagious disease causes the eruption of small blisters on the face or body. The blisters then develop into weeping, oozing ulcers, which are finally covered by yellowish scabs. The infection not only spreads from one person to another but also from one part of the body to another. It is essential that any youngster suspected of having impetigo be excluded from school and referred for medical treatment. Treatment effectively controls the infection in a few days, and excluded students may be readmitted on the basis of a note from the physician.

Boils or *carbuncles* are swollen, usually painful infections that arise around hair follicles. They are usually caused by staphylococcal or streptococcal bacterial infections. As long as the skin that covers a boil or carbuncle remains unbroken, it poses no danger to others. When the skin eventually bursts and drainage occurs, there is immediate risk that the infection will spread to others. Attempts to induce early rupture and drainage by squeezing a boil or carbuncle present a risk that the infection may invade the bloodstream and be spread to other parts of the body. These twin dangers dictate that persons with boils and carbuncles be referred for medical treatment and advised neither to pick or squeeze the area nor to attempt self-treatment by hot compresses or any other means.

Bellyaches. In the case of any individual who complains of pains in the belly, regardless of location, *appendicitis* should always be suspected. No food, water, or medication of any kind should be given. In appendicitis, the pain typically shifts from one location to another and is accompanied by acute soreness and muscle rigidity. Nausea, vomiting, and either diarrhea or constipation sometime accompany appendicitis. Those with acute appendicitis usually prefer to lie on one side with the legs drawn up.

Cessation of pain may signify a ruptured appendix. It is not easy to rule out appendicitis, and it is not a school health service function to attempt to do so. Any student or staff member with suspected appendicitis belongs under the care of a physician who is equipped to conduct blood tests and other diagnostic procedures and to arrange for surgery if indicated. The risk of failing to remove an inflamed appendix is much greater than that involved in removing a normal appendix.

Recurrent bellyaches are sometimes the result of chronic appendicitis and sometimes are psychosomatic in origin. The latter is almost a sure bet when the ache recurs daily at the same time that a hated class is scheduled. Careful questioning may identify such cases. ("What is it that you hate about school?")

Other bellyaches are due to a variety of food or waterborne infections or poisons. Food infection or poisoning is almost always the source of an epidemic of bellyaches that occur among school members. Singly occurring cases have usually acquired their illness from food or water obtained outside the school.

Primary prevention of school-based food or waterborne infections or poisons is discussed in Chapter 12. The prompt removal from service of any food handler who is suffering from diarrhea, a sore throat, or a boil or carbuncle is an important aspect of prevention. When suspected outbreaks of school origin do occur, immediate notification of and investigation by public health authorities is a must.

The specific diseases discussed below are illustrative of the food and waterborne gastrointestinal diseases.

Infectious hepatitis is caused by a specific virus (A type) that is different from the virus (B type) that causes serum hepatitis. Unlike serum hepatitis, which is ordinarily spread by injections, infectious hepatitis is usually acquired by the oral ingestion of food or water that is contaminated by human fecal matter. In schools and families the possibility that direct or indirect transfer may occur, such as through kissing or sharing a beverage, has not been ruled out. Disease onset is characterized by nausea and/or vomiting, loss of appetite, abdominal discomfort, and headache. Jaundice may appear later. The disease is prolonged, and relapses tend to occur during convalescence. There is no specific curative treatment. Some persons have the disease in such a mild form that it is not recognized. Occurrences of the disease among family contacts of patients may be prevented or modified by injections of immune serum globulin.

Salmonella infections occur so frequently that most of us have probably suffered at least one episode without recognizing it as such. There are several different *Salmonella* bacteria, ranging from those that produce relatively mild forms of the disease to those that produce typhoid and paratyphoid fever. The onset is abrupt and is characterized by diarrhea, abdominal cramps, nausea, vomiting, and sometimes fever. Onset usually occurs between 12 to 24 hours after ingestion of contaminated food. Most cases require little or no treatment; usually only replacement of lost body fluid is required. In typhoid fever and other severe forms, specific drug therapy may be helpful. Sources of infection include ill food-handlers, inadequately cooked food (especially poultry, meat, milk, and eggs), food that is kept warm for several hours before serving, and food that is contaminated by insect or rodent feces.

Staphylococcal food poisoning is caused by food that has become contaminated by staphylococcal bacteria, often by food-handlers who have boils or carbuncles who fail to wash their hands thoroughly, or who use their bare hands instead of gloves in the preparation of foods to be served raw. If the contaminated food is kept at room temperature instead of under refrigeration for some hours before it is served, the bacteria produces a toxin (poison) that causes abrupt onset of nausea, abdominal cramps, vomiting, and diarrhea. Body temperature is frequently below normal, and blood pres-

sure may be reduced. The poisoning is rarely fatal, and victims usually recover in a day or two. The types of food most commonly implicated include pastries, salads, dressings, custards, cold meats, and meat products, all of which should be kept under refrigeration from the time they are prepared until they are served.

Botulism, like staphyloccal food poisoning is caused in a toxin produced by a bacterium growing in contaminated food. The causative bacillus is one that grows and produces its poison most efficiently in a non-acid environment from which air is excluded. The foods most commonly implicated are fruits and vegetables that have been canned under conditions of inadequate heat and steam pressure, and smoked or preserved meats and fish, especially those encased in tight plastic wrappings. The organism produces gas; thus, any can of food that bulges should not be served. The toxin is destroyed by boiling. Twelve to 36 hours after consumption of contaminated food, the victim will have headaches, dizziness, vomiting, diarrhea, and weakness. As the toxin invades the central nervous system, hoarseness, difficulty in speech, and double vision are observed. A majority of the victims die, although early recognition and treatment with a passive vaccine is effective. Any suspected case should be immediately reported to public health authorities. Persons who have eaten food suspected of contamination must be located and given treatment.

QUESTIONS FOR STUDY AND DISCUSSION

1. What are the respective responsibilities of schools and health departments in regard to communicable disease control in schools?
2. List and describe each of the four basic communicable disease control procedures that are applicable through school health and health education.
3. What are the general characteristics of syphilis and gonorrhea?
4. What basic and effective procedures for the control of VD can be applied in schools?
5. Which of these VD control procedures are likely to arouse community opposition, and why? What ways can you suggest of overcoming community opposition?

6. What control measures are applicable to respiratory tract diseases generally?
7. What specific school procedures are applicable to control of each of the respiratory tract diseases discussed in the text?
8. What control measures are applicable to skin infections and infestations?
9. What specific school procedures are applicable to each of the skin infections and infestations described in the text?
10. What noncommunicable causes of bellyaches are suggested? In what ways and how accurately can school professionals distinguish any of these causes from the others?
11. If you were a student who came to the school nurse with a probable noncommunicable bellyache, what procedures would you prefer that the nurse follow?
12. What school-community procedures help prevent communicable gastrointestinal diseases in general?
13. What specific procedures are applicable to the control of each of the communicable gastrointestinal diseases discussed in the text?
14. Given extremely limited time in which to teach students about communicable diseases, what general concepts would you emphasize, and why? What two or three specific diseases would you choose to teach about at the elementary and secondary levels, and why?

REFERENCES

Benenson, A. S., editor: *Control of communicable diseases in man,* ed. 11, New York, 1970, American Public Health Association.

Eisner, V., and Callan L. B.: *Dimensions of school health,* Springfield, Ill., 1974, Charles C Thomas, Publisher.

Hanlon, J. J.: *Public health administration and practice,* ed. 6, St. Louis, 1974, The C. V. Mosby Co.

Henderson, J.: *Emergency medical guide,* ed. 3, New York, 1973, McGraw-Hill, Inc.

Kogan, B. A.: *Health: man in a changing environment,* ed. 2, New York, 1974, Harcourt Brace Jovanovich, Inc.

Mayer, J.: *Health,* New York, 1974, D. Van Nostrand Co.

The medicine show, ed. 4, Mt. Vernon, N.Y., 1974, Consumers Union.

Nemir, A., and Schaller, W. E.: *The school health program,* Philadelphia, 1975, W. B. Saunders Co.

Sartwell, P. E., editor: *Maxcy-Rosenau preventive medicine and public health,* ed. 10, New York, 1973, Appleton-Century-Crofts.

CHAPTER 16 ❧ Other departures from normal physical health

Many children and young people are handicapped in learning or in other aspects of life by a variety of long-lasting, or non-infectious, health problems. Among these, problems of vision and hearing and learning disabilities have been discussed in Chapter 14. This chapter is devoted to discussion of several other common chronic physical health problems.

NUTRITION PROBLEMS

In our discussion of growth and development we attempted to distinguish between the concepts of overweight and fatness. Individuals may weigh more than average for their age and height and still be in excellent health if their excess weight is largely composed of muscle. Conversely, healthy individuals may weigh considerably less than average if this is dictated by genetic predisposition rather than by inadequate dietary intake or disorders of metabolism. Nevertheless, there are individuals who are much too fat or too thin to be described as healthy.

Fatness. Mayer* estimates that about 10% of the school population may be too fat and notes that the prevalence of fatness ranges up to 20% in some high schools. Children tend to be less fat in the elementary grades than they do at later ages. Many healthy boys put on fat during the year or so before puberty, but this fatness usually disappears with the adolescent growth spurt. Normal skinfold thicknesses for girls, on the other hand, are greater than those for boys at every age and increase steadily with age. There is no doubt that many adolescent girls who believe

themselves to be too fat really are not. There is a general tendency to fatness among lower socioeconomic groups, perhaps because high carbohydrate foods are traditionally cheaper than high protein foods, and perhaps because the poor have learned to eat whenever and whatever food is available.

It is an oversimplification of the problem to say that fatness is caused by overeating and a lack of exercise and to conclude from this that the solution is simply to exert will power and thus eat less and exercise more. We pointed out earlier that tendency to fatness is associated with genetic body types, specifically with endomorphy and mesomorphy. There are also environmental factors, such as the kind of food available, social conditioning with respect to the kinds of food and eating patterns that are valued, and the potential for exercise available, that influence obesity. In addition, complex physiological and psychological factors play a part in the control of eating habits and metabolism; there are, for example, persons who are fat (or thin) because of endocrine gland disorders, although such cases are rare. We know that fat parents produce fat babies who grow up to be fat adults.

Epidemiological studies have demonstrated that associations exist between obesity and a variety of health problems; for example, as a group, those who are obese are more likely to develop cardiovascular disease and diabetes than those who are not obese. Recent evidence suggests, however, that these ailments are not necessarily the result of fatness alone but are caused by interactions of fatness with other factors. For example, those who are both obese and have high blood pressure are more susceptible to heart disease than those who are merely fat,

---

*Mayer, J.: *Health,* New York, 1974, D. Van Nostrand Co., p. 145.

and those who are both obese and have a family history of diabetes are more likely to develop diabetes than those who are fat only. Still, fatness imposes dreadful social and psychological consequences upon its victims. In our society, for example, fatness is considered repulsive, and fat people tend to be rejected not only as potential sex partners but also as friendship and job candidates.

Prevention. There are three approaches to the primary prevention of fatness to which school health and health education can make what may prove to be significant contributions. One is the promotion of healthful dietary practices through the kind of integrated nutrition education and school feeding program described in Chapter 13.

This must include an absolute prohibition against the empty calorie snacks too frequently made available to youngsters via vending machines, candy sales, and the like, and the substitution for these of fruit and other items that are relatively low in calories and high in vitamins and minerals. The second approach is the development of joy and skills in lifetime physical activities that can be promoted through a sound program of physical education, recreation, and sports for the many rather than sports for the few. The importance of this last admonition should be obvious to anyone who has observed the high prevalence of potbellies among former athletes. Finally, it is essential that the future mothers of America be taught that a big baby is not necessarily

Table 16-1. Ninetieth percentile skinfold thickness measurements for U.S. youth (in millimeters) by age, race, and sex and site of measurements

Age, race, and sex	Site of measurement	
	Triceps	Subscapular
White males		
12 years	19.8	14.0
13 years	19.7	16.5
14 years	17.4	14.6
15 years	16.4	14.8
16 years	16.5	15.0
17 years	15.8	17.1
White females		
12 years	22.1	18.6
13 years	22.7	21.3
14 years	23.5	20.4
15 years	25.4	24.4
16 years	25.5	24.0
17 years	25.3	23.4
Black males		
12 years	15.3	9.4
13 years	15.6	11.6
14 years	14.2	10.5
15 years	10.6	9.4
16 years	11.7	11.2
17 years	14.0	11.9
Black females		
12 years	22.5	20.5
13 years	23.9	18.7
14 years	22.1	18.1
15 years	22.7	21.5
16 years	26.4	26.6
17 years	23.3	22.1

Adapted from Skinfold thickness of youths 12-17 years, United States, DHEW Publication No. (HRA) 74-1614, Jan. 1974.

a better baby, that it is a great mistake to stuff food down an infant until it runs out of his or her mouth. They should come to understand also that desired toys, trips, or activities are as effective rewards for good behavior as slabs of cake or candy bars and that these are far healthier than calorie-laden goodies. This reasoning is based on studies that indicate that overfeeding in infancy results in large numbers of fat cells in the body and that fat babies become fat children who grow to be fat adults.

Identification. Many obese individuals can be readily identified as such by observation of the rolls of the fat that surround them, particularly about the upper arms, chest, belly, and thighs. If we accept Mayer's estimate that 10% of the school population are too fat, then other less obvious cases may be identified by assuming that those with skinfold thicknesses at or in excess of the ninetieth percentile for U.S. youth may be so classified. Table 16-1 shows the ninetieth percentile values for U.S. youth for both triceps and subscapular measurements.

Skinfold measurements are not reliable if carelessly made. Those who take the measurements must be trained to do so. The subject must be placed in a standard posi-

tion, which for most measurements is relaxed and standing. The skinfold, which consists of two layers of skin and its underlying fat, is grasped firmly between the thumb and forefinger, and the calipers are then applied. Special skinfold calipers, which are so constructed as to exert a constant pressure against a skinfold of any thickness, are used. The reading should be checked against one taken at the same site on the opposite side of the body. The reading taken is then compared with a table of norm values.

Treatment. Weight reduction is a fertile field for quacks of all kinds, because so many persons wish to lose weight and because there is no quick and easy method of doing so. Teenage girls are particularly susceptible to weird and unsafe published diets, many of which are authored by individuals with legitimate medical degrees but without scientific or ethical sense. Those whose families are well-to-do are, like their parents, fair game for pill-happy "fat doctors," purveyors of weight reduction devices, and operators of so-called health spas, who not only rob them of their money but often of their health as well. That no one of these approaches is at once quick, safe,

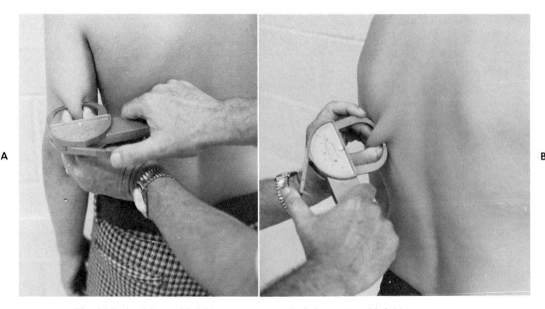

Fig. 16-1. A, Triceps skinfold measurement. **B,** Subscapular skinfold measurement.

and effective is demonstrated by the fact that so many of them exist and prosper.

Safe and effective approaches to obesity reduction must start with a medical health examination and interview that are designed to determine any medical problem that may be present, such as endocrine disorders and high blood pressure, as well as the extent of the obesity and the individual's family health history, dietary, and exercise habits. A diet is prescribed that is designed to provide all recommended nutrients for health and activity with the total caloric intake (from carbohydrates, fats, and protein) lessened to one that will produce a weight loss of about 2 pounds a week when combined with a medically safe exercise program. But all this is not enough. There must also be concurrent psychological support to assist the individual in acquiring a new set of eating and exercise behaviors that must be maintained for the rest of his or her life.

Such support may be provided through group therapy. Behavior modification techniques are sometimes employed. In some schools group therapy of this kind is provided through the joint effort of school dietitians, nurses, and health and physical educators in cooperation with the personal sources of health care of the participants. One of the in-school sponsors should be a person trained in behavioral therapy, if this approach is used.

Obese students should be referred to their physicians for preparticipation evaluation and dietary and exercise prescriptions. Such groups should meet regularly throughout the year. The procedures used are often patterned after the techniques used by such relatively successful programs as TOPS or Weight Watchers.

Anorexia nervosa. A disturbing number of cases of anorexia nervosa are observed among adolescent girls. These girls have apparently been so aversely conditioned against food that they are literally starving themselves. A number of deaths have been reported. Their plight suggests that the American antifatness crusade may have been too vigorous. In many cases, hospital-ization for forced feeding is medically required. Psychotherapeutic intervention is essential though not always successful. As early as this condition is suspected, the parents should be urged to seek medical and psychotherapeutic assistance. School counseling without referral is useless and only delays possibly effective treatment.

DENTAL DEFECTS

The most common dental health problems among school-age children and youth are dental caries (tooth decay), malocclusion (misaligned teeth), and periodontal diseases (diseases of the gums and other tissue surrounding the teeth). Caries is the most common cause of tooth loss among children, while periodontal disease causes most loss among adults. Collision sports and accidents also cause significant loss among active persons.

Preservation of healthy teeth and gums and restoration of damaged or missing teeth are important for several reasons. Sound teeth improve personal appearance, contribute to effective speech, and are necessary to digestion. In addition, tooth decay and periodontitis frequently cause both bad breath and dental pain or discomfort.

Few if any of us are able to achieve and maintain good dental health without regular dental care. Yet National Health Survey data for 1973 indicate that 33% of U.S. children and youth under the age of 17 years have never visited a dentist. Fig. 16-2 shows that both dental health and dental care are correlated closely with family income. Even if the poverty aspect of the problem were eliminated, as it has been to some extent through Medicaid and other welfare programs, most authorities agree that the present number of professionals is inadequate to meet the need for preventive and restorative care. Some progress is being made by training dental hygienists and other auxiliaries to assume some of the work traditionally performed by dentists. Thus, it is essential that everything possible be done through school health and health educa-

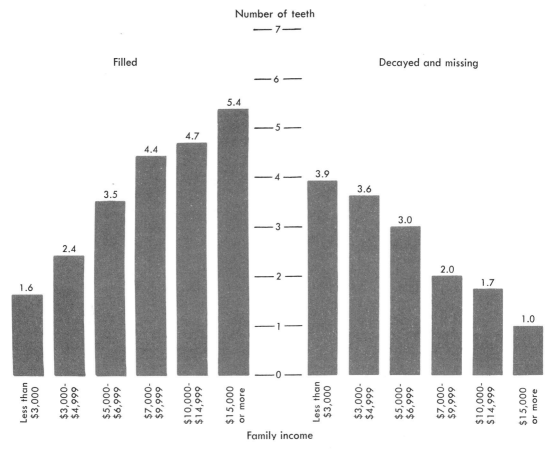

Number of teeth

Filled   Decayed and missing

Fig. 16-2. Average number of filled and of decayed and missing permanent teeth per person among youths 12 to 17 years of age, by family income, United States 1966-1970. (Source National Health Survey.)

tion to prevent dental problems and promote dental health.

Tooth development begins in early prenatal life and continues until the roots of the third molars are developed, usually between the ages of 18 and 25. Development of the crowns (those portions of the tooth above the gum line) is complete by about age 8. All twenty primary (baby) teeth have usually erupted by the age of 2 years. These teeth are gradually shed between the ages of about 6 and 11. The first permanent teeth, usually the first molars, appear at about age 6 or 7. Many parents neglect the care of these teeth either because they do not know that they have erupted or because they mistake them for baby teeth. Other permanent teeth, except for the third molars

(wisdom teeth), appear between the ages of approximately 8 and 13. The third molars usually appear during the late teens or early twenties. Thus, the protection and promotion of dental health throughout the school years, and especially through middle or junior high school, influences dental health throughout life.

Another important general dental health protective and promotional factor during development is nutrition. Dreizen* states that the nutrients known to contribute to dental development are fluorine, calcium, magnesium, protein, and vitamins A, C, D, and E.

---

*Dreizen, S.: The importance of nutrition in tooth development, J. Sch. Health **43:**114-115, Feb. 1973.

Caries. Tooth decay is a process of tissue destruction that requires the presence of a susceptible tooth surface, certain bacteria, and carbohydrates. *Plaque,* the rather soft sticky material that coats the teeth each day, holds the bacteria and carbohydrates against the enamel. Bacterial action on the carbohydrates produces acids that destroy tooth enamel. The decay process, if unchecked by early identification and professional repair of the enamel, may proceed to involve the soft inner tissues of the tooth. The infection may cause inflammation of the inner tissues and result in toothache. It may totally destroy these tissues and eventually cause tooth loss.

Surveys indicate that the average prevalence of cavities among U.S. school children is approximately three per child in the elementary grades and four in senior high school. Prevalence increases through the twenties, and declines thereafter.

Appropriate school management of instances of decay is referral for professional dental care. Some decay is observable. Much of it, particularly in the early stages, is not. Although toothaches sometimes result from food decay, they may also be caused by periodontal disease. In any case, such signs and symptoms indicate a need for professional dental care. Poor families will require assistance in meeting this need—assistance that is all too frequently unavailable. Uneducated parents, affluent or poor, may also require interpretation of the problem. Treated or untreated, toothaches disappear with time, although the basic cause persists. Relief of pain pending dental care may be provided by applications of eugenol (oil of cloves) to the decayed tooth surface. The danger of this procedure is that it may tend to discourage the needed visit to the dentist. For that reason, school policy may prohibit use of eugenol or limit use to a single application. Use of gum that contains aspirin or of an aspirin tablet held against a decayed surface or gum boil only further damages soft tissues and is ineffective as a pain killer.

The single most effective school-community procedure for the prevention of caries is the provision of adequate amounts of fluoride. The single most effective means of providing fluoride is to adjust the fluoride content of the community water supply to 1.0 part per million in the northern part of the country or to 0.7 parts in the south. Above a level of four parts, fluoride may produce unsightly mottled tooth enamel. This procedure is cheap and safe, and reduces decay by about two thirds. Other methods that are somewhat less effective and usually more expensive include fluoridation of water in school only, distributions of daily doses of fluoride in tablet form, topical application of fluorides to the tooth surfaces of children and youth by dentists and dental hygienists, and regular use of toothpastes that contain fluorides. There is some additional advantage to topical applications or the use of fluoride toothpastes even in areas where water supplies are fluoridated. Applications of protective sealants to cleaned tooth surfaces by a dentist or dental hygienist are also useful in prevention.

Restriction of the frequency of carbohydrate intake by the substitution of such foods as raw vegetables, fresh fruits, and sugarless gum and soda for high carbohydrate snacks is also of preventive value. In some elementary schools, classroom birthday parties are restricted to one a month. Daily toothbrushing and flossing is of some value in preventing caries. These processes remove the colonies of bacteria essential to the decay process; a day or two is required for colonies to reform. Cleansing, however, is never as thorough as it needs to be to prevent all decay. Colonies hide in the grooves of tooth surfaces, which are best protected by fluorides and sealants. Use of so-called antiseptic mouthwashes has not been shown to prevent tooth decay or to combat bad breath effectively.

Malocclusion. Misaligned teeth, like tooth surfaces that are susceptible to decay, are sometimes inherited and sometimes acquired. The prevention and early restoration of decayed surfaces or of tooth loss help prevent the occurrence of malocclusion.

When a primary tooth is lost too early or when a permanent tooth is lost, the other teeth shift to fill the empty space and misalignment results. Other causes of acquired malocclusion include pressure habits such as tongue thrusting or thumb-sucking prolonged past babyhood, enlarged tonsils, and teeth that fail to erupt on schedule (impacted teeth). Most causes, including such congenital problems as cleft palate, are correctable. Another cause of malocclusion is mouth breathing, which may result from allergies or structural defects of the nose.

The possible effects of severe malocclusion include not only poor appearance and difficulty in biting and chewing, but also pain, poor speech, and susceptibility to caries and periodontal disease. These, in turn, may result in peer rejection and a poor self-image.

National Health Survey examination and health history data indicate that among U.S. children aged 6 to 11, 5.5% have malocclusion for which correction is mandatory, correction is highly desirable among another 8.7%, and correction is elective for an additional 22.0%. Only about 2.5% of the children had received orthodontic care. The percentage of those who had received corrective care ranged from 1.6% in those from families earning less than $7,000 per year to 7.3% in those from families earning $15,000 per year or more.*

Correction of severe malocclusion and its effects and underlying cause is complicated, time-consuming, and expensive. The services of an orthodontist are required. Those of an oral surgeon, plastic surgeon, pediatrician, and speech correctionist may also be needed for cleft palate correction. Even with the assistance of all available community resources, some cases may never receive needed care. Dental school faculty members are usually eager to find and provide treatment for the more complicated cases of malocclusion, because they are useful in teaching and research. Also, the state crippled children's service may be a useful resource. Less complicated cases are of little interest, and the motivation to obtain care is less. It is these borderline cases that are most likely to be neglected by both their parents and the community.

Periodontal disease. Gingivitis, or inflammation of the gums, is identifiable by the presence of red, swollen, bleeding gums. Perhaps half of all school-age children and youth have gingivitis, and probably most if not all of us have it at one time or another in our lives. Although a transient gingivitis is typical of adolescence and may be associated with the hormone imbalances that occur at that stage of development, most gingivitis appears to be caused by poor oral hygiene and to be preventable by good personal and professional dental care.

Health instruction should therefore aim to promote routine professional care, daily brushing and flossing, and to develop brushing and flossing skills. Excellent teaching resource materials are available through the American Dental Association.* Toothpaste companies make available to schools low-cost kits consisting of a toothbrush and tube of paste. The effectiveness with which students brush and floss can be assessed by use of a disclosing dye and special lamp available as a kit in many drugstores. The dye adheres to plaque but not to clean tooth surfaces.

Although plaque is largely removable by brushing and flossing, the hard calculus or tartar that forms from it is not. Plaque tends to migrate and form calculus between the gum and lower tooth surfaces as well as between the teeth. This may result in the formation of pockets in which other debris and bacteria accumulate. If the calculus is not removed, gum tissue may grow over the pocket, resulting in an infected abscess that may cause pain or gum boil formation.

*U.S. Health Services and Mental Health Administration: *An assessment of the occlusion of the teeth of children 6-11 years, United States,* DHEW Publication No. (HRA) 74-1612, Washington, D.C., 1973, U.S. Government Printing Office, pp. 12-13.

*211 East Chicago Ave., Chicago, Ill. 60611, and through state dental associations.

Thorough cleaning, scaling, and polishing of teeth (called prophylaxis) by a dental hygienist or dentist, usually twice a year, is thus not only helpful in the prevention of periodontal disease, but is also part of the standard treatment procedure. In some schools dental hygienists provide prophylaxis as a service to students. Such service is needed most in poverty areas and in localities remote from sources of regular professional care. It is inappropriate in affluent areas where dental care is readily available.

Periodontitis, or pyorrhea, is often the end result of neglected oral hygiene or of gingivitis. This severe form of gum tissue infection spreads and may, if unchecked, invade and destroy the bony tissues (alveolae) that hold the teeth in place. Professional dental care—the sooner the better—can control periodontitis and prevent tooth loss from this cause.

Tooth injuries. Involvement in accidents, fights, and collision sports is a frequent cause of broken or knocked-out teeth. Such injuries are emergencies that require immediate dental care. A knocked-out tooth can frequently be successfully reinserted in its socket; therefore, it should be taken with the youngster to the dentist's office. Reimplantation is most likely to be successful prior to adolescence.

Properly fitted mouth guards are highly effective in preventing tooth injuries among athletes. Most states and school systems require their use. They may be fitted by either school dental health service staff members or by dentists in the community under a plan developed jointly by practitioners and school staff. Some other accidental injuries may be preventable by teaching students not to bite hard objects. Many teeth are broken in attempts to open bottle caps or crack nuts with the teeth.

HEART PROBLEMS

Only about one school-age youngster in every 100,000 dies each year from a disease of the heart. Yet any indication of a heart defect is profoundly disturbing to most parents and teachers. Their usual reaction is to limit physical activity and to overprotect the youngster in other ways. Individuals labeled as having a heart problem are inclined to use the label as an excuse for avoiding activity. Proper home and school management depends on careful medical evaluation of each case, the development of recommendations suitable to both the nature of the problem (if a real problem does, in fact, exist), and the personality of the individual.

Detection and follow-up. The recording of a heart murmur by the examiner on a school medical health examination is a frightening indicator. It is essential that all concerned recognize that a heart murmur is an abnormal heart sound that may or may not indicate that a true heart problem is present. Perhaps half of all elementary-age children have such murmurs, many of which disappear as they mature and most of which are of no medical significance. A heart murmur means that medical evaluation by the child's personal physician is indicated. If the personal physician remains in doubt as to whether the murmur is significant or innocent, then further evaluation by a heart specialist (cardiologist) is in order. The school health examination is a useful means of detecting possible heart disease if care is taken in its reporting and follow-up of findings.

In some localities students are screened for heart murmurs by technicians. In one procedure, technicians tape-record the heart sounds of students, and the sounds are then evaluated by heart specialists. In another procedure, heart sounds and heartbeat timing are evaluated immediately by a portable computer. The latter technique, utilizing a test-retest procedure, resulted in referral of 11 fourth graders of about 800 screened for medical evaluation in one city. Of these, 7 youngsters were found to have definite heart disease.*

Teacher observation is a third means of

---

*Dennison, D., and Fennimore, J. A.: A heart-sound screening program for elementary children, J. Sch. Health **41**:349-350, Sept. 1971.

detecting possible heart problems in need of evaluation. Children with heart problems may show such signs of inadequate blood oxygenation as breathlessness, pallor, or bluish lips, especially after mild physical activity. They tend to limit their own activity.

To prevent overanxiety, any indication to youngsters or parents that a heart problem is suspected should be avoided when referrals are made for medical evaluation. Instead, observations and other relevant information gathered by school professionals should be made known directly to the student's source of medical care. School management should include interim activity restriction until medical recommendations are received. Such limitations should be reviewed at that time and periodically thereafter. Many youngsters need no activity restriction at all; others may require only partial or temporary limitation. Some may have their heart damage surgically repaired.*

Prevention. The two most common causes of heart damage among school-age youngsters are congenital heart defects (defects that arise before birth) and rheumatic heart disease, which occurs primarily in the northern states. Prevention of birth defects will be discussed later in the chapter.

The first step in the prevention of rheumatic heart damage is the early detection and treatment of cases of strep throat and scarlet fever. Victims of these infections should be excluded from school until treated, for the protection of themselves and others. Fewer than 5% of those who have untreated streptococcal infections develop rheumatic fever, however.

The second step in prevention is the early recognition and adequate treatment of those cases of rheumatic fever that do occur. Rheumatic fever is not a communicable disease. It is usually detected through observation of signs and symptoms, such as unexplained fatigue, migrating polyarthritis,

and chorea (also called St. Vitus' dance). In migrating polyarthritis, several different joints are painful or inflamed, and the pain and inflammation moves from one joint to another. These pains are sometimes brushed off as growing pains, but growth is not painful. Muscle pain, which is usually the result of exercise, is sometimes mistaken for rheumatic fever pains, which are located in the joints. Chorea is an involvement of the central nervous system. Muscle coordination deteriorates, there is muscular weakness, and speech may become indistinct. Emotional instability is common. The distressing signs and symptoms peculiar to chorea disappear with time and bed rest.

The risk of rheumatic heart damage is not as high in first attacks as in subsequent episodes. To prevent subsequent strep infections and thus subsequent attacks of rheumatic fever and risk of heart damage, prophylactic doses of penicillin are administered routinely for a number of years or for life. Other drugs are substituted for those who are sensitive to penicillin. Rest at home during acute episodes of rheumatic fever and convalescence from them is standard practice. Patients may receive homebound instruction during their prolonged school absence.

ACNE

Most teen-agers have acne, and most of them worry too much about it. Their worries are exacerbated by the negative attitudes of adults toward "pimply faced kids" and by the numerous myths that have been invented and perpetuated about it. The myths include the beliefs that acne is caused by masturbation or other ways of having orgasms, that it is caused by sexual abstinence, that it is caused by inadequate personal cleanliness, that it is preventable by a good diet, and that it is caused by any and every food that teen-agers like to eat, including chocolate, nuts, and pizza.*

---

*Informational and instructional materials are available through local affiliates of the American Heart Association, 44 East 23rd St., New York 10010.

*Fulton, J. J., Plewig, G., and Kligman, A. M.: Effect of chocolate on acne vulgaris, J.A.M.A. **210:**2071-2074, Dec. 15, 1969.

Teen-agers need to know that none of these myths is supported by sound research evidence. They need to know that most normal, healthy teen-agers develop acne by about age 13 and that it usually disappears by the age of 23. It is caused by an excess production of androgens, or male hormones, which are normally produced by the bodies of both boys and girls, and for which nothing in the way of hormone therapy should normally be attempted. They should know that frequent thorough washing of the face and a healthful basic four diet are helpful. In mild acne, nongreasy over-the-counter acne medications that are designed to promote skin peeling are often helpful, as are short hair and frequent shampooing if one's hair is inclined to be oily. In severe acne, characterized by numerous severely inflamed lesions, advice and treatment by a physician, especially a dermatologist, is indicated.

POSTURAL PROBLEMS

Good posture is evidenced in good body alignment and balance as an individual sits, stands, walks, or runs. Defective posture sometimes reflects underlying defects of skeletal development or injuries that may require assessment and possible treatment by a medical specialist in orthopedics. Often it results from body muscle imbalances or weaknesses that are correctable or preventable by exercises and by the development of skills in walking, running, standing, or sitting correctly. Other causes include mental depression or anxieties, poorly fitted shoes, and postural fads that may be assumed by adolescents.

Postural problems may be identified by medical health examiners, by the use of screening devices such as that shown in Fig. 16-3, or by observation. It is important to distinguish between true postural problems and apparent problems that are really manifestations of a growth stage. For example, up until about the age of 12 most healthy youngsters have protruding stomachs and shoulder blades and knock-knees.

Thus, *lordosis,* a postural condition in which the lower back sways in and the stomach protrudes, is usually a normal condition during the elementary grades and is abnormal later on. Abnormal lordosis is usually both preventable and treatable by exercises that strengthen the abdominal muscles. Referral to an orthopedist is not usually appropriate.

Kyphosis, in which the upper vertebrae and shoulders tilt forward, should always be referred to an orthopedist if pain accompanies a youngster's efforts to straighten up. If pain is not present, then climbing, rope skipping, and carrying books balanced on the top of one's head are helpful. Individuals with nonpainful kyphosis who recog-

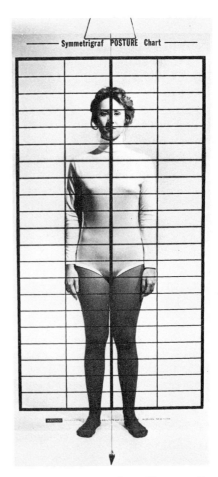

Fig. 16-3. Posture screening. (Courtesy Reedco, Inc.)

nize their problem and wish to correct it are often able to do so.

Scoliosis, in which the spine is curved from one side to the other when viewed from the rear and in which one shoulder droops below the level of the other, is a condition that should always be referred to an orthopedic specialist, and the sooner the better. Early professional treatment and diagnosis are essential, because scoliosis becomes worse with age.

DIABETES MELLITUS

Susceptibility to diabetes mellitus is usually inherited, and many parents of diabetic children therefore develop guilt feelings. They often tend either to overprotect their children or to ignore the problem. The disorder is much more severe when its onset occurs in childhood or youth rather than in adulthood; diabetic youngsters invariably require daily insulin injections to live. This opens them up to risk of insulin reactions as well as the diabetic acidosis to which all diabetics are at risk. The prospect of either emergency may be disturbing to teachers and to the diabetics themselves. Anxieties of diabetic children and their parents may be alleviated by participation in the activities of the American Diabetics Association and its local affiliates. The Association publishes helpful literature, and many affiliates conduct educational meetings for diabetic youngsters and their families. Summer camps for diabetic children and youth are located throughout the United States.*

The school management of diabetic emergencies (acidosis and insulin reaction) is not complicated. It is helpful to distinguish between the two:

Cause of acidosis	**Cause of insulin reaction**
Insufficient or omitted insulin dose	Too much insulin, too little food, too much exercise

---
*Information may be obtained from the American Diabetes Association, 18 East 48th St., New York 10017.

Signs of acidosis	**Signs of insulin reaction**
Gradual onset	Sudden onset
Flushed face	Pale, ashen face
Dry skin	Moist, clammy skin
Odor of acetone on breath (like cheap wine)	No odor of acetone on breath
Looks and acts like a drunk	Faintness, unconsciousness

The appropriate school management of acidosis is to transport the youngster immediately to a hospital emergency ward together with the information that he or she is diabetic and the name of the personal physician. Experienced diabetic individuals recognize the faintness that precedes insulin reaction. Most of them carry candy or sugar with which to ward off impending reactions. If the victim does not have candy or sugar and is conscious, it should be administered orally. A sugar-laden soda or orange juice is a convenient source. If the victim is unconscious, a retention enema of sugar solution may be administered. If the condition is, in fact, insulin reaction, recovery should occur in about 10 minutes and should be followed by a period of rest. The parent and/or physician should be notified. If rapid recovery does not occur, the diabetic should be taken to a hospital emergency room with complete information.

Appropriate routine school management depends on the nature of the case. If the diabetic youngster has frequent episodes of acidosis or insulin reaction, it may be wise to avoid hazardous activities such as machine shop, rope climbing, or swimming alone or in a crowded pool. If the diabetes is well controlled, there is no reason to apply such restrictions. In general, there is no reason to limit vigorous physical activity or athletic participation. Exercise is most safely scheduled shortly after a meal or snack, and the teacher or coach should have a soda or orange juice on hand. There are many diabetic professional athletes, among whom is Bobby Clarke, captain of the Philadelphia Flyers.

Detection of juvenile diabetes is important but rarely a problem. In the young, diabetes occurs as an explosive serious disease that is obvious to any informed adult. The insulin insufficiency results in inability to metabolize carbohydrate calories. Undiscovered and untreated, diabetic youngsters therefore consume enormous quantities of food and water. Yet they are fatigued and lose weight. They urinate frequently. Because they burn fat instead of carbohydrate for calories and because their fat metabolism is abnormal, their bodies produce the toxins that lead to acidosis. The standard screening test for detecting early diabetes is a blood sugar test following a snack or meal heavily loaded with carbohydrate calories. Its use among students is unnecessary and unproductive. Its use among adult school staff members, particularly those who are middle aged, overweight, and who have a family history of diabetes, is both helpful to them and productive. In adulthood, the onset of diabetes is usually undramatic and easily missed.

EPILEPSY

As in the case of diabetes, epilepsy arouses anxiety among parents, teachers, and its young victims. Although diabetes carries some social stigma, epilepsy carries more. Individuals who are epileptic are discriminated against socially and in the job market to a greater extent than are those with diabetes. Parents of epileptic children are more likely than those of diabetic children to withhold from the school the information that their child has epilepsy—information that is essential to humane school management of the case. Yet with appropriate continuous drug therapy, seizures occur rarely or not at all in about 80% of the cases.

Epileptic seizures take a variety of forms, among which the most frightening is a severe grand mal attack. Severe grand mal attacks frequently include unconsciousness, rigidity, and spasmodic jerking. The tongue may be severely bitten, and the bowels and/or bladder may empty. Breathing may be suspended. The proper management of such an attack is, first, to ease the student to the floor and remove any furniture that may

cause injury. Clothing should be loosened. The victim should be turned on his or her side so that saliva or vomitus will run from the mouth and not cause choking. It is undesirable to force anything hard between the teeth; it may cause choking or broken teeth. A cut tongue will heal; broken teeth will not. When consciousness and rationality return, the individual will need to rest. The parent and/or the youngster's personal physician should be notified.

Petit mal seizures, on the other hand, frequently pass unnoticed and require no emergency management. Seizures usually last less than 1 minute and are characterized by failure to respond to questions, eye and lip movements, or trembling. Teachers need to be aware of the reason behind the behavior so that they may respond sympathetically.

There are other types of epileptic seizures, but these two illustrate the extreme forms seizures may take. Mixed forms of epilepsy are common. Some epileptic individuals have a forewarning, called an aura, that a seizure is about to occur. Some have seizures only at certain times, most frequently during nonschool hours. These patterns and the extent to which each case is controlled by drugs need to be known and considered in planning school management on an individual basis.

Most epileptic students require no modification of school program, but those who may have a seizure during school hours and who do not have a reliable aura need to avoid potentially dangerous situations, such as certain shops and physical education activities. One grand mal epileptic student loved to swim, but her seizures were neither well enough controlled nor predictable enough by aura to permit her to do so in school physical education classes. In addition, the swimming classes were overcrowded. Her physical education teacher proposed a happy and acceptable solution; the girl would be permitted to join the synchronized swimming group, which was small and met after school. The nature of the activity permitted close teacher observation, and the teacher was fully qualified in water safety.

Many cases of epilepsy are first discovered when a seizure occurs at school. It is essential that school professionals follow through to be sure that epileptic students are under continuing personal medical management. Some epileptic students may be required to take their medication during school hours, and provisions may be required to be sure that the prescribed drugs are available and taken as directed. Safe keeping is essential, because the drugs used to control seizures are among those subject to abuse such as phenobarbital and diphenylhydantoin. Parents and students may require counseling to help them to come to accept and deal sensibly with the condition.

The question of whether or not classmates should be informed that a fellow student has epilepsy and taught how to deal with seizures in advance is difficult to answer. On the one hand, the epileptic student has a right to expect that his or her diagnosis will be held in confidence. On the other hand, advance information may help to promote proper management and minimize classroom disorder if a seizure does occur. The right answer for any given case is likely to be the one that emerges from a parent-student-teacher-nurse conference in which decisions are based on the nature of the individual case rather than on generalizations about epilepsy. The occurrence of one seizure in school makes the question moot, of course.*

ALLERGIES AND ASTHMA

Allergies affect many of us. They vary widely in nature and severity. Following initial exposure to an ordinarily harmless substance of any kind, an individual may develop a sensitivity to any future reexposure to that substance. The substance becomes an allergen to the sensitized individual. Future contact between the allergen and sensitized body cells results in release of body substances called *histamines,* which in turn cause tissue inflammation, muscle spasm,

---

*Further information and instructional materials are available through the Epilepsy Foundation of America, 1828 L St., N.W., Suite 406, Washington, D.C. 20036, or its nearest local chapter.

and dilation of blood vessels. Essentially any substance may become an allergen to someone, and allergens may enter the body and cause trouble in any conceivable way. Frequently, allergic reactions mimic the signs and symptoms of communicable diseases.

Some allergens appear only seasonally or sporadically in the environment, and attacks are therefore seasonal and sporadic, as in the case of pollen-induced hay fever or skin rashes that erupt after one eats strawberries. By trial and error or logical processes of eliminating possible causes, some individuals are able to identify the substances to which they are allergic and can simply avoid contact with them. Those who can do so are fortunate. Others who may be unable to identify or avoid contact with sporadic or seasonal allergies may be able to alleviate their distressing symptoms by taking antihistamine drugs. This approach carries with it some degree of risk, for these drugs cause drowsiness, which may lead to accidents. In addition, they do not prevent the cell damage that allergies cause or prevent the progression of a simple respiratory allergy to asthma.

When the allergen cannot readily be identified and avoided at least most of the time, the allergic individual faces an expensive, time-consuming, and not always productive series of tests that allergists use to try to identify allergens. Again, once identified by such tests, the allergen may prove to be one that can be avoided. If not, a time-consuming and costly series of desensitization treatments is indicated.

Asthma is the most serious of all the allergic diseases. It may or may not be seasonal. Attacks may be triggered not only by exposure to allergens but also by psychological or social cues or stresses. An acute attack of bronchial asthma can be frightening. The youngster wheezes, chokes, and gasps for half an hour or longer until the mucus that plugs the respiratory system is expelled. Many asthmatic youngsters carry medication, usually in the form of an inhaler or pills, that helps them through an attack. They breathe better sitting up. Attacks are likely to leave them exhausted, and they may need to rest or go home afterward.

We can best help asthmatic students and those with other allergies at school by being aware of the allergens and psychological cues or stresses that precipitate each individual's attacks and by helping avoid them. At the same time, allergic and asthmatic youngsters should not be allowed to utilize their problem as a convenient excuse for avoiding school tasks. Exercise is to be encouraged, but alternate exercises may have to be substituted for those that involve exposures to allergens or stresses that might precipitate an attack.

BIRTH DEFECTS

Some infants are born with birth defects. Such defects range from ludicrous malformations, such as having six toes, to those that result in severe handicaps or early death, such as mongolism or Tay-Sachs disease. The possible types of birth defects are too numerous and complex to discuss each one here. Instead, this section is focused on birth defect prevention through school health and health education.

Some birth defects result from inherited defective genes, while others are caused by defects in the intrauterine environment in which babies grow and develop before they are born. Thus, one approach to prevention is the identification of potential inherited defects before pregnancy occurs or early in the pregnancy, coupled with the prevention of high-risk pregnancy or its termination through abortion. A second approach is directed to improvement of the health of prepregnant and pregnant teen-age girls and to change of behavior potentially harmful to their offspring.

Preventing inherited defects. Screening tests are now available that may be used to identify carriers of certain heritable birth defects. These include tests for sickle cell anemia traits, which are present in about one in every ten black Americans, and for Tay-Sachs disease, which is prevalent among Jews of Central or Eastern European ancestry. These serious diseases result when both parents carry the recessive trait. Each pregnancy carries with it a 25% risk that the child will be born with the disease. Given advance knowledge of this risk through screening test results and genetic counseling, trait-carrying individuals can then decide whether to assume the risk of having a defective infant, to prevent the risk by mating with noncarriers only, to practice birth control, or to abort pregnancies that do occur. Genetic counseling, which can be provided on a group as well as on an individual basis, is an essential component of any school or school-community detection program.

Some other inherited defects can be detected only by tests of amniotic fluid during pregnancy, as a result of which parents are limited in their choice to either abortion or acceptance of the fact that their child will be defective. Mongolism is an example of a disease in this category. Other such disorders are identifiable only at birth or later; these include phenylketonuria, a metabolic disorder that causes mental retardation but that fortunately can be controlled by diet.

Preventing environmentally caused defects. The role of rubella occurrence in early pregnancy as a cause of birth defects has been noted. Other diseases can also cause birth defects, and the prepregnant teen-ager should therefore be protected against as many infections as possible. Each pregnant girl or woman should have a blood test for syphilis and should be treated if she has it.

Pregnancy before the age of 17 and after 35 carries with it an increased risk of a defective baby. Most Planned Parenthood and other community birth control clinics today serve teen-agers regardless of whether or not they are married or have parental consent. School professionals are increasingly doing whatever they can to make local community services and their policies known to young people.

Education about pregnancy and childbirth can help to reduce the risk of birth defects by emphasizing the importance of an adequate and nutritious diet before and during pregnancy. Pregnant teen-agers need additional milk (a total of at least 3 cups daily) and added protein from other sources. Early identification of pregnancy through pregnancy tests and adequate prenatal care through clinical services are available in some communities. Except as directed by a physician who knows of the pregnancy, *all* drug use should be discontinued during the prenatal period. This includes the use of self-prescribed supplemental vitamins, aspirin, alcohol, tobacco, and all other non-prescription drugs, as well as those that have been prescribed but that are not essential to maternal health.*

TERMINAL ILLNESSES AND THE SCHOOL

Some children have congenital malformations, heart conditions, or types of cancer that end in death during their school years. Some of them come to realize that they will not live long, while others are taught to believe that they will get better soon. Those who are destined to live with debilitating handicaps face a future that seems worse than death to many adults. The parents and teachers of fatally ill and severely handicapped children tend to pamper them. Not infrequently, community groups provide funds for a trip to Disneyland or for a last Christmas.

If we were able to explore the feelings of fatally ill or severely handicapped children openly with them, we might be better able than we are to provide school and other experiences more in keeping with their real needs and desires. We hesitate to do so, however, because we are overwhelmed by our own feelings, and perhaps because we are afraid to learn how they feel. We probably are not far off the mark if we settle for and act on the belief that they would wish to be treated as all children wish to be treated by caring adults. All normal children do wish for a trip to Disneyland,

and they also wish to have the same pleasant and productive learning experiences as their peers. If this reasoning is correct, then we should set for them the same school tasks and expectations as we set for others. These, of course, must be modified in accordance with limitations imposed by their handicaps, which may include frequent and prolonged school absences.

QUESTIONS FOR STUDY AND DISCUSSION

1. What useful and effective school procedures can be used in the prevention, identification, and treatment of fatness?
2. What is anorexia nervosa? What are the implications of the condition for school health and health education?
3. What is the most effective school-community approach to the prevention of dental caries? What other in-school procedures are useful in prevention or amelioration of caries?
4. What school procedures are helpful in preventing or managing cases of malocclusion, periodontal disease, and tooth injuries?
5. What are the two most common types of heart problems among school-age children and youth?
6. How can and should heart defects be treated and followed up in the school setting? What is the significance of heart murmur?
7. What can be done to prevent heart problems in children and youth through school health and health education?
8. What are some of the common myths about acne? What useful and valid advice can school professionals give young people about acne?
9. How can lordosis, kyphosis, and scoliosis be identified? Which of these can be prevented or corrected through nonmedical in-school intervention, and how? Which should always be referred for nonschool medical advice?
10. How can diabetes mellitus best be discovered early among students and among adult school members?
11. What procedures are recommended for the identification and first-aid management of diabetic emergencies? What procedures are recommended for the general nonemergency school management of diabetic students?
12. What procedures are recommended for the general and emergency management of epileptic students?
13. What procedures may be helpful to allergic or asthmatic school members?
14. What intervening school health and health education procedures can be utilized to help prevent inherited or environmentally caused birth defects?
15. How do you think most children with terminal illness or severe handicaps prefer to be treated at school, and why?

---

*The material in this section was adapted from several of the excellent free and low-cost educational materials available for school use through the National Foundation–March of Dimes, P.O. Box 2000, White Plains, N.Y. 10602.

REFERENCES

Eisner, V., and Callan, L. B.: *Dimensions of school health,* Springfield, Ill., 1974, Charles C Thomas, Publisher.

Hanlon, J. J.: *Public health administration and practice,* ed. 6, St. Louis, 1974, The C. V. Mosby Co.

Henderson, J.: *Emergency medical guide,* ed. 3, New York, 1973, McGraw-Hill, Inc.

Kogan, B. A.: *Health: man in a changing environment,* ed. 2, New York, 1974, Harcourt Brace Jovanovich, Inc.

Mayer, J.: *Health,* New York, 1974, D. Van Nostrand Co.

The medicine show, Mt. Vernon, N.Y., 1974, Consumers Union.

Nemir, A., and Schaller, W. D.: *The school health program,* ed. 4, Philadelphia, 1975, W. B. Saunders Co.

Weiner, F.: *Help for the handicapped child,* New York, 1973, Mc-Graw-Hill, Inc.

CHAPTER 17 ❧ School injury control

Injuries occur to children and youth not only in school but also at home and in the community. They occur as a result of both accidents and premeditated attempts of individuals to harm others or themselves. Their effects range from minor inconvenience and pain to extended disability and death. It is probably beyond the ability of school professionals to eliminate all injuries that occur within school jurisdiction, let alone those that occur in homes and the community, but their ability to reduce the incidence and severity of injury has been proven. Effective injury control depends on planned programs that involve school staff members and students, parents, and relevant community resources.

SCOPE AND TRENDS

Injuries are the leading cause of death among school-age children and youth, as shown in Table 17-1. Males are much more likely to die from violence than are females, and youth are much more likely to die from violence than are children. For all sex and age groups, except 5- to 14-year-old females, violence accounts for more than half of all the deaths that occur. Of the violent causes, accidents are the most common assigned cause. Of these, about half are the result of automobile accidents. Between 1955 and 1970 the accident and suicide death rates for the total U.S. population remained essentially the same. Homicides, however, increased from 4.5 per 100,000 of population in 1955 to 8.3 in 1970.*

Injuries, on the other hand, are relatively unimportant as a cause of school absence. Of the 4.38 days of school absence reported on average for U.S. youngsters 6 to 16 years old in 1973, only 0.36 occurred as a result of injuries.* By the senior high school years, about 19% of all youngsters have suffered broken bones, and 12% have been knocked unconscious, with a higher proportion of such injuries occurring among boys than girls.†

These and other injury data should be accepted and interpreted with caution. Except in the presence of contrary evidence, investigators tend to assign traumatic deaths to a more socially accepted cause such as accidents rather than to homicide or suicide. We really do not know how many injuries are the result of accidents and how many result from fights, attempted homicides or suicides, or parental abuse. We can be fairly certain, however, that more injuries occur than are reported.

SCHOOL SAFETY PROGRAM

Schaplowsky‡ postulates that five phases are involved in controlling injuries resulting from accidents. The first is *investigation* of accidents that do occur and of those reported in published literature to determine factors that might cause injuries. The second is *analysis and interpretation,* in which causative human and environmental factors are inferred from the data gathered. The third is *control program planning,* the objective of which is to make decisions about

---

*U.S. National Center for Health Statistics, *Facts of life and death,* DHEW Publication No. (HRA) 74-1222, Washington, D.C., 1974, U.S. Government Printing Office, pp. 34-35, 44-46.

*U.S. Department of Health, Education, and Welfare: *Current estimates from the health interview survey,* DHEW Publication (HRA) 75-1522, Washington, D.C., 1974, U.S. Government Printing Office, p. 24.

†U.S. Department of Health, Education, and Welfare: *Examination and health history findings among children and youth,* DHEW Publication No. (HRA) 74-1611, Washington, D.C., 1973, U.S. Government Printing Office, pp. 12-13.

‡Schaplowsky, A. F.: Community injury control: a management approach, Am. J. Public Health **63:**252-254, March 1973.

Table 17-1. Violent death rates per 100,000 population in selected sex and age groups by cause, United States, 1970

Cause	Sex and age group	Rate
Accidents	Males 5 to 14 years	27.4
	Females 5 to 14 years	12.5
	Males 15 to 24 years	110.5
	Females 15 to 24 years	27.6
Homicide	Males 5 to 14 years	1.0
	Females 5 to 14 years	0.7
	Males 15 to 24 years	19.0
	Females 15 to 24 years	4.6
Suicide	Males 5 to 14 years	0.5
	Females 5 to 14 years	—
	Males 15 to 24 years	13.5
	Females 15 to 24 years	4.2
Total rates from violence	Males 5 to 14 years	28.9
	Females 5 to 14 years	13.2
	Males 15 to 24 years	143.0
	Females 15 to 24 years	36.4
Total rates from all causes	Males 5 to 14 years	50.5
	Females 5 to 14 years	31.8
	Males 15 to 24 years	188.5
	Females 15 to 24 years	68.1

Data from National Center for Health Statistics.

preventive measures that will be undertaken. The preventive measures selected should be feasible and should not cost more than they are worth. For example, one could eliminate physical education accidents that are caused by falls from climbing apparatus by eliminating climbing as an activity, but physical educators would rightly object to such a procedure because of the benefits that climbing provides in terms of developing good posture and potential lifesaving skills. Programs may include education and environmental adjustments to control the energy exchanges that cause accidents. For example, climbing accidents may be controlled by careful step-by-step instruction in safe climbing and by placing an energy-absorbing surface beneath climbing apparatus. The fourth step is *implementing the control measures* selected. This step always costs effort, often costs money, and may involve changes in the ways in which people do things. This step, therefore, is often the most difficult. The fifth step is that of *evaluating program success,* which simply means determining whether the incidence of injuries or the

seriousness of the injuries has been reduced, and inferring from accident data how the program could be modified to make it more effective.

Accident reports and surveys. An adequate system of reporting accidental injuries is clearly essential to Schaplowsky's scheme. The widely used accident report form developed by the National Safety Council is shown in Fig. 17-1 by permission of the Council. Note that the form provides for the reporting of home and community accidental injuries as well as those that occur under school jurisdiction. Items are included that are useful in pinpointing where, when, how, and why the accident occurred, and what might be done to prevent the occurrence of similar accidents. Other items provide data that can be used to measure the severity of the injury.

Although some schools require that all school jurisdiction accidents be reported, however slight, we recommended in Chapter 10 that reporting might well be delimited to those injuries resulting either in medical care or in at least half a day of school absence. Although reporting nonschool accidents may be useful in education for home safety and community safety improvement, local planners may also decide to delimit reporting to school jurisdiction accidents only. The rationale for these delimitations is that reporting of minor injuries is unlikely to be scrupulous and that the reporting of these and nonschool injuries adds greatly to the burden of data collection and analysis.

In smaller schools, data may be hand tabulated. In larger schools, coding and keypunching for machine analysis becomes worthwhile. Either way, the data should be

(check one) ☐ School Jurisdictional ☐ Non-School Jurisdictional	**RECOMMENDED** **STANDARD STUDENT ACCIDENT REPORT** (See instructions on reverse side)	(check one) Recordable ☐ Reportable Only ☐

School District:

City, State:

General

1. Name | 2. Address

3. School | 4. Sex   Male ☐   Female ☐ | 5. Age | 6. Grade/Special Program

7. Time Accident Occurred   Date: Day of Week: Exact Time: AM ☐   PM ☐

Injury

8. Nature of Injury

9. Part of Body Injured

10. Degree of Injury (check one)   Death ☐   Permanent ☐   Temporary (lost time) ☐   Non-Disabling (no lost time) ☐

11. Days Lost   From School: From Activities Other Than School: Total:

12. Cause of Injury

Accident

13. Accident Jurisdiction (check one)   School: Grounds ☐   Building ☐   To and From ☐   Other Activities Not on School Property ☐   Non-School: Home ☐   Other ☐

14. Location of Accident (be specific) | 15. Activity of Person (be specific)

16. Status of Activity | 17. Supervision (if yes, give title & name of supervisor)   Yes ☐   No ☐

18. Agency Involved | 19. Unsafe Act

20. Unsafe Mechanical/Physical Condition | 21. Unsafe Personal Factor

22. Corrective Action Taken or Recommended

23. Property Damage   School $ Non-School $ Total $

24. Description (Give a word picture of the accident, explaining who, what, when, why and how)

Signature

25. Date of Report | 26. Report Prepared by (signature & title)

27. Principal's Signature

Fig. 17-1. Accident report form. (Courtesy National Safety Council.)

analyzed to reveal the school's grade levels, times, sites, and activities associated with the most common and most serious injury occurrences. Such analysis reveals the parameters within which control program planning is most needed. Within these parameters the recommendations of reporters may then be reviewed and sites visited to obtain information more specifically helpful in program planning. Analyses and subsequent planning should be conducted at least annually. Some safety directors follow the wise procedure of making an on-site investigation upon receiving a report of any injury that results in either permanent impairment or death. In these cases, serious hazards in immediate need of correction are likely to exist, and there is a possibility that a liability suit may be filed.

In addition to surveys of accidental injuries, some school professionals utilize surveys to collect input data for safety program planning. These surveys are designed to discover environmental defects that constitute safety hazards, such as broken or worn playground equipment and stairways in need of repair. Survey instruments, usually in the form of check lists, have been designed by some local and state school authorities. It is fairly easy to develop such forms locally by utilizing data collected by means of accident report forms and the expertise of such school professionals as driver training teachers, physical educators, and shop and science teachers. Student assistants may be used to collect environmental data. In many states and communities, fire marshals survey school buildings periodically for fire hazards and compliance with fire safety laws.

Student and community input. The importance of student input in the planning of safety programs has been emphasized by Martin and Heimstra,* who conclude that the involvement of children in the development and evaluation of child safety pro-

grams is likely to be a productive means of improving child safety. They argue that programs designed by adult experts frequently fail because child and adult perceptions of the environment are likely to differ and because adults often overestimate the abilities of children as bicyclists or pedestrians. In kindergarten and other early grades, the perceptual abilities of children are not as well developed as they will be later. In the past, adults have invented safety slogans and rhymes, which children dutifully memorize and repeat in the mistaken belief that these rituals somehow prevent accidents without further actions on their part.

In Baltimore, a joint health department–school committee established a comprehensive set of guidelines for handling animals in classrooms.* The guidelines include instructions for preventing infections and bites, handling of bites if they do occur, and other precautions. For example, it is recommended that handling of animals be avoided and that hands be washed with soap if animals are handled. Biting animals should be kept alive and in isolation for observation, and the health department should be notified of the incident. Cages for animals should be so constructed that wooden parts are protected from gnawing by wire mesh, which should be sufficiently close-knit to prevent children from inserting their fingers.

Parent input in planning is important to home-school cooperation in safety programs. For example, where youngsters ride bikes to and from school, parent-school agreement as to the grade level at which the practice first becomes appropriate is essential. In some locations joint parent-school planning has resulted in the identification by means of signs of homes in which children who are threatened with attack or who are injured may find safe haven or assistance. Effective methods of safety education include pupil inspection of their own homes for safety hazards and the correction

---

*Martin, G. L., and Heimstra, N. W.: Consumer input for safety programs, J. Sch. Health **44:**80-82, Feb. 1974.

*Gordon, J., and others: Classroom ecology and safety, J. Sch. Health **42:**178-181, March 1972.

of problems thus discovered. Without pre-planning involving parents, such projects may result in more home-school resentment than they do in education.

These inputs can best be routinely obtained and correlated with the information obtained from injury reports in the process of program planning and evaluation through either a school health council or a specialized safety committee or council, as described in Chapter 4. Students may also be involved in conducting school safety programs through building-level committees or councils, safety patrols, and the like. Their involvement not only contributes directly to the safety of school members but also serves an educational function.

Program segments. School safety programs have evolved into a number of segments, some of which are common to nearly all schools. Each segment is usually designed to deal with a particular problem by changing behavior through safety education or by changing the physical or social environments to reduce or eliminate hazards. One such segment, addressed to the prevention of eye injuries in school shops and labs, has already been discussed in Chapter 14. Others are presented below.

Traffic safety. Accidents involving motor vehicles account for approximately half of all accidental deaths that occur in the United States. School safety programs that are designed to aid in controlling deaths and injuries from this cause include pedestrian and bicycle safety instruction and traffic control during the lower grades, school bus safety at all grades, and driver education at the senior high school level. As a result of school-community efforts in the past, traffic death rates per 10,000 registered vehicles has declined steadily over the years from over 40 in 1910 to about 5 today.*

When young children enter school, their perceptual-motor abilities are not yet well enough developed to enable them to cross streets safely. Most are unable to judge the

distance and speed of an approaching automobile and therefore either hesitate to cross when crossing is safe or dash across the street when it is unsafe to do so. One approach to the problem is through training children to cross streets safely. Another is the provision of supervision at crossings.

Skill in crossing streets is best taught in the same way as any other skill, through demonstration, supervised practice, and feedback to the learner. Supervised practice and feedback need to be continued until the skill is mastered. An elementary school staff that wishes to do an effective job of pedestrian safety education might therefore set up simulated street crossings on the school grounds for initial demonstration and practice. Real situations near the school may also be used if carefully selected and guarded during instruction. This training may be supplemented by classroom instruction in which films may be used as a form of demonstration, together with explanations of the reasons behind such recommended behaviors as crossing with the green light.

Adult crossing guards and upper grade level safety patrol students provide continued supervised practice and feedback under real conditions. Adult guards are provided and trained by the local police department in most states and localities and placed at hours and crossings that are determined jointly by school and police officials. Adult guards in most states have the police power to direct both vehicular and pupil pedestrian traffic; student safety patrol members can direct only pupil traffic. In most localities adult and student patrol persons work together at the more hazardous crossings, while student patrol members may serve at less hazardous ones. Neither guards nor patrol personnel should have the right or duty of punishing pupils who disobey their signals or instructions. Their obligation is to identify and report recalcitrant students to a designated school official for disciplinary action.

The effectiveness of guards and patrol members is increased when all school members are instructed with respect to the loca-

---

*Accident facts 1974, Chicago, 1975, National Safety Council, pp. 40-41.

tions of guarded crossings and the duties and obligations of those who supervise them. Adult school members should set an example to youngsters by obeying guard and patrol signals. Every pupil who walks or bicycles to and from school should learn and be expected to follow a relatively safe and direct route. One common duty of safety patrol members is to assist teachers and parents in such safety instruction.

A publication of the National Safety Council, *Policies and Practices for School Safety Patrols,** sets forth standards developed by representatives of the Council, the U.S. Office of Education, the National Education Association, the International Association of Chiefs of Police, the National Congress of Parents and Teachers, and the American Automobile Association. Local branches of the American Automobile Association and the PTA, as well as police departments, usually work with school professionals in organizing, instructing, and equipping patrol members.

In some schools, safety patrol members also serve on buses to assist the driver in supervising loading, checking to see that all who should be on board are present, maintaining order during trips, and assisting those who must cross a street or highway at a bus stop to do so safely. In other schools, adults are employed to fulfill these functions. One or the other of these plans is essential. The primary role of the driver is

*This and other helpful materials relevant to school safety are available from the Council, 425 North Michigan Ave., Chicago, Ill. 60611.

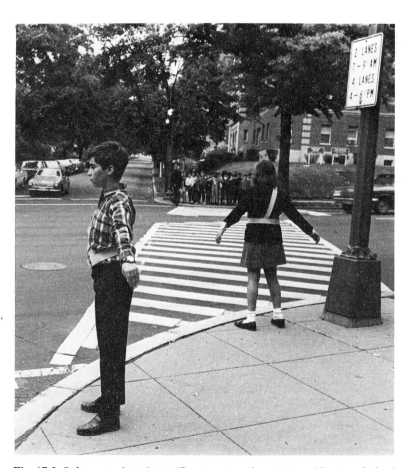

Fig. 17-2. Safety patrol students. (Courtesy American Automobile Association.)

to drive safely and to stop at the right places. He or she cannot reasonably be expected to keep track of individual youngsters and maintain discipline without assistance. Minimum, sensible rules of bus behavior should be democratically developed and understood by all.

In a minority of states anyone with a valid driver's license is considered qualified to drive a school bus. In times when the unemployment rate is low, school administrators are forced to employ any minimally qualified persons who apply. Desirably, drivers should be emotionally mature and stable persons who are either experienced bus or truck drivers or who will receive on-the-job training. Health examinations should be required to weed out those with defective eyesight or hearing or those with defects that predispose them to mental confusion or loss of consciousness, such as inadequately controlled epilepsy, diabetes, high blood pressure, or certain heart diseases.

American school buses cannot now be regarded as representing any great feats of safety engineering. Regulations—and the extent to which they are enforced—vary from state to state and school system to school system. Clearly, a safe school bus provides a seat for every rider. The seats should be firmly anchored and equipped with fully padded backs and with restraints, just as automobiles are. Any protruding metal parts such as grips or rails should also be padded. Interior panels should be so designed that they do not splinter during accidents. Doors and windows should be designed so that passengers are not thrown out of them during accidents.* Such a school bus may exist somewhere; we have never seen one. Periodic thorough checks conducted by a mechanic, including a check when a bus is first delivered, plus daily checks by drivers, are essential. Maintenance workers and drivers alike are plagued by defective transmission and brake systems from the time

buses are delivered until they are finally retired.

School bus routes are usually selected, as they should be, with economy of operation as a goal. Safety should, but does not always, receive equal consideration. Some roads that might be economically desirable to use may present hazards from cross traffic or from poor road maintenance, both of which should be avoided. Stop locations that minimize the necessity for backing and turning the bus or for children to cross highways under unsafe conditions should be selected.

Typical safe operating practices require bus drivers to do more than simply observe general state traffic laws. Many states require school buses to travel at lower speeds than other vehicles, prohibit filling the gasoline tanks while children are on the bus, and prohibit the driver from allowing anyone else to occupy the driver's seat or operate the bus. Most states have enacted legislation requiring other drivers to stop when approaching a school bus that has stopped to load or unload passengers. Unfortunately, these regulations are not uniform throughout the states. Strict police enforcement is essential to compliance.

Driver education is another school program designed to contribute to traffic safety. Automobile insurance rates reflect the fact that drivers in their teens and twenties, especially males, have a much poorer accident record than any other age group.* Given evidence that a young driver has successfully completed a school driver education course, companies will generally lower the cost of insurance slightly. Driver education courses ordinarily include both classroom instruction and supervised practice. Classroom instruction may include units on vehicle and highway safety engineering, relevant state laws, the relationship of alcohol and drug use to traffic accidents, the driver-pedestrian responsibilities. A recent trend has been to place emphasis on defensive

---

*U.C.L.A. Trauma Research Team. Cited in *Accident facts 1974*, p. 92.

Accident facts 1974, pp. 42, 54.

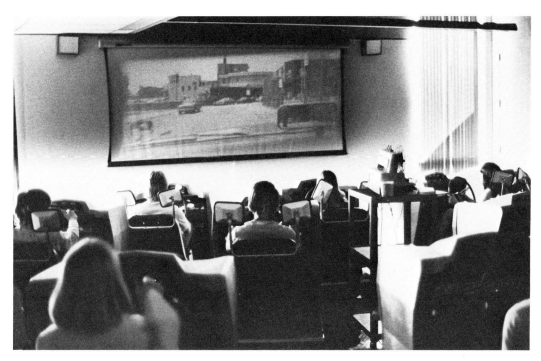

Fig. 17-3. Simulated driver training. (Courtesy David Spilver.)

driving, the basis of which is the notion that one must expect other drivers to behave irresponsibly. Practice may involve the use of simulated automobiles in which students are expected to react in correct ways to traffic conditions shown on a screen (Fig. 17-3). On-the-road supervised practice is generally regarded as an essential part of driver training in addition to or in lieu of simulation. The primary objective of driver education is to equip students with the knowledge, attitudes, and skills required for safe driving. Skills alone are not sufficient, but they are essential. Safe drivers must also learn and scrupulously obey the rules of the road. They must learn the meaning of social responsibility, come to regard automobiles as the lethal weapons that they are, and be able to keep calm under the frustrations they must endure under modern traffic conditions.

Driver education courses increased in number and in the importance assigned to them throughout the 1950's and 1960's. Given the present necessity of fuel conservation and the high cost of automobile insur-

ance and maintenance, driver education may be subject to reappraisal. Many parents may come to feel that they cannot afford to have young licensed drivers in their families.

Fire safety. As we have indicated previously, school building codes and periodic inspections by state or local fire marshalls are helpful in school fire prevention. When modern schools are well planned, constructed, and maintained, the risk of fire occurrence and fire-related injury and death is relatively small. However, old, non–fire resistant buildings remain in use, and even new buildings are not always well kept; a false sense of security may be engendered by fire-resistant construction.

Construction and maintenance practices that are helpful in fire prevention and control include the removal of unused flammable material or its storage in places that are separated from heat sources by appropriate insulation. Each floor should have two or more exits, and exit doors should swing outward. Exterior and corridor exit doors should be equipped with panic bars, that is, bars the width of the door that need only be pressed against to release the latch. In some schools, exit doors are often chained shut to prevent entry by unauthorized persons. This practice is never justifiable. Panic hardware is designed so that it can be locked against entry and still not bar exiting. Multistoried buildings should be equipped with adequate fire escapes that provide access to open grounds, not to enclosed courtyards. Inexpensive, wireless electronic smoke and heat detectors are now available that can easily be installed in both old and new buildings. These may be connected directly to the central fire-warning system.

Most fire deaths result not from heat but from toxic fumes. It is therefore essential to be able to empty any school building in 3 minutes or less. This ability depends not only on school planning that provides adequate means of egress but also on the development of plans and procedures for evacuation and on frequent fire drills. In most states the minimum number of fire drills required each year is specified by law; one a month is not too frequent. Drills should never be announced in advance. Students should not be allowed to take coats with them; if this is allowed in practice, it is likely to be followed in real situations. At least one exit, a different one on each occasion, should be blocked, the better to simulate real situations.

Fire-fighting equipment within the school should be placed at strategic locations and periodically checked and renewed to be sure that it is operable. School professionals should be aware, however, that their first obligation is to evacuate pupils from the building, not to put out the fire. No building is worth the life of a school member.

Safety in physical activity. A majority of the accident injuries and deaths that occur in school are associated with physical activities. We accept the risks inherent in vigorous activity as a reasonable trade-off for the enjoyment and health benefits that activity provides, but we attempt to control the incidence and severity of such injuries.

Well-planned and maintained physical facilities and the selection and maintenance of appropriate exercise equipment and supplies are important environmental approaches to exercise safety. Areas of the school grounds that are open to vehicular traffic should be located apart from those devoted to physical activity. Playground equipment should be isolated from playing fields. Playground areas should be marked with lines to denote safety warning, as well as marked with those lines that are specified by game rules. For example, softball or baseball diamond markings might include lines around the batter's area in addition to foul lines. Facilities, equipment, and supplies should be designed or selected for hard wear, safety, and for their appropriateness to the maturity and skill of those who will use them, as well as cost. Protective equipment should be available in a quantity and range of sizes that permit it to be properly fitted to individual participants. Facilities, equipment, and supplies should be periodically inspected for the hazards that result from wear, and unsafe things should be retired from use until they are repaired. All students and faculty should be made aware of their responsibility to observe and report hazards.

Educational approaches include direct teaching of the specific hazards and preventive measures associated with each activity. Progressive development of skills from the simple to the complex is recommended, and consideration should be given to the growth and development characteristics of the group as a whole and to the stamina and abilities of individuals within the group. Conditioning appropriate to the nature of complex vigorous activities should be provided before instruction or participation in such activities. Development, explanation, and enforcement of safety rules governing any hazardous activity are essential. This applies not only to organized formal activities but also to unorganized free play. As might be expected, unorganized and unsupervised activity is associated with higher risk of injury than organized and supervised play. For this reason, it is strongly recommended that each school provide supervision of all free play periods.*

Many of the above recommendations apply to school athletic programs and to physical education and informal recreation. But athletics poses special problems that are caused, at least in part, by the fact that athletes play for keeps, while nonathletes play to learn and for fun.

The American Alliance for Health, Physical Education, and Recreation conducted its first National Sports Safety Congress in 1973.† Two of the papers presented dealt with medical restrictions to athletic presentations. A basic principle enunciated by both authors is that few if any defects should result in total restriction from all sports; the nature of the defect or defects present, the physiological and psychological nature of the individual, and the nature of the sports available must all be considered in determining which sports should be proscribed and which permitted. One of the authors (Russell Lane) stated that a minimally acceptable medical screening examination for athletic participation should include a complete medical history and physical examination, a complete blood cell count, and urinalysis. He also suggested that better quality examinations might result from a policy of examining athletes every 2 years rather than annually. He proposed also that individual athletes and competing teams be matched on the basis of parameters revelant to the sport. For example, wrestlers might be matched by weight taken at the beginning of the season, rather than preceding each match, to control the potentially hazardous practice of attempting to make a given weight. Football teams might be matched by the number of reserve players each has. Both emphasized that acute

conditions such as infections and dislocations call for temporary removal from participation, again based on the risks and circumstances involved.

Another concern expressed in papers presented at the conference dealt with product safety. The safety of artificial turf, for example, is open to serious question. Football helmets vary widely in quality, and modern hard plastic helmets are legally used as battering rams against opponents. These and other potentially hazardous products are now under the legal purview of the Consumer Products Safety Commission, which is now developing standards. In addition, a National Operating Committee on Standards for Athletic Equipment, representing both consumers and manufacturers, was established in 1970 to conduct athletic equipment safety research. Future activities of these two groups should do much to alleviate the problem. Betty Hartman pointed out that protective rules rather than protective equipment have traditionally been used in women's athletics. She favored keeping sports in which deliberate collisions occur out of the female repertoire and recognized the need for better injury data and improved training and conditioning for female athletes.

Other areas of concern in athletic safety include the need for properly prepared sports physicians, whose training cuts across the boundary lines of general practice, orthopedics, pediatrics, and neurology and provides a knowledge of sports, nutrition, rehabilitation, and physical medicine. The National Athletic Trainers Association has prepared well-considered curricular and certification requirements for athletic trainers, but it will be some time before adequately prepared sports physicians and trainers are available to fill the needs that exist for their services. In the meantime, it appears essential that both coaches and school health service professionals become as well versed in sports safety as they can through reading current literature and attending conferences in the field.

Liability. In our litigious society, no dis-

*The specific suggestions cited are adapted from *School safety policies,* Washington, D.C., 1968, American Association for Health, Physical Education, and Recreation, pp. 12-21.
†Craig, T. T., editor: *Current sports medicine issues,* Washington, D.C., 1974, American Association for Health, Physical Education, and Recreation.

cussion of school safety would be complete without some attention to ways in which school professionals can protect themselves against the risk of liability suits arising out of injuries to students. Tort law is not the least complicated legal subject, and jury and judicial rulings are not altogether predictable, but some principles have emerged on which one may base protective actions.

A tort arises whenever one acts or fails to act in such a way that real injury to another person results. One common test of whether or not a tort has been committed through negligence by a school professional is whether or not the professional acted as a reasonably prudent member of his or her profession would act under like circumstances. Another test has to do with the question of how foreseeable the accident was. If it could reasonably have been foreseen, then the professional should have taken some appropriate action to prevent its occurrence. Still another test is whether the accident resulted largely through the fault of the injured person, but children and young people are not considered as accountable for their own actions as are adults.

Protective actions, most of which have been stated earlier in this section, arise out of those principles. As school professionals, we are obligated to recognize hazardous environmental factors and to do whatever we can to neutralize them. Before exposing students to whatever risk an activity involves, it is our obligation to inform them of the risk and to reduce the risk through safety education, physical conditioning of the students, the provision of protective equipment, or any other appropriate means. When we observe students acting in such a way that an injury might result, we are duty bound to at least attempt to stop them. If an injury does occur, we must provide appropriate first aid and other relevant care to avoid aggravation of the injury. No reasonable judge or jury expects us to be omnipresent, but they do expect us to be reasonable human beings and to act somewhat more reasonably and knowingly than nonprofessionals.

Some states permit school districts to assume the legal costs associated with negligence suits or to pay judgments assessed against school professionals, but most do not. Some professional associations, AFT and NEA, for example, provide professional liability insurance at reasonable cost to their members. It is a good investment for any school professional.

HOMICIDE AND SUICIDE

As we have seen, homicide and suicide deaths occur as school problems largely at the senior high school age levels and are nowhere near as common as are accidental deaths. These tragic events rarely occur on school property and are probably rarely the sole result of school-related events. We believe, however, that a desirable school climate, as described in Chapter 11, may be of preventive value, just as certain specific actions by school health service professionals and teachers may also be.

Homicide. We observed earlier that homicide, or at least reported homicide, is much more common among high school age youths than it is among children and that victims are more often males than females. The homicide rate (1972) for nonwhite U.S. males is roughly 10 times that for white males, and the rate for nonwhite females is about 6 times that for white females. The 1968 U.S. homicide rate for males was 13.4 per 100,000 population (6.6 for whites), as compared with rates of 2.2 for Canada, less than 1.0 in the Scandinavian and Western European countries, and 1.8 in Japan. In 1972, two thirds of all murders in the United States were committed with guns.*

These data only describe the scope of the problem; they do not explain or tell us how to deal with it. They strongly suggest that one approach that is likely to be effective is meaningful gun control legislation, strictly

---

Statistical abstract of the United States, 1974, U.S. Department of Commerce, Bureau of the Census, Washington, D.C., 1974, U.S. Government Printing Office, pp. 150-151.

enforced. Hanlon* quotes a number of authorities in support of this position, including the late J. Edgar Hoover and a representative of the International Association of Chiefs of Police. Thus far the National Rifle Association and other components of the pro-gun lobby have successfully blocked any attempt to pass such legislation at the national level and in most states and localities. Another approach suggested by Hanlon is that of social conditioning. He points out that we live in a society in which comic books, television shows, and movies glamorize guns and murder, and in which toy guns are regarded as appropriate gifts for little boys. Deglamorization of guns and violent aggression would require turning all these societal influences around.

Early in this book we noted Jan Fawcett's contention that hopelessness breeds violence and that if we can maintain in young people a realistic sense of hopefulness that they can achieve their life goals, then violence may thereby be prevented.†

Meninger and Modlin‡ state that violence-prone individuals frequently indicate their disturbance by expressing the fear that they are losing control, by seeking help from a variety of other people, by buying a gun, or by doing a variety of other subtle and not so subtle things. They suggest that counselors may intervene by providing an opportunity for the person to talk about and think through his or her problems or by suggesting that he or she leave the stressful situation for a while.

Berkowitz§ cites evidence to dispute the notion that catharsis (smashing a vase or playing football) successfully relieves aggressive impulses, and he suggests instead that the mere presence of guns or other weapons, in fact, stimulates aggression. One successful act of aggression breeds further acts of aggression.

To summarize, we may best be able to reduce homicides committed by young people by supporting gun control legislation, deglamorizing guns and violence in our culture, producing a society in which young people, particularly young black males, have some reasonable hope of achieving the appropriate life goals that they set for themselves, and by offering mental health counseling to individuals who give us any indication that they may be about to commit an act of violence. What does not work is kicking ashcans, playing aggressive games, or watching violent movies as ways of relieving violent impulses.

Suicide. Suicides, like homicides, occur more frequently among people in their teens and twenties than among children, and more frequently among males than females. Unlike homicides, they occur somewhat more frequently among white males than among nonwhite males, and rates are essentially equal for white and nonwhite females. Among males, firearms and explosives are the means most frequently used, poisoning ranks second, and hanging third. Among females, poisoning ranks first, firearms and explosives second, and hanging third. In comparison with other countries, the U.S. suicide rate is a modest 11.1 per 100,000 population. Sweden's rate is high, at 22.0; and Ireland's is low, at 1.8.* These last data suggest that in some cultures suicide is an accepted way of dealing with personal problems and that in other cultures it is not acceptable. Hanlon† cites data that indicate that in adolescence the suicide attempt ratio may be as high as one attempt per 100 persons.

Hanlon also states that women attempt

*Hanlon, J. J.: *Public health administration and practice,* ed. 6, St. Louis, 1974, The C. V. Mosby Co., pp. 500-504.

†Fawcett, J., editor: *Dynamics of violence,* Chicago, 1972, American Medical Association, pp. 193-198.

‡Meninger, R. W., and Modlin, H. C.: Individual violence: prevention in the violence prone individual. In Fawcett, J., editor: *Dynamics of violence,* pp. 71-73.

§Berkowitz, L.: Experimental investigation of hostility catharsis. In Fawcett, J., editor, *Dynamics of violence,* pp. 139-144.

Statistical abstract of the United States, 1974, pp. 64, 144, 150, 151, 818.

†Hanlon, J. J.: *Public health administration and practice,* p. 449.

suicide more frequently than men, but are not successful as often. He also notes that among young people, suicide frequently follows perceived mistreatment or failure.

In retrospect it is easy to recognize the cries for help that usually precede a suicide attempt, which in itself is a cry for help. These include talking or writing about suicide. The belief that those who talk about committing suicide do not do it is a myth. Depression, especially depression that is worse than its cause justifies, is another common danger sign. Suicidal individuals are not always psychotically disoriented or addicted to drugs, but many are. Pain and rejection by loved ones are frequent precursors of suicide, as hypochondria, insomnia, and hopelessness also are.

Suicidal individuals need, above all else, to have someone to talk to. This need can be met by anyone with whom the suicidal person feels comfortable. Medical intervention is highly desirable, because antidepressant drugs may be helpful in the late teens, and tranquilizers may be useful at younger ages.* These drugs are useful in warding off suicide attempts until a more hopeful attitude toward life can be developed. Professional help can be obtained through community mental health centers. Suicide prevention centers exist in many large cities. Some of them provide a 24 hour a day hotline service that not only offers the suicidal individual an opportunity to talk with someone but also furnishes advice to those attempting to block a suicidal attempt. Such centers may provide followup services directly or by referral. Followup is essential because repeated attempts are common.

There are those who believe that any person who wishes to commit suicide should be allowed to do so. This position is especially untenable when it is applied to children and young people. Adolescence is a time of emotional storms not unrelated to the endocrine hormone imbalances typical of the teens and to the adolescent's search for identity. Time and maturation heal many of the insults that lead young people to attempt suicide, and many of those who attempt suicide are talented, lovable, sensitive persons.

CHILD ABUSE

An unknown number of children are frequently and severely beaten or otherwise tortured by one or both parents, and many of them are crippled or killed as a result. Parents of all socioeconomic levels are among the perpetrators, and children and youth of both sexes and all ages are among the victims. From the accumulated evidence it appears that nearly all abusing parents were themselves abused as children and that many if not most of the abused children were unwanted or have been rejected by their parents. Many abusive parents give the child's need for discipline as the reason (or rationalization) behind their abusive behavior.*

From these and other observations it may be inferred that school health and health education can contribute to the primary prevention of child abuse by providing instruction in family planning to prevent the birth of unwanted children and in the art of parenting and nonharmful discipline of children. Part of this education includes an absolute prohibition against the use of corporal punishment in the school.

Laws have now been enacted in all states that provide for the detection and treatment of cases of child abuse. These laws vary in detail from state to state but are based on two model codes, one of which was proposed jointly by the Children's Bureau and the American Humane Association and the other by the American Academy of Pediatrics. The statutes generally require the reporting by physicians and often by school professionals of all suspected cases of child

---

*Renshaw, D. C.: Suicide and depression in children, J. Sch. Health **44:**487-489, Nov. 1974.

*Lystad, M., editor: *Violence at home,* National Institute of Mental Health, DHEW Publication No. (ADM) 75-136, Washington, D.C., 1974, U.S. Government Printing Office.

abuse to a single legally designated agency. There is usually a provision exempting those who report such cases from legal action for making reports that are not proven to be well founded. The agency that receives the report is authorized to take such action as may be necessary to protect abused children, either on its own authority or with court approval. Actions may include hospitalization, removal of the child from the home, or continuation of placement in the home under court or social agency supervision. Emphasis is placed on rehabilitation rather than on criminal prosecution of abusive parents.

Although these statutes have resulted in increased numbers of cases reported, there remain a number of nonlegal barriers to early detection. First among them is the reluctance of all of us to interfere in family matters and our inclination to accept at face value the usual parental explanation that the child was injured in an accident. We also tend to accept punishment of children. One survey revealed that 80% to 90% of all American adults have spanked a child and that half of them approve of in-school spanking of children.* In addition, many abused children hide their injuries and at least state that their punishment is deserved. Nonabusive spouses likewise tend to protect their abusive mates. Injured or dead children are frequently taken to hospital accident wards by one or the other parent, who cites accident as the cause of injury and who may also try to hide the situation by patronage of a different hospital on subsequent occasions.

Teachers, nurses, and other school professionals should be aware of the provisions of the child abuse statute in their state, especially as they relate to their own actions in detecting and reporting cases. They should suspect abuse in the case of any child who appears at school with frequent fresh injuries, who dresses in a manner designed to hide arms and legs, and who avoids undressing in the presence of others for physical activity or shower. Such suspicions should always be investigated by some designated school professional (such as the nurse), and a report should be filed as is legally and morally required. Contact with and joint action by school professionals and the family physician may be required. The goal of reporting is not further punishment but the prevention of crippling and murder.

Adequate follow-up of reported cases always requires the cooperation of school professionals with the legally responsible agency, especially in cases dealt with by continued supervised placement in the home. Many abusive parents are no better able to control their cruel behavior than alcoholics are able to control their drinking. The problems that abusive parents face are complex and not subject to easy or quick solutions, and injury may therefore recur. Still, many if not most abusive parents have been and can be rehabilited through mental health and social casework intervention. Parents Anonymous chapters, patterned after Alcoholics Anonymous, have emerged in many communities to assist in the rehabilitation of abusive parents through peer support.

The difficulty in obtaining reports and the uncertainty of the effectiveness of treatment of abusive parents may lead to revision of statutes. As this is written a revision of the Pennsylvania law is under consideration that provides legal penalties for those who should report cases but fail to do so.

QUESTIONS FOR STUDY AND DISCUSSION

1. Among which school-age and sex groups are accidental deaths, homicides, and suicides most common? Which of these causes of violent death is most common? What is the relative importance of violence as a cause of school-age deaths compared with all other causes combined?
2. What are the five phases proposed by Schaplowsky for the development of injury control programs?
3. What are the main values of school accident reports and surveys? How would you proceed in establishing an accident-reporting and survey system for a school or school system?
4. Why are student and community input important in school injury control? In what

---

*Lystad, M., editor: *Violence at home*, p. 49.

way, if any, are these inputs obtained in a school or school system with which you are familiar?

5. What means are usually chosen to attempt to achieve the goals established for school safety program segments?
6. Develop a check list of desirable school practices in promoting traffic safety, fire safety, and safety in physical activity. Which of these practices are or are not followed in a school system with which you are acquainted?
7. In what ways can you as a school professional best protect yourself against the possibility of successful suit for negligent injury to a student?
8. What can schools do to prevent homicides?
9. What provisions, if any, would you propose to be included in federal gun control legislation? Defend your position.
10. Debate the issue of censorship of violence in the media.
11. What signs of suicidal intent should you as a school professional look for among students and peers? What should you do about it if you observe such signs?
12. What characteristics of abusive parents and abused children are described in the text?
13. What should you as a school professional do about it if you suspect that a student is being abused by his or her parents?

REFERENCES

Anderson, C. L.: *School health practice,* ed. 5, St. Louis, 1972, The C. V. Mosby Co.

Hanlon, J. J.: *Public health administration and practice,* ed. 6, St. Louis, 1974, The C. V. Mosby Co.

Miller, D. F.: *School health programs: their basis in law,* Cranbury, N.J., 1972, A. S. Barnes & Co., Inc.

Nemir, A., and Schaller, W. E.: *The school health program,* ed. 4, Philadelphia, 1975, W. B. Saunders Co.

Oberteuffer, D., Harrelson, O. A., and Pollock, M. B.: *School health education,* ed. 5, New York, 1972, Harper & Row, Publishers.

Wilson, C. C., and Wilson, E. A., editors: *Healthful school environment,* ed. 2, Washington, D.C., 1957, National Education Association and American Medical Association.

CHAPTER 18

❧ Sexuality and the school

Both social and individual concerns underlie school health and health education activities related to sexuality and sex problems. One social concern is that the burgeoning world population may soon exhaust the capacity of planet earth to provide sufficient food and other resources, a topic discussed in Chapter 1. Other social concerns have to do with illegitimate births and teenage mothers, and what some perceive to be a general breakdown in morals and family solidity. More personal concerns include the hang-ups and guilt feelings that make the realization of a satisfying and fulfilling sex life difficult or impossible for many.

NATURE AND SCOPE OF SEX-RELATED PROBLEMS

Fig. 18-1 shows the relationship between world food production and population. It suggests that we are not yet in much more serious difficulty than we have been in the past, but we must realize that at some future time human reproduction is very likely to outstrip agriculture and technical ability to feed humans. The fact that a world Food Conference was held in Rome in November 1974 and that its accomplishments were meager attests to the reality and complexity of the problem. The third world nations (the small, developing countries) sent representatives to the conference to beg for immediate delivery of the food grains required to stave off starvation, and they left with precious little. Efforts to create substantive long-term plans failed in large part.* While population control programs have been quite successful in the affluent nations, they have been less so in the third world nations. The latter are unable to grow, buy, or beg enough food to prevent starvation,

and they retain ties to cultures in which children grow up to be the sole source of support of their elderly parents.

Population control progress in the United States is illustrated in the first column of Table 18-1. From the low of the depression year 1940, our birth rate climbed to its post–World War baby boom peak around 1960. Since then, the birth rate has steadily declined. It was during the 1960's that the pill became popular and that significant federal support of birth control programs began. The provisional birth rate for 1972 (detailed data for that year are not yet available as this is written) was 73.4, well below the depression low. This does not mean that our total population is shrinking or is about to do so. One reason is that 1972 births exceeded 1972 deaths by a ratio of about three births for every two deaths. Another reason is that the 1960 bumper crop of babies will be producing babies of their own around 1985. But enough progress (if you favor zero population growth) has been made so that some school buildings and hospital maternity wards are being closed for lack of customers.

With respect to teen-age and illegitimate births, the remaining data in the table present a mixed picture. The rate of illegitimate births has climbed steadily since 1940. The rate for 10- to 14-year-old mothers remained fairly constant from 1940 to 1970, while that for 15- to 19-year-olds has followed the general curve.

Mothers below the age of 17 and their babies have been shown in numerous studies to be high-risk mothers and babies. The risks are medical, educational, and social. They specifically include higher maternal and infant mortality, a higher incidence of obstetrical complications, and a higher rate of prematurity than are found among mothers in their twenties and their babies.

*Rothschild, E.: Short term, long term, *The New Yorker,* May 26, 1975.

Teen-age mothers are more likely to drop out of school than their nonpregnant peers, and their babies tend to be mentally and neurologically retarded. Marriages of pregnant teen-agers or of teen-agers who have recently gave birth are three or four times more likely to end in divorce than are marriages in later life. Repeated pregnancies tend to follow the first, and a high proportion of teen-age mothers and their babies must be supported by public welfare programs.*

*Osofsky, H. J., and Renga, R.: The adolescent pregnancy. In Wallace, H. M., Gold, E. M., and Lis, E. F., editors: *Maternal and child health practices, problems, resources, and methods of delivery,* Springfield, Ill., 1973, Charles C Thomas, Publisher, pp. 886-889.

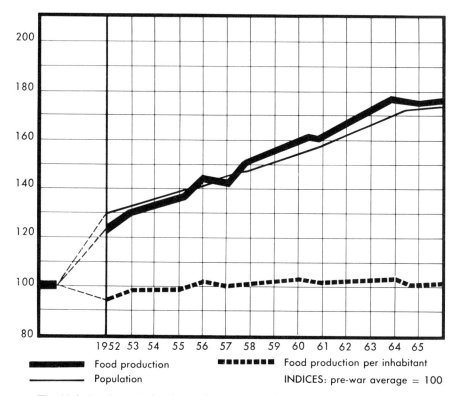

Fig. 18-1. Food production in relation to population. (Courtesy *World health.*)

Table 18-1. Birth rates by age of mother per 1,000 women in age group, and estimated illegitimate birth rates per 1,000 unmarried women, United States, 1940-1970

Year	All births 15 to 44 years	10 to 14 years	15 to 19 years	Illegitimate births 15 to 44 years
1940	79.9	0.7	54.1	7.1
1945	85.9	0.8	51.1	10.1
1950	106.2	1.0	81.6	14.1
1955	118.5	0.9	90.5	19.3
1960	118.0	0.8	89.1	21.6
1965	96.6	0.8	70.4	23.5
1970	88.0	1.2	68.3	26.4

Data from National Center for Health Statistics.

We live in a pluralistic society in which there is no general consensus as to what does or does not constitute morally acceptable sexual behavior. Some maintain that sexual intercourse outside marriage is always a sin; others maintain that it is no sin if there is mutual affection; and still others feel that it is no sin at all if there is mutual consent. Some believe that illegitimacy is a sin; others believe that it is worse to enter a bad marriage than none at all. This lack of consensus places a terrible burden on young people; most of them want to know and do what is right, but the adults and peers to whom they turn for help are not in agreement. Some therefore conclude that the data presented here indicates a breakdown in individual sexual mores and morals, others that society is at fault, and still others that we are in the process of trading in an old unworkable set of mores and morals for a new and better set.

The prevalence of hang-ups that result in inadequate, unfulfilling, or distorted sex lives is not known. The success of the Masters and Johnson clinic and its imitators suggests that it may be quite high. Katchadourian and Lunder* state that most cases of sexual malfunctioning result from conflicts and problems that arise out of past experiences. Among these they list anxieties and depressions, some of which arise out of situations in which a couple may find themselves, and others for no rational reason. Other sexual malfunctioning may result from past learning experiences, such as being taught that sex is immoral and dirty, or from defective psychosexual development. Katchadourian and Lunder suggest that many such problems are not only preventable through sex education but may also be correctable through education and through psychotherapeutic intervention. They note that Masters and Johnson combine counseling and education in their highly successful approach to the treatment of such problems. Although not all divorces result from sexual hang-ups, many of them do. The 1971 United States divorce rate was 15.7 divorces per 1,000 marriages, more than double the rate of 7.5 for 1930, and higher than the rate of 14.4 recorded in 1945 when couples were breaking up as a result of wartime stresses and experiences.*

School health and health education cannot prevent or solve all the sex problems of children and youth. Psychosexual development is primarily a learning process that requires us to encounter and solve problems —a process that, by its nature, cannot be painless. But it can help children and youth sidestep some of the problems and help them cope with some of those problems that do arise. A successful approach must heavily involve parents and community agencies as well as schools, and contributions by school health service professionals as well as educators.

SEX EDUCATION

The general principles and guidelines for health education explicated in Chapters 5 through 8 apply as much to sex education as they do to other health education topics. Some aspects of it, however, are controversial and threatening to teachers. The discussion below may prove helpful.

Developing a philosophy. Except in some isolated areas and among certain religious groups there is no longer any question that schools can and should play an important role in sex education. Numerous recent surveys indicate that the majority of parents, students, and school professionals favor in-school sex instruction.† The storm centers focus instead on issues of objectives, content, and method.

One of these areas of controversy has to do with the issue of whether and how sex-

---

*Katchadourian, H. A., and Lunder, D. T.: *Fundamentals of human sexuality*, New York, 1972, Holt, Rinehart and Winston, Inc., pp. 310-318.

Statistical abstract of the United States, Washington, D.C., 1974, U.S. Department of Commerce, Social and Economic Statistics Division, Bureau of the Census, p. 66.
†Conley, J. A., and Hoff, R. S.: The generation gap in sex education: is there one? J. Sch. Health **44:**428-437, Dec. 1974.

related morals and values should be dealt with in school. Hoyman* states that there is now little expert dissent from the position that young people must have both facts and values, that an ethical framework is essential. He identifies sexual permissiveness as the key issue, pointing out that no culture, not even that of Sweden, is totally permissive and that a number of different value systems coexist in the United States today that range from puritan abstinence to complete permissiveness. He identifies a number of American core value issues that need to be resolved by and with young people if a new and commonly accepted code of sexual behavior is to emerge. These include our need for human survival and our desire for individual self-fulfillment, our commitment to individual freedom and need for social responsibility, and the preservation of our rights of freedom of speech and religion. We can best help youth, he concludes, if we openly discuss issues of values and morality with them, helping them make sound judgments without indoctrination. We do not necessarily need to be neutral, but we do need to be objective. We need to impart accurate biological and other scientific information relevant to value development and behavioral decision making, but values and behavior are of primary importance.

Another philosophical issue relevant to the development of school curricula is that posed by the feminist movement. Levy and Stacey† charge that sexism pervades elementary schools, citing sex-role stereotyping and put-downs of girls in elementary text readings as well as sex segragation for instruction and pupil school housekeeping task assignments. They cite evidence from research with children to back their contention that boys accept superior and girls inferior roles early on, but the authors deplore what they regard as overdependence

on such quickie solutions as nonsexist textbook selection guidelines and role-reversal classroom games. They call for change based on careful analysis instead. Trecker* identifies similar problems in secondary school curricula and textbooks. She calls for reforms that go beyond textbook and course-offering revision to include specific attention to such female needs as those for instruction in self-defense and contraception.

These and other philosophical issues must first be resolved before proceeding to sex education curriculum development. Philosophy guides the selection and statement of objectives, the selection of content and the means by which it is presented, and the development of evaluative procedures. If the subject is ignored, the lack of a guiding philosophy will return to haunt teachers and administrators. A soundly based philosophy can best be developed through the active involvement of parents, students, and the community religious leaders as well as educators and sex education specialists. It is not to be expected that all groups will agree on all issues; parents are likely to espouse somewhat more conservative attitudes than students or experts, for example. More areas of agreement than of disagreement, however, are likely to be found.†

Content and objectives. The same groups that were involved in the development of a statement of philosophy should also be called upon in the development of objectives and selection of content, not only because their support is needed, but also because peers, parents, clergy, and other social segments share responsibility for and provide a large part of the sex instruction that youngsters receive. Some possible content areas are considered below.

Cognitive aspects. Gordon‡ suggests that

---

*Hoyman, H. S.: Sex education and our core values, J. Sch. Health **44**:62-69, Feb. 1974.
†Levy, B., and Stacey, J.: Sexism in the elementary school: a backward and forward look, Phi Delta Kappan **55**:105-109, 123, Oct. 1973.

*Trecker, J. L.: Sex stereotyping in the secondary school curriculum, Phi Delta Kappan **55**:110-112, Oct. 1973.
†Dearth, P. B.: Viable sex education in the schools: expectations of students, parents, and experts, J. Sch. Health **44**:190-193, April 1974.
‡Gordon, S.: What place does sex education have in schools? J. Sch. Health **44**:186-189, April 1974.

in schools where student distrust, low morale, or apathy is present, an unbiased presentation of essential cognitive information is likely to be the most realistic approach and that this may be supplemented through outside agencies. If, however, opposite conditions are present, then a curriculum may be developed that is designed to help students develop greater awareness and understanding of their sexuality. In any event, there is need for a certain amount of factual information. The kind of information selected should vary with grade level and should be designed to provide youngsters with an acceptable vocabulary so that they can ask intelligible questions. It is also important that they acquire information essential to the development of desirable sexual attitudes and behavior, whether or not this is a part of the school curriculum. It is equally important to avoid the presentation of information that youngsters perceive as irrelevant to them. It serves no useful purpose to require them to memorize the names and complex interactions of the hormones that affect sexual development and activity, for example. This sort of information is more useful to physiologists and physicians than to others.

Children usually come to school having acquired some names and explanations of the purposes of their own external genitalia and organs of elimination and sometimes of those of the other sex. These names and explanations often are in terms of either family vocabulary that is usually not understood by others, or street vocabulary that is considered obnoxious in most schools. We used to believe that everyone ought to trade off family and street vocabulary for clinical Latin, but some of us are having second thoughts about this. Clinical Latin is useful because meanings are precise and because it is acceptable in polite society, but it is also difficult to spell and pronounce, especially in early childhood. Outright rejection of family or street vocabulary may only serve to convince youngsters that there really is something dirty or sinful about sex organs and their function.

Shortly before or after school entrance, most modern children acquire a reasonably accurate notion of what pregnancy is and how babies are born. They are likely to become aware that their version of these events differs somewhat from that of others, and they will probably want to review and check the accuracy of the information they possess. But they may not know what sexual intercourse is, or, if they do, they may not know how conception does and does not occur.

We have pretty much rejected Freud's notion of a sexual latency period, and we are aware that some youngsters begin sexual activity of some sort around age 10. Sometime around grade 5, if not before, children therefore begin to need to know what sexual intercourse is and how pregnancy occurs. In many schools, related information about menstruation is taught to girls at about this time, but often not to boys. Also, boys are less likely than girls to be taught about it at home and therefore need to acquire their information at school at or about the same time girls are taught.

Soon after, boys and girls begin to have orgasms in various ways, if they have not yet begun to do so. They need to know that nearly all boys and perhaps two thirds of all girls masturbate, that some have erotic dreams that for boys may or may not result in having nocturnal emissions, and that myths about the harmfulness or significance of these events are only myths. If they choose to have intercourse, they need to know how to avoid pregnancy and VD, and what it is possible to do when they suspect that these problems have occurred. Instruction should also be designed to uncover and replace with facts whatever myths are current about impregnation, VD, birth control, abortion, homosexuality, and other areas of concern.

Attitudinal aspects. Jane Woody* has proposed a scheme, based on behavioral theory and ordered by developmental stages, that encompasses the development of seven

*Woody, J. D.: Contemporary sex education: attitudes and implications for child rearing, J. Sch. Health **43:**241-246, April 1973.

successive basic attitudes. Each of these is accompanied by several guidelines for teaching that is addressed to parents. The attitudes and some of the guidelines are restated and revised below since they seem logically to apply to in-school teaching and guidance. The attitudes are closely correlated with the cognitive aspects described above.

The first attitude is that there is nothing inherently bad or dirty about sex organs and their functions. This attitude (or its undesirable converse) is largely developed in early (preschool) childhood. Some parents help develop the desirable attitude by acceptance of their own nudity and that of their children under acceptable circumstances in the home. They name and explain the functions of external genitalia. They use praise and rewards for successful toilet use rather than punishment for soiling. They accept childhood sexual exploration and expressions of concern as outgrowths of normal curiosity rather than sins or sinlets. In school we have not yet come to accept heterosexual nudity, and it is doubtful if we should. But we can present this and the art of toilet training to senior high school students as part of their preparation for parenthood. We can name and explain the genitalia and their functions, beginning early with simple explanations of the external components. We can accept and give straightforward answers to questions, and we can recognize and at least attempt to correct the error when giggles and blushes suggest that parents or some other source has instilled the idea that sex is bad or dirty.

The second attitude is that we adults should consciously attempt to ensure that boys develop as boys and girls as girls. Members of gay liberation groups may quarrel with the validity of this, and by a majority vote the American Psychiatric Association has decreed that homosexuality is not an illness. Nevertheless, most parents prefer that their children grow up as heterosexuals because they wish them not to be social outcasts, if for no other reason. It may therefore be useful to provide school opportunities for interactions with the same and opposite sex. We can recognize that many youngsters engage in same-sex exploratory play as part of learning what they are, and we should neither overreact to such play nor label it as homosexual. Better male-female balance on elementary school teaching staffs would provide more male models for boys. School curricula in general need reform to avoid giving superior-inferior ratings to sex-related roles. Whether or not the teacher and school attitudes and behaviors cited above will have much effect on the incidence of homosexuality is open to question, but they should at least foster sexual egalitarianism.

Woody's third attitude is that masturbation is a normal way of expressing sexual need for both sexes in a variety of circumstances and at different age levels. She and most other modern authorities view it as perhaps necessary to the development of healthy sexual response. Punishment and displays of anger or disgust are inappropriate responses to instances of masturbation that occur in public. The appropriate response is to try to divert the youngster's attention to another activity. Youngsters probably need to be told directly that masturbation is acceptable in private but not in public and that we believe it to be normal and harmless.

The fourth attitude is that sex education is a continuing process and that youngsters need accurate and complete information about sexual anatomy and physiology, sex-related behavior, birth control, VD, and psychological factors related to sexual behavior before puberty. One implication of this attitude is that all teachers should be prepared to give accurate information geared to children's levels of understanding in response to questions asked at any time. We need to be sensitive enough to recognize and deal with any problems that underlie the questions. For example, a boy might ask how often it is normal to ejaculate. This may not be simple curiosity, but reflect the boy's concern that something may be wrong because he does it more or less frequently than his peers. The answer is that perfectly normal, healthy individuals vary greatly in frequency, that sexual need is an individual matter. We also need to have resolved our own conflicts to the point where we are able to discuss sex openly with children. We need to be able to integrate values with facts and to do so in an unemotional way. For example, most of us believe that there is nothing right about an 11-year-old child having sexual intercourse, but we may be able to recognize that it is better for them to do so with some degree of knowledge and protection than without it. To achieve this kind of balance we do not have to give up our own values, but we do need to recognize that different social and cultural groups have different expectations. We need to be aware of what these are, of differences in male and female sexual response, and of the various sex games that people play.

The fifth attitude is that the advantages and disadvantages of possible premarital sex behaviors must be evaluated by each individual in terms of his or her own personal characteristics and values, subgroup mores, and environment. These characteristics are apt to be similar to those of a youngster's parents if a good child-parent relationship exists. The fact that it frequently does not exist impels us to engage in value clarification and behavior evaluation strategies in school. In doing so we need to recognize and accept individual and group differences. We need to develop a climate in which youngsters can discuss these things openly. We do not need to hide our own values, but we must not try to impose them on our students; any attempt to do so would be futile, anyway.

The sixth attitude is that adolescents ought to have access to birth control methods and information. The romantic preference of many teen-agers is that their first act of intercourse be spontaneous and unplanned—an attitude that leaves them open to the risks of VD and pregnancy. Many responsible teen-agers still choose to delay the onset of sexual intercourse until they feel that they are mature enough to accept the emotional and social responsibilities that go with it. Those who choose otherwise must be made aware of their responsibilities for the health and emotional well-being of themselves, their partners, and their potential babies. Sexually active teen-agers must be helped to define a moral code that they can live with comfortably, without guilt feelings. This will usually include conscious planning to prevent VD and unwanted pregnancy, but it implies also a rejection of promiscuous sex in favor of an emotional commitment to one's partner. The development of such a code is a difficult task that involves deep, open, and frequently uncomfortable discussion and thought.

The seventh and final attitude is that open and clear communication about sex is of great importance in developing and maintaining not only good sexual relationships but also other kinds of rich interpersonal relationships. Again, a few parents are able to achieve such openness with each other and their children, and we in school can perhaps help future parents to improve intimate communication skills. Adolescents, whether or not they are able to communicate at home, depend a great deal on open discussion with their peers as they attempt to develop their sexual identities, their abilities to be open and intimate with a loved partner, their emotional independence from their parents, their own value systems, and career goals. We in school can provide opportunity for such discussions under skilled leadership. We can provide the essential background information for such discussions. We can stress the importance of honest communication about sexual needs and feelings between partners and the importance of accepting one's partner as a whole person, not only as a sex object.

Some teaching strategies. Burt and Meeks* present some specific content and

---

*Burt, J. J., and Meeks, L. B.: *Education for sexuality: concepts and programs for teaching,* Philadelphia, 1975, W. B. Saunders Co., pp. 191-391.

strategies for sex education. We have abridged and adapted a few of these for presentation, with the caution that they are here meant to serve as examples only. Those who are called upon to provide sex instruction should consult this or another of the excellent resource books now available.

At the kindergarten or first grade level, pupils can prepare family albums that identify family members, their roles in family work and recreation, and their social roles. A tour of boys' and girls' bathrooms will reveal differences in equipment that can be related to the names and functions of the visible body parts of boys and girls.

At about grade 4 or 5, detailed information about the anatomy and physiology of human reproduction can be presented by use of overhead transparencies. Students can work out simple problems in human genetics. Using pingpong balls for ovaries, straws for the fallopian tubes and vagina, and a paper cup for the uterus, they can construct a schematic model of the female reproductive system and can place a small rubber doll in a plastic bag in the "uterus" to represent a fetus.

At the junior or senior high school level, students can prepare individual posters advertising what of their own traits they con-

sider to be most appealing to others. Peers can then try to identify which posters refer to whom. A study of homosexuality might culminate in the preparation and debate of legislative proposals relating to homosexuals. They can list the various kinds of sexual activities that they have read about or discussed in class, ranging from kissing to sexual intercourse, and make moral decisions about the appropriateness of each activity for each of several levels of intimacy ranging from casual acquaintance to marriage, and for persons of varying age levels. Methods of contraception can be examined in relation to effectiveness, availability to unmarried teen-agers, possible side effects, and personal acceptability. Structured and unstructured rap sessions are particularly valuable during adolescence.

Lochner and Gotta* have proposed a logical choice model that could be presented to junior or senior high school students as a guide to behavioral decision making (Fig. 18-2) with respect to the specific problem of premarital pregnancy. The first step or level is a simple dichotomy: to have premarital heterosexual intercourse

---

*Lochner, J. W., and Gotta, J. M.: Premarital pregnancies and the choice process, School Health Review 3:18-22, Jan.-Feb. 1972.

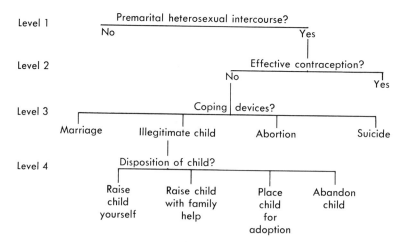

Fig. 18-2. Premarital pregnancy choice model. (Adapted from Lochner, J. W., and Gotta, J. M.: Premarital pregnancies and the choice process, School Health Review 3:18-22, Jan.-Feb. 1972.)

or not to have it. If the choice is not to have it, then premarital pregnancy is not a problem. If the choice is made to have intercourse, then a second-level choice must be made: to use effective contraception or to use ineffective or no contraception. If effective contraception is not used and if pregnancy results, then one of several third-level coping devices must be selected: marriage, the bearing of an illegitimate child, abortion, or suicide must be chosen. A girl who chooses to bear an illegitimate child is faced with one of several fourth-level choices: raising the child herself or with family help, placing the child for adoption, or abandoning the child.

Many of the strategies described above are difficult for beginning teachers to manage. Most new teachers are more comfortable if they begin sex instruction with a presentation of anatomy and physiology and with extensive use of visual and audiovisual aids. They can then advance to discussion of psychosocial factors by use of the old and effective device of having students submit questions that concern them in written form. Cards may be passed out for this purpose and collected in a box. The teacher can then compile and organize the questions by topic. Those that call for straightforward answers can be handled in that way. Others may require further study and/or discussion.

Who should teach sex education? Psychologists, nurses, and physicians, health educators, and other groups of professionals all lay claim to being best qualified as sex educators. Some colleges and universities today are beginning to prepare sex educators as such through curricula that provide a broad interdisciplinary background. Perhaps the most important qualification is that whoever teaches it should be comfortable in dealing with sex-oriented material. Another is that the teacher should be one who will not be shocked by four-letter words or blue jokes presented by students. Most students who engage in such behavior do so in an effort to shock the teacher and will continue to do so if the teacher reacts in the desired way. On the other hand, most of us would

agree that dirty jokes told by teachers have no place in a class devoted to sex education.

The basic principle that teaching should be done by fully qualified regular members of the school staff is a third guideline that should be followed to the extent possible. At present there are many schools that lack a qualified staff member. Such schools sometimes utilize the services of outsiders or of noncredentialed school physicians or nurses. The instruction thus provided is usually conducted in one or two sex-segregated sessions that are frequently held after school hours. There are numerous obvious disadvantages to arrangements of this sort. Those who teach may or may not be effective teachers. They may or may not have good rapport with the students. If sessions are segregated, boys will always wonder what the girls are being taught and vice versa. The time allotted is usually sufficient only for the presentation of basic information. Groups are too large for any meaningful interactions to occur. However, if such sessions are well planned and well managed, they are often more useful than no instruction at all. If they are reasonably successful, they may serve to demonstrate the need for a reasonably complete sex education curriculum taught by well-qualified teachers.

Sex education for exceptional students. Highly talented students have the same sex-related needs and interests as those within the so-called average range. They are handicapped, however, in the sense that some of them are so brilliant that it is difficult for them to find equally talented members of the same or other sex with whom they can establish meaningful and satisfying interpersonal relationships. Relatively large school districts sometimes help solve this problem by identifying highly talented children and young people from a number of schools and bringing them together for special projects. Here they may develop the kind of mutual work and play relationships that, as Erikson points out in *Childhood and Society,* are essential to the fulfillment of intimacy.

Retarded children also have need of sex

instruction. They are often more trusting of others than those of average or higher intelligence and are thus susceptible to sexual exploitation. As Shindell* reports, they have the same sexual interests and desires as others. Those who are sex-segregated in institutions frequently develop homosexual relationships, as would logically be expected, while those who are unable to relate to others logically meet their needs through masturbation. Noninstitutionalized retarded persons sometimes marry, and those marriages in which effective birth control methods are used are often successful. The content and nature of sex education can be very much like that provided for other students except that the difficulty of retarded persons in managing abstractions must be recognized and provided for, and their need for effective birth control services must be met. In instruction, use of physical models that can be seen and touched is recommended. For many retarded persons, appropriate birth control methods are limited to intra-uterine devices and vasectomies or tubal ligations.

Blind students are deprived of many of the formal and informal visual experiences that contribute importantly to the sex education of others, as Cataruzolo and Ennis† point out. They learn largely by hearing and feeling. Therefore, presenting educational dolls with genitals, using a stethoscope to listen to the fetal heartbeat in a pregnant woman, and passing around sanitary napkins, tampons, and contraceptive devices that may be felt are recommended. Tape recordings, braille materials, and readings by volunteers can be useful.

TEEN-AGE PREGNANCY AND THE SCHOOL

A decade and more ago teen-age pregnancies were managed in ways designed to

keep the girls involved out of school, out of sight and out of mind, and to punish them for their misbehavior in a variety of ways. The boys involved were largely ignored except when they were forced either to marry their girls or to provide money for back-alley abortions. Most such marriages ended in divorce. The babies were sometimes reared with less than adequate support from welfare sources and sometimes sold on the baby market to any couple who wished to adopt them for whatever reason, good or bad.

Pregnant girls were almost routinely kicked out of school and sometimes kicked out of their homes. Some districts provided homebound instruction, but most of the girls never returned to school and never graduated. They were thus ill prepared to support either themselves or their babies, and most of them became welfare dependents. In some cases those with affluent parents were sent out of town to bear their babies and sometimes were provided with illegal abortions of perhaps better quality than poor girls could afford. Those poor girls who were fortunate in their family relationships usually bore their babies who were then raised with the aid of adult women in the home. Others were often left to their own devices, which might include poor-quality abortions, often self-induced. Some, rich and poor, received more or less decent care in homes and hospitals for unmarried mothers. Perhaps the best of these were those provided by the Salvation Army. Birth control services, however, were rarely provided, and many once-pregnant girls found themselves pregnant again and repeating the whole miserable cycle of events.

The indefensible practices cited above and their predictable and unfortunate consequences are still with us in many localities. But much more humane and sensible practices together with supportive programs now exist in many schools and communities and are being planned and implemented in others. In the remaining sections of this chapter, national forces that have stimulated these changes and the nature of emergency

---

*Shindell, P. E.: Sex education programs and the mentally retarded, J. Sch. Health **45:**88-90, Feb. 1975.
†Cataruzolo, M. J., and Ennis, C. A.: Sex education and/or family living in the residential school for the blind, J. Sch. Health **51:**563-566, Dec. 1971.

programs and policies will be discussed.

National influences. Braen and Forbush* have reviewed national trends and developments that have influenced change in practices and programs. These include the increased numbers of teen-agers during the 1960's, which resulted in increased numbers of teenage pregnancies, and the civil rights movement and antipoverty legislation of those years. Another force was the success of pioneer programs for pregnant teen-agers. Many of these were interagency programs. Those in over 300 communities were linked together in research and information-sharing groups now called The Consortium on Early Child Bearing and Child Rearing. This group together with a membership organization, the National Alliance Concerned with School-Age Parents, now promotes the development of useful programs.

Federal and some state legislation and policy, notably California's, have also contributed to local policy and program improvement. For example, the Offices of Education and Child Development have supported local school programs of education in parenting for both boys and girls, including as one of their objectives the postponement of parenthood. Improvements in health education and in school health services and feeding programs, particularly in schools serving low-income populations, have occurred as a result of support provided through recent amendments to the Elementary and Secondary Education Act. Many of these improvements are directly related to the problem of teen-age parenthood. Recent amendments to the Social Security Act provide for broadened social services to teen-age parents, among others. Other new laws, regulations, and court decisions prohibit discrimination against teen-age parents in respect to the provision of educational and health services.

Recent court decisions, among them Stanley versus Illinois (U.S. Supreme Court, 1972), have established that unmarried

*Braen, B. S., and Forbush, J. B.: School-age parenthood: a national review, J. Sch. Health **45:** 256-262, May 1975.

fathers have the right to provide for their children and to give or withhold consent in adoption proceedings. It is significant that in the case cited the father wished to continue to provide for his children after the mother died, rather than to have them placed in foster homes without a hearing as to his fitness to care for them. Many professionals have long believed that it is not only socially desirable for unwed fathers to help in the solution of the problems they helped create, but it is also of benefit to the father's own development as a human being.

Programs and policies. The extent and nature of programs for pregnant teen-agers and policies relating to them vary widely. Some are based in schools, others in hospitals or other community agencies. Some include pregnancy prevention and abortion services; others do not. Whatever their scope and nature, it seems obvious that they should result from cooperative planning involving both potential providers and consumers of the services offered, as well as community opinion leaders, and that the services offered should be as comprehensive as possible.

A truly comprehensive program will include at least the following: (1) the services of physicians and/or nurse practitioners prepared in both obstetrics and pediatrics, educators, and psychologists and/or social workers, and (2) the active participation of agencies and schools providing laboratory, abortion, maternal and child, family planning, and welfare services. In small communities the services available will usually be more generalized.

Early detection. Early detection of pregnancy is important. One reason is that the earlier pregnancy is discovered the less risk there is of complications arising out of abortion, if this option is chosen by the girl. If the girl chooses to bear her baby, the provision of early prenatal care and education can greatly enhance her chances of bearing a healthy baby and of preventing damage to her own health. The psychological stress imposed by anxiety about whether she is or is not pregnant is lessened by early provision of a yes or no answer and by taking positive coping actions if the answer is yes.

In one large city high school, all girls are informed that pregnancy tests are available at no cost through the school nurse to any girl whose menstrual period is 2 weeks or more overdue. The tests are run in a co-operating hospital laboratory and are paid for by funds provided by the school parent-teacher organization. Other means of providing tests have been developed in other schools and communities.

Girls are unlikely to utilize a testing service unless they are assured not only by school authorities but also by other girls who have used the service that they will receive nonjudgmental and helpful counseling and services.

Counseling. The aims of counseling should include not only decision making of the sort outlined in Fig. 18-2 but also assistance in informing and establishing good relationships with parents, the boyfriend, and other individuals important in the girl's life. Another goal of pregnancy counseling is to identify and refer the girl to appropriate sources of assistance. The need for counseling is not necessarily confined to the period immediately following identification of pregnancy but is likely to span the entire time period from identification until a satisfactory postabortion or postdelivery adjustment has been achieved. Each of the possible phases of counseling described in Chapter 9 is likely to be called into play.

Girls whose pregnancy test is negative are likely to be in need of birth control counseling. Such counseling is not available in all schools, and it is probably better in any case that it be provided by an agency able to furnish the equipment or supplies appropriate to the method chosen. Good birth control counseling addresses itself to the girl's feelings about her sexual activity as well as to the selection and use of an appropriate method. Some girls are uncomfortable about the pattern of sex behavior that they find themselves drifting into and need help in resolving either their behavior or their guilt feelings about it. In many such cases

it may be helpful to include boyfriends in counseling sessions.

Those who prove to be pregnant must decide between abortion and continuing the pregnancy. This is a choice the girl must make for herself, based on her own set of ethics and values, not those of her counselor. The role of the counselor is to assist the girl in defining the likely consequences of both choices, including guilt feelings and practical difficulties that may arise. Although abortion without the consent or knowledge of the girl's parents is possible in some states and localities, they must sooner or later be informed and involved if the decision is to continue pregnancy. When and how they are to be informed is also a decision the girl must make for herself. The counselor may become directly involved in communicating with the parents at a time and in ways agreed to by the girl, and the counselor may be helpful to both the girl and her parents by keeping the attention of all of them focused on the problem and possible solutions. Youngsters in trouble are usually aware that parents are likely to have strong feelings and may dread the prospect of ventilation. They are often unaware that after an initial outburst, most parents can then become supportive and sympathetic.

A well-planned school-community program makes referral to other agencies for needed medical and social services much easier than it would otherwise be. Methods helpful in assuring successful referral were reviewed in Chapter 9.

Continued academic education. Over the past few years we have seen rapid movement away from school policies and programs that forced pregnant teen-agers to leave school. This movement is based on the recognition that all those of school age have a right to an education and that continued education is likely to reduce the risks faced by these young mothers and their babies. Those who continue in school are less likely to have repeated pregnancies. Comprehensive programs not only recognize this right but also offer a choice between continuance in the regular school academic program and enroll-ment in a special program conducted in a location apart from the regular school during pregnancy.

Regular school placement permits the girl to keep pace with her classmates and often to graduate with her classmates. She may continue to participate in most if not all extracurricular activities. A full cur-riculum is available to her. Special school plans, on the other hand, often operate on a 12-month basis, permit greater flexibility, provide easier access to counseling and health and welfare services, and may also provide a special feeding program based on the needs peculiar to pregnancy.*

Those who opt for abortion will, of course, have no need for special placement. Those who choose to continue their preg-nancies will need to choose between the options offered and may need counseling assistance to arrive at an intelligent deci-sion. Following the teen-ager's abortion or delivery, opportunity and encouragement must be provided for continued education. Those who deliver and keep their babies may require day care services for their in-fants. In-school day care services may be offered that not only meet the needs of the mother but that also provide a laboratory for education in parenting.

Education for parenthood. Although preg-nant girls have an immediate need for parenthood education, instruction of this kind opened to all may be helpful in pre-venting a wide range of health problems in the next generation. Desirably, the scope of the subject includes preconception health and family planning; prenatal, delivery, and postnatal maternal health; infant and child health; and child rearing. It should also in-clude instruction in interpersonal relation-ships, including budgeting and other mun-dane skills that may help prevent many of the conflicts related to family disruption and divorce.

*Washington, V. E.: Models of comprehensive service: special school based, J. Sch. Health **45:** 274-277, May 1975.

Medical services. Those girls who opt for abortion after counseling will need referral to an abortion service. Counselors need con-siderable information concerning available services if they are to make intelligent re-ferrals. Quality of service is of primary consideration; services provided in teaching hospitals (those either associated with medical schools or that train physicians in internships or residencies) are likely to be of the highest quality. Eligibility require-ments such as the amount charged and the humaneness with which patients are treated are other important factors. Interviews with girls who have had abortions may be helpful in judging the services available. If school policy prohibits direct abortion counseling and referral, other agencies such as Planned Parenthood may provide it.

Those who choose to continue their preg-nancy will require early and continuing prenatal care, delivery service, and post-natal care. Those who keep their babies will need routine pediatric services in all cases, and those whose babies are born with defects may need specialized habilitative services. Those whose family financial re-sources permit them to do so may obtain these needed services from private sources of their own choice. The high medical risks involved indicate that specialized obstetrical and pediatric care is desirable. For those without adequate funds, high-quality ser-vices are available through health depart-ments and clinics in many communities. Since labor may begin when the girl is in school, the hospital in which delivery is scheduled should be known to the school. It is desirable that school nurses be prepared to manage deliveries that occur in school. The training and supplies required for nor-mal delivery are minimal.

Birth control services are essential fol-lowing delivery or abortion to prevent re-peated pregnancies. It is unrealistic to expect those who have begun sexual activity to give it up just because a pregnancy has occurred. Data from existing programs indi-cate that girls who remain in school are less likely to become pregnant again than those who drop out, but school continuance does not eliminate repeat pregnancies.

Social services. If adequate counseling services are not available in school, they may be replaced or supplemented by services provided by community agencies such as a family service agency or mental health center. In addition, many girls are likely to require financial assistance of some kind for medical and hospital expenses and child support. Many girls are malnourished to the point where iron deficiency anemia and other problems are apparent, and their babies are also likely to be malnourished. Many of them are eligible for U.S. Department of Agriculture food stamps or other nutrition programs and need guidance in utilizing these sources of help. If the baby is to be offered for adoption, it is essential that the girl be guided to a legitimate social agency for this service. Physicians and attorneys who agree to arrange adoption and provide the girl with money in return must be considered to be black marketeers in babies, no matter how good their reputations are.

QUESTIONS FOR STUDY AND DISCUSSION

1. What social and individual problems related to human sexuality justify school sex education and sex-related services?
2. What are the specific implications of each of these problems for sex education and sex-related services?
3. Why is a statement of philosophy of particular importance in the development of a sex education program?
4. What specific issues should be resolved in developing a statement of philosophy? Who should be involved in developing a philosophy, and why?
5. List some of the objectives and content areas that might be included in a sex education program. What grade levels are most appropriate for each of these? Suggest a teaching strategy appropriate for each in terms of both content and the grade level selected.
6. If you were a school administrator, what qualifications would you consider most important in hiring a sex education instructor, and why? What instructions and advice would you give to a new teacher employed for sex education?
7. Why do exceptional children need sex education? How might sex education be varied to best suit the needs of the gifted, the retarded, and the blind?
8. In what ways are school policies and programs associated with teen-age pregnancy changing, and why?
9. Describe desirable school policies and programs for (a) early detection of pregnancy, (b) counseling, (c) continued academic education, (d) education for parenthood, (e) medical services, and (f) social services for pregnant teen-agers.
10. How can comprehensive services be provided in the presence of laws or school policy prohibiting the provision of one or more essential components in the schools?

REFERENCES

Burt, J. J., and Meeks, L. B.: *Education for sexuality: concepts and programs for teaching,* Philadelphia, 1975, W. B. Saunders Co.

Hanlon, J. J.: *Public health administration and practice,* ed. 6, St. Louis, 1974, The C. V. Mosby Co.

School-age parents, J. Sch. Health **45:**253-296, May 1975.

Teen-age pregnancies and the school, School Health Review **4:**3-23, May-June 1973.

Wallace, H. M., Gold, E. M., and Lis, E. F., editors: *Maternal and child health practices, problems, resources, and methods of delivery,* Springfield, Ill., 1973, Charles C Thomas, Publisher.

CHAPTER 19 ❦ Psychoactive drugs and the school

Nearly all of us use one or more psychoactive drugs. We do so to obtain mental stimulation, relaxation, heightened perception, imagery, or euphoria. The drugs we choose may be legal and socially acceptable or illegal and socially unacceptable. Their potential for producing dependence or harm to health varies with the drug, dose, and pattern and frequency of use but bears little relationship to the legality or social acceptability of the drug.

Our society has attempted to control the use and abuse of psychoactive substances largely through restrictive laws, propaganda or education that focuses on their ill effects, and treatment programs designed to cure dependence. With some exceptions, none of these approaches has been conspicuously successful. Our response to failure has been largely to try more of the same. A few innovative approaches to education and treatment, however, are at least logical, and some show evidence that they may be partially successful.

NATURE AND SCOPE OF THE PROBLEM

Survey data indicate that the psychoactive drug most commonly used in the United States is caffeine, which most of us use in the form of coffee, tea, cola drinks, and cocoa. A 1971 study indicates that over 80% of U.S. adults drink coffee, 20% drink five cups or more a day, and over half of them drink tea. Some 43% of the men and 34% of the women smoke cigarettes. Only 22% of the men and 37% of the women classified themselves as nondrinkers of alcohol, while 35% of the men and 14% of the women stated that they were heavy or very heavy alcoholic drinkers. At least some marijuana use was reported by about 15%

of those who were 12 to 17 years of age and by 20% of those aged 21 through 24. Marijuana use decreased sharply after age 25.* A more recent survey of marijuana use among students at a school of public health showed that half of them reported using marijuana up to three times a week, and 6% use it three times a week or more.†

Caffeine, alcohol, and nicotine are legally and socially accepted in the United States. All states place legal age restrictions on the sale of alcohol, which are not always strictly enforced, and some place age restrictions on the use of cigarettes, which are seldom if ever enforced. Marijuana is a socially accepted drug among youth, but legal prohibitions exist. Penalties that are out of proportion to the minimal dangers associated with its use are frequently imposed.

The study by Perry and associates revealed that psychoactive prescription drugs (sedatives, stimulants, sleeping drugs, and antidepressants) were used daily by 7% of the men and 17% of the women in their sample. The extent of the use of these and other types of drugs illegally obtained is not well documented. A study of persons who had been using heroin for only one year and who had been admitted to treatment centers in Washington, D.C. over a period of several years is instructive in terms of *relative* incidence if not absolute incidence or prevalence. This study showed incidence rates rising from a low of 0.2

---

*Perry and Cisin. Cited in Brecker, E. M., and the editors of Consumer Reports: *Licit and illicit drugs,* Mt. Vernon N.Y., 1972, Consumers Union, pp. 475-481.
†Seiden, R. M., Tomlinson, K. R., and O'Carroll, M.: Patterns of marijuana use among public health students, Am. J. Public Health **65:**613-621, June 1975.

cases per thousand in 1960 to a high of 4.2 cases in 1969, and declining to a low of 0.2 again in 1973. Rates for young persons were three- to fourfold those for the population as a whole, and those for blacks seven to nine times higher, although these groups followed the historical general trend. Noting a prior heroin use epidemic associated with the years following World War II, as well as other evidence from the literature, Greene concluded that heroin addiction follows a pattern similar to that of communicable diseases. The agent is heroin. The reservoirs of disease and victims are both humans (supplier and user, respectively). The vectors (disease carriers) are usually not pushers but well-intentioned friends of the new users.*

From a longitudinal study of drug use among a national sample of U.S. youth during and following their high school years, Johnston† concluded that nonaddictive illegal drug use is much less common than news reports would lead one to suppose. Further, drug use short of addiction has no significant effect on academic grades. Although delinquency was more common among users than nonusers, the data indicated that the delinquency preceded drug use and therefore that nonaddictive drug use did not cause the delinquency. His data did not include reports of caffeine use, but 80% of the youth used alcohol at some time during high school and a third of them used it weekly; about two thirds smoked cigarettes at some time, and one third smoked at least weekly. Marijuana was used at some time by one of five youths, and weekly by 6%. Other drugs (hallucinogens, amphetamines, barbiturates, and heroin) were each used weekly by only 1% to 2% of the sample, and at some time by 10% or less. Only 2% had ever used heroin, but 10% had tried amphetamines. Use generally increased only slightly in the post–high school years and followed the same general pattern.

It is thus clear that the favorite drugs of youth include those favored by their parents —caffeine, nicotine, and alcohol. Marijuana and hashish tend to be youth drugs, more popular in the post–high school years than in high school.

Drug dependence. The National Commission on Marihuana and Drug Abuse* has identified five different patterns of drug use:
1. Experimental drug use
2. Social or recreational drug use
3. Circumstantial-situational drug use
4. Intensified drug use
5. Compulsive drug use

Experimental use is usually motivated by curiosity, is usually shared with friends, and the risks involved are usually low. Frequency of use is low, although the amounts of drugs used may vary. Risk of dependency is low.

Social or recreational use assumes patterns, as in ritualized pot parties, for example. Such use is still voluntary; there is still no real dependence on the drug. Risks remain relatively low but vary with the drug. For example, the risk that dependence might arise out of social use is greater for heroin than for most other drugs.

Circumstantial-situational use is related to a specific task or situation. Such use is self-limited but may vary in frequency, intensity, or duration. For example, students a generation or so ago often used amphetamines only at examination time to enable them to stay awake and study. Another example is the person who always gets drunk on New Year's Eve and on certain other holidays, and only then. Users of this sort are at somewhat increased risk of becoming dependent.

Intensified use is long-term regular daily

*Greene, M. H.: An epidemiologic assessment of heroin use, Am. J. Public Health (Suppl.) **64:**1-10, Dec. 1974.
†Johnston, L. D.: Drug use during and after high school: results of a national longitudinal study, Am. J. Public Health (Suppl.) **64:**29-37, Dec. 1974.

*National Commission on Marihuana and Drug Abuse: *Drug use in America: problem in perspective,* second report, Washington, D.C., 1973, U.S. Government Printing Office, pp. 94-98.

use. It is prompted by a need to escape from pressing problems. Use of this type is exemplified by the business person who requires one or more martinis to unwind before lunch each day. These persons may succeed in maintaining their normal social and family lives and in meeting their job responsibilities, at least for a time, but they are at high risk of dependence and other problems.

Compulsive use is a pattern in which use of large doses occur at high frequency. If the drug is withheld, the individual suffers acute physical and/or mental discomfort. The user becomes preoccupied with obtaining a sufficient supply of the drug. This category includes not only skid row alcoholics and street junkies but also secret users who succeed in maintaining a front of respectability.

The Commission* postulates that drug dependence is the result of the interaction of a number of different forces. One of these is the *psychological importance* of drug use to the individual. It is not unusual, for example, for golf to become such an important activity to a person that family life is neglected. The mere fact of repetition serves to reinforce golf playing as dependent behavior. In drug use, however, continued use may be directly reinforced by the effects of the drug on the brain. If these effects are seen as desirable, psychological dependence is more likely to result from initial drug use.

A second force is the reinforcement potential provided by the *pharmacological action* of the drug itself. Drugs vary widely in pharmacological reinforcement potential, as indicated by survey data cited previously showing differences in the proportion of people who use a drug frequently and in high doses from those who use it infrequently and in relatively low doses. Thus, marijuana appears to have a rather low potential for pharmacological reinforcement, while the potentials for nicotine and heroin

are higher. Mode of administration has some effect; amphetamines (a class of stimulant drugs) are less capable of producing dependency when consumed orally than when they are injected, for example.

Pharmacological reinforcement potential is related to two contributing phenomena. One of these is the development of *tolerance* to a drug. Heroin or alcohol users, for example require more frequent and higher doses of their drugs to produce the same effects as they become more and more accustomed to their use. The other phenomenon is that of *withdrawal sickness* or symptoms. A compulsive, dependent drinker, for example, may suffer hallucinations and other distressing symptoms when his or her supply of alcohol is withheld. Fear of withdrawal sickness can be a powerful reinforcer. It is possible, in the case of some drugs, to develop *cross-tolerance* and *cross-dependence* between the drug that is used and another one quite like it in its pharmacological characteristics. This phenomenon makes it possible to use methadone to replace heroin in the treatment of heroin dependence.

Psychosocial reinforcement is also heavily involved in the development of drug dependence. Numerous studies have shown, for example, that youngsters whose parents and peers smoke cigarettes are more likely to become smokers than those who do not associate with smokers. Psychosocial reinforcement may work in the opposite direction as well. Studies have shown that drinkers who come from homes in which alcohol is only used with meals or in rather elaborate religious or family rituals, and in which drunkenness is frowned upon, are less likely to become alcohol dependent than those who come from homes in which total abstinence is practiced or alcohol is misused. Another type of psychosocial reinforcement is that provided when drug use permits a person to escape temporarily from an unpleasant marriage or from feelings of social inadequacy.

Thus, drug dependence is characterized by compulsive, continuous use of a drug in

---

*National Commission on Marihuana and Drug Abuse: *Drug use in America,* pp. 130-138.

high doses. If the drug is withdrawn, illness and discomfort occur. The drug selected is one whose pharmacological effects meet some physical or psychosocial need. A behaviorist would say that the person has become conditioned to use of the drug through repeated use and a variety of learning reinforcements.

COMMONLY USED DRUGS

Caffeine. Caffeine, as most of us know from experience, is a central nervous system stimulant. We wake up with it in the morning. It keeps students awake over their studies and term papers at night. It keeps long-distance drivers awake behind the wheels of their vehicles and typists awake behind their keyboards. No one has been able to estimate how much good work has been accomplished and how many motor vehicle accidents have been prevented with its help.

Yet caffeine has its dark side. Many individuals develop such a sufficiently high tolerance to it that they require many cups of coffee or tea each day—amounts that would lead to insomnia, heartbeat irregularities, and upset stomachs in others. Take away caffeine from a dependent person and he or she will suffer headaches, nervousness, and inability to work; thus, dependence may occur. Moreover, caffeine has been implicated as a possible cause of peptic ulcers and certainly as an aggravating agent. Heart patients must limit or eliminate caffeine if they wish to avoid irregular heart rhythm. Its lethal dose in humans has been estimated at the equivalent of 70 to 100 cups of coffee—an amount unlikely to be consumed in that form but that can be ingested in the form of caffeine tablets.

Nearly two thirds of all coffee or tea drinkers limit their consumption to three cups a day or less. The risk of ill effects is small and is no doubt outweighed by the many benefits most of us obtain from it. (What do you think would happen if a federal law were passed outlawing the sale and possession of all caffeine-containing beverages?)

Nicotine.* Nicotine is an obliging drug; it relaxes users when they wish to be relaxed and stimulates them when they wish to be stimulated. It is, in fact, a stimulant. Most users, however, use it because they have become dependent on it.

That it is extremely dependency producing has been demonstrated in a number of laboratory experiments. New smokers usually find the effects of nicotine obtained through one or two cigarettes unpleasant, but if they continue, they quickly develop tolerance to the point that they can easily consume quantities exceeding half a pack or more each day. Withdrawal is accompanied by unpleasant symptoms, among them nervousness, drowsiness, lightheadedness, headaches, fatigue, and gastrointestinal disturbances. Fewer than half of all smokers who quit with the aid of smoking clinic attendance remain abstinent for as long as 6 months, and the abstinence tapers off to less than 20% 4 years after treatment.

Most of the social concern about smoking evolves primarily from the incontrovertible body of evidence that has accumulated over the years that shows that smoking, particularly of cigarettes, is a major cause of lung cancer, heart disease, bronchitis, and emphysema and, in general, that it shortens life. Smoking mothers are more likely than others to bear low birth weight babies and to have spontaneous abortions or stillborn babies. Lung cancer is now believed to be the result primarily of the tars inhaled rather than nicotine, while nicotine has been more clearly implicated as a cause of heart disease.

Most smokers begin to smoke and develop dependency in childhood and youth. Most adult smokers are aware of and accept the adverse health effects of smoking but are unable to quit because they are dependent. We tend to reach youngsters about the effects of smoking on health, but we do not usually teach them that nicotine is high

---

*Most of the information in this section is derived from Brecker, E. M., and editors of Consumer Reports: *Licit and illicit drugs,* pp. 209-240.

in its ability to produce dependence. In fact, we lead them to believe that anyone who wants to quit can do so, and they believe it.

Alcohol. Beverage (ethyl) alcohol is a central nervous system depressant. Moderate consumption of it reduces anxiety and tension and relieves pain. It aids digestion. One of its initial effects is to relax inhibitions and thus stimulate conversation and social interaction. We do not know how many good friendships, love affairs, and marriages have been promoted and maintained by the moderate use of alcohol. Moderate use also has some adverse effects. For example, beyond one or two drinks—and this varies with individual factors and the circumstances and manner in which alcohol is consumed—reaction time and coordination are affected, and the risk of having an automobile or other type of accident increases. In addition, lowered inhibitions may result in behavior one may regret later.

Acute alcoholism (drunkenness) fosters complete, if temporary, escape from reality. Drunkenness (the legal definition of which varies somewhat from state to state) is associated with further increase in risk of accidents of all kinds, homicides, other crimes, suicides, and child abuse. Confusion and hallucinations may occur. Moods vary; some drunks are quiet, others happy or silly, and still others aggressive, argumentative, and abusive. Nausea and vomiting are frequent. Hangovers temporarily incapacitate many individuals after drunkenness.

Many of those who drink do so in moderation and in ways that demonstrate responsible behavior. Others get drunk on occasion without apparent lasting ill effects. Some heavy drinkers who are not necessarily dependent on alcohol develop rather high levels of tolerance to it. They, like chronic alcoholics, may suffer from brain and liver damage at some time in their lives. They may become less skillful and productive on their jobs, and personal interactions may suffer. Eventually, they may suffer

from withdrawal symptoms that not only include the nervousness, headache, and loss of appetite associated with hangovers, but also the frightening hallucinations and loss of motor control of delirium tremens. Another hazard is posed by the cross-tolerance and cross-dependence of alcohol and certain other drugs, notably barbiturates. Although barbiturates may be used to suppress alcohol withdrawal symptoms, when the two are taken together the effect of the two drugs is synergistic (greater than the sum of their effects taken separately). Fatalities are therefore common among those who have access to both drugs.

Chronic alcoholism involves a commitment to alcohol that supersedes that to one's family and other loved ones, career, self-respect, and dignity. The destruction of physical, mental, and social health is nearly complete. Still, significant numbers of alcoholics are able to attain and maintain a state of abstinence with the continued assistance provided in a number of treatment programs, of which Alcoholics Anonymous (AA) is perhaps the most successful. Recently, AA has begun to sponsor programs for alcoholic youths.

Marijuana. Marijuana, its derivative hashish, and other sources of cannabis are taken to reduce fatigue and depression and to produce a state of euphoria and heightened sensation by means of intoxication that is usually mild. Although less popular than alcohol among youth, and although many marijuana users also consume alcohol, others have found it to be an acceptable and intrinsically less harmful substitute for alcohol.

The effects of marijuana appear to be highly associated with the expectations of the user. Those who believe that one does not lose control with marijuana use are not likely to do so, while those who do believe thus may do so. It can cause brief loss of memory and impairment of attention; thus there is some increase in risk of accidents with use. Heavy use appears to produce some physical laziness.

The Commission on Marihuana and Drug

Abuse* states that the only apparent increase in criminality associated with its use is in the area of marijuana law violations. Its capacity to produce dependence is low. Abstinence produces little, if any, physical discomfort. It is not an aphrodisiac. There is no credible evidence at this time to support the belief that use, or at least moderate use, causes serious physiological harm. Although individuals who use any one drug tend also to use one or more others (such as caffeine and alcohol), there is no basis in fact or logic for believing that marijuana use per se leads to heroin addiction.

Heroin. Heroin is one of a number of drugs derived from opium. Opiates are used to relieve pain and to induce a state of tranquility or relaxation. It is now believed that their pain-relaxing effect is due largely to their ability to relieve worry and anxiety about the pain. The pleasure ascribed to heroin use by some addicts may be due to the feeling of warmth ("rush") felt by some users. Or, it may result from the alleviation of withdrawal sickness.

Heroin is one of the most, if not the most, dependency producing of all drugs. Casual users are believed to be few compared with the number of dependent users. Tolerance appears to develop over a brief period of time and with it a distressing withdrawal sickness. Runny nose, increased tear production, yawning and sweating, fitful sleep, dilated pupils, loss of appetite, irritability, and tremor occur. Other effects include weakness, depression, nausea, vomiting and diarrhea, alternate chills and flushing, body pains, involuntary muscle spasms, and kicking. In general, however, the direct effects of opiate dependence on physical health cannot be considered to be severe. Unlike alcohol, continued use of heroin does not appear to produce brain damage. Most dependent persons do not lead productive lives. It does appear to interfere temporarily with sexual function and to produce

menstrual irregularities. Many female users conceive and bear healthy babies. Although some defects and problems are noted, such as low birth weight, it is uncertain whether these are the direct result of heroin use or of the kind of life users lead to support their dependence. Some degree of constipation is common. Aside from severe and distressing withdrawal sickness, the major problems associated with heroin dependence are those caused by the heroin control laws and their enforcement. Dependent persons must pay a high price for their drug supply, and many of them neglect health care and nutrition and engage in stealing or prostitution to buy it. Hepatitis and other infections are common, because illegally sold supplies and the equipment used to inject the drug are often contaminated.

Many methods of controlling heroin dependence have been attempted in the past. Present legal restrictions and enforcement programs in the United States have not been proven to be more effective than was alcohol prohibition. They seem to have created more problems than they have solved, and psychotherapeutic approaches have not been significantly effective. The most effective present mode of treatment is methadone maintenance. By various standards this approach is effective in 65% to 90% of those treated. Basically, dependent persons are switched from heroin to methadone, a drug somewhat like heroin, but that permits heroin-dependent persons to function normally and usefully in society without the deleterious effects of heroin previously described. Other advantages are that methadone is taken by mouth, is effective in one-a-day doses, and does not produce increased tolerance.

APPROACHES THAT DO NOT WORK

From the foregoing discussion it is apparent that a number of school-community programs designed to prevent or control the use of psychoactive drugs or the alleviation of dependence have not been effective and that some of them have only created

---

*National Commission on Marihuana and Drug Abuse: *Drug use in America*, pp. 158-159.

graver problems. Some approaches that have not been effective are:

1. The discouragement of coffee and tea drinking by young children while permitting them to consume caffeine in the form of cocoa and cola drinks.
2. Attempts to convince young people that cigarettes are harmful while permitting or instilling the belief that tobacco is relatively nondependency producing.
3. Attempts to deal with the alcohol problem and to control marijuana and heroin use by means of prohibition. This is not to say that restrictive drug legislation has no useful role to play; 75 years ago opium could be purchased without restriction in drug or grocery stores, and that did not work either.
4. The presentation of abstinence as the only personal alternative to any kind of drug use or dependency. Many use caffeine, alcohol, and marijuana in responsible ways and are able to avoid dependency; the same cannot be said of tobacco or heroin use.

Louria* has cited other noneffective or countereffective approaches, including:

1. Crash programs designed to make instant drug experts out of public school teachers by teaching some teachers who are then expected to teach their colleagues.
2. The use of deeply personal small group discussion techniques, especially those involving marathon sensitivity sessions or techniques designed to shatter the personal defenses of participants. These may be of some value (this has not been proven) to mentally healthy participants, but they can be shattering to those with problems. Such devices should therefore *never* be used by inadequately trained leaders. Some small group techniques are useful if they do not involve deep probing.

3. "Turn in a pusher" programs and the use of student informers designed to identify drug users and sellers by organized vigilante action. These approaches are violative of individual rights, are likely to get out of hand, and create guilt feelings and other psychological problems among the vigilantes. *Individual citizens* acting as individuals are, of course, obligated to inform responsible legal authorities of violations.
4. Instilling hatred of pushers. Hate is destructive of the hater.
5. Programs designed and conducted without built-in evaluative procedures. Approaches that are intuitively attractive and even logically defensible (such as national prohibition) are often continued simply because they are appealing and logically based, even though they may be useless or worse than useless in effect.

DEVELOPMENT OF NATIONAL POLICY

Recognizing the need to reconcile the American desire for personal freedom of choice with the need for collective restraint to prevent social harm, the National Commission on Marihuana and Drug Abuse* has proposed a set of goals and premises for the development of national policy. The first of these is the recognition that drug use in itself is not an irresponsible act, as in the case of medical or bona fide religious use. Risk of harm increases with freedom of choice and also varies with the specific drug chosen. Secondly, the Commission states that "the primary goal of drug policy must be to minimize irresponsible drug-using behavior." Specifically, irresponsible behavior is defined as occurring (1) "when the manner or circumstances of use pose a threat to the safety or welfare of others," or (2) "when the pattern of use substantially impedes or risks the impairment of the indi-

*Louria, D. B.: A critique of some current approaches to the problem of drug abuse, Am. J. Public Health **65**:581-583, June 1975.

*National Commission on Marihuana and Drug Abuse: *Drug use in America,* pp. 205-225.

vidual's social and economic functions," or (3) "when the pattern of use reduces the individual's options for self-fulfillment by impairing his faculties or retarding his development." Third, the Commission states that "a secondary aim of public policy must be to discourage the use of drugs for self-defined purposes" by removing social pressures that motivate use and by encouraging choice of relatively risk-free means of self-fulfillment.

In addition, the Commission urges that institutions (such as schools) should "motivate and assist the individual to make responsible choices . . . Public policy can reduce or stop drug use by relieving some of the environmental pressures that motivate people to use them." In promoting responsible individual decision making, the Commission urges that alcohol use and other forms of self-medication with psychoactive drugs be included along with so-called street drugs by teachers and others as they assist individuals in understanding their needs and personal responsibilities. It states that credible dialogue with young people about drugs must point out the perceived advantages as well as the risks associated with drug use. The Commission also urges that policy reflect "the complexity of drug-using behavior," and states that "the major thrust of policy should be to minimize the incidence and consequences of (high risk) intensive and compulsive use."

The Commission makes a number of specific recommendations with respect to the control of alcohol, marijuana, the opiates and a number of other types of drugs. It concludes that although the social costs of long-term heavy use of alcohol are higher than those for any other problem drug, it is unrealistic to reconsider prohibition. Instead, they urge that the public be taught that alcohol is a powerful psychoactive drug and should be treated as such and that nonprohibitory means of controlling its availability be developed. Although the Commission recommends that marijuana not be made legally available at this time, it does propose that possession of small amounts for personal use be decriminalized. Because of the high dependence liability of the opiates, the Commission urges that restrictions on availability and possession be maintained and that methadone maintenance be continued with a good deal of flexibility.

Brecker* reaches a somewhat different set of conclusions with respect to marijuana and heroin, based on the demonstrated failure of highly restrictive and punitive legislative and enforcement approaches. He agrees that methadone maintenance should be continued and emphasized but that something akin to the British system be substituted for prohibition, at least temporarily and experimentally. Under this system, narcotic-dependent persons obtain maintenance supplies of their drug through legal sources, thus eliminating the opportunity for criminal black market profit. Based on a recent review of the marijuana literature,† Consumer Reports recently reiterated support of decriminalization of marijuana use.‡

The establishment of a more rational national drug policy is essential to the development of appropriate school health and health education policies and programs. Schools cannot be in the position of violating or tolerating violations of laws, but neither can school professionals maintain credibility with the young if they support irrational legislation and enforcement policies.

DRUG EDUCATION FOR PREVENTION

With respect to drug education in the schools, the Commission§ made this rather shocking recommendation: "In recognition of ignorance about the impact of drug education, the Commission recommends that policy makers should also seriously con-

---

*Brecker, E. M., and editors of Consumer Reports: *Licit and illicit drugs,* pp. 529-539.

†Brecker, E. M., and the editors of Consumer Reports: Marijuana: the health questions, Consumer Reports **40:**143-149, March 1975.

‡Marijuana: the legal question, Consumer Reports **40:**265-266, April 1975.

§National Commission on Marihuana and Drug Abuse: *Drug use in America,* pp. 346-366.

sider declaring a moratorium on all drug education programs in the schools, at least until programs already in operation have been evaluated and a coherent approach with realistic objectives has been developed. At the very least, state legislatures should repeal all statutes which now require drug education courses to be included in the public school curriculum."

This recommendation was not capriciously based. In support of it, the Commission noted that there is no clear consensus regarding what it is we are trying to prevent or how to go about it. The Commission points out that much effort has been expended on proposals to reform society and thus presumably to prevent the need for drug abuse. The proposals, however, have had little apparent effect on attempts to stop all use of illegal drugs. In addition, much school drug education ignores the perceived benefits of drug use while emphasizing deleterious effects through propaganda. The federal government and the states have provided funds for drug education to be conducted without credible evaluative procedures. A number of studies have shown that most of the educational materials in the field contain scientifically fallacious material and that most programs disregard basic communications theory. A 1972 review of drug education films, for example, concluded that only 16% of those rated were factually and conceptually acceptable.

Drug education goals. The Commission recommends that drug educators reject attempts to persuade people not to use psychoactive drugs in favor of emphasis on offering nonchemical alternatives to their use. By what means other than drug use can people attain stimulation, relaxation, heightened perception, imagery, or euphoria? How can people, especially adolescents, better cope with life's problems than through the use of drugs?

The Commission did not reject the notion that information about drugs should be provided. It states, however, that it "should be incorporated into more general programs, stressing benefits with which drug consumption is largely inconsistent."

If these two goals were to be achieved fully, there would be little or no use of psychoactive drugs, even including relatively innocuous substances such as coffee and marijuana. It seems likely that they can be achieved for many but not all persons and for many but not all psychoactive substances. We have not and are unlikely in the foreseeable future to develop a totally mentally healthy population and a totally mentally healthy social environment. While there can be essentially no responsible use of either tobacco or heroin because of their high potential for dependency production, there are and will probably continue to be responsible users of coffee, marijuana, and alcohol. For these reasons many authorities believe that a sensible and realistic drug education policy should include a third goal: the responsible use of *selected* psychoactive substances by those who choose to use them.

Approaches. Many of the approaches used in attempts to achieve the above goals have little if any apparent direct connection with the use of drugs, and some of them are taken not in the classroom but in other aspects of school life. For example, Louria* notes that the Outdoor Games Council has obtained evidence that free play experience helps children develop their value systems and improve their self-image. He also suggests that students and the administration in each school might jointly select a teacher to receive training and serve as an ombudsman whose role would be to assist students in dealing with their problems while maintaining confidentiality except in life-threatening situations.

Winn† suggests that we can help young people become better decision makers through use of value clarification strategies

*Louria, D. B.: Am. J. Public Health **65**:581-583, June 1975.
†Winn, M.: *The drug alternative,* Washington, D.C., 1974, American Alliance for Health, Physical Education, and Recreation.

and experiential learning. Some of the techniques used have been described in Chapter 7. One experiential strategy, called bragging, is designed to help students identify things about themselves about which they feel good and to learn to feel comfortable in telling these good things to others. In groups of three to five, each person is given 1 minute to tell the others good things about himself or herself (brag). The others then ask questions about what each one has bragged about. In whole group discussions, the class then discusses what society's attitudes about bragging and humbleness are, whether bragging helps one feel good about himself or herself, and whether or not telling something good that is true about oneself is really bragging.

Other approaches are more obviously directly related to drug use. One of these is a small group role-playing situation such as a party in which one participant attempts to persuade someone who is assigned the role of saying "no" to try a given drug. Through discussion following this experience, and perhaps postdiscussion repetition of it, students may arrive at a better understanding of some of the factors that are important in making choices and sticking to them. These include a well-considered rationale for one's choice of behavior, asking for some alternate form of refreshment (such as a soda) instead of the proffered drug, respecting the right of the person offering the drug to make his or her own decision, and expecting that the person offering the drug will respect another's decision not to do so.

Approaches designed to achieve the third objective, that of responsible use, are probably best focused on a given drug, such as alcohol. After discussion of reasons why some individuals drink and others do not, unbiased material might be presented concerning the risks and benefits of alcohol use and ways in which the risks may be reduced. These include:

1. Setting a personal limit, based on body weight, on the amount of alcohol to be consumed.

2. Setting a limit on speed of drinking (an hour or more per drink is the safest).
3. Selecting a relatively safe form of alcohol (the safest is a diluted, uncarbonated form such as unfortified wine).
4. Consuming food before and during drinking.
5. Avoiding the use of other drugs before, during, and for several hours after drinking.
6. Avoiding drinking at times of emotional upset.
7. Avoiding driving until the alcohol consumed has been oxidized by the body.

Finally, each student may be assigned the task of choosing and defending his or her own pattern of drinking behavior. Those who choose to abstain might develop a rationale and set of techniques for saying "no." Those who choose to drink might develop a set of drinking behavior rules for their own use that are consistent with the material presented and to which they feel certain they can adhere. Both groups may also be asked to defend their choices in terms of their life goals.

These and other approaches require evaluation, and appropriate evaluative techniques are difficult to apply in school settings. The central questions include: Do they result in improved self-esteem? Do they result in the use of nonharmful, nondrug means of coping with life problems? Do they result in less drug use and less drug dependency? Do they result in more responsible use of those substances that can be used responsibly? If so, how long do these desirable behaviors last?

Resource materials. Many accurate and useful resource materials are now available. Unfortunately, many biased and inaccurate resources are also available. Therefore, any of the materials selected for use should be evaluated by competent authority. The National Commission* has recommended that national standards for evaluating materials

---

*National Commission on Marihuana and Drug Abuse, pp. 354-355.

be developed and that some central agency such as the National Clearinghouse for Drug Abuse Information provide evaluative lists to government and private agencies.

The Commission has also recognized the importance of selecting materials in conformance with communications theory. It is important, for example, that materials relate to the views, knowledge level, and other aspects of the nature of the group to which it is addressed. In urban high schools, for example, many students already use drugs and know or think they know a great deal about them. Materials that assume a state of abstinence and naivety would clearly not be suitable for them.

By whom and how should drug education be taught? Many writers favor a program of drug education that is integrated into a number of school subjects (such as biology, social studies, health) rather than a single course labeled drug education. This view is shared by the National Commission. Like sex, it is too important, complex, and sensitive a subject to be taught by persons not specifically and intensively prepared to do so. The state and federal governments together with selected colleges and universities throughout the country are now offering formal coursework and workshops designed to prepare teachers for this responsibility.

OTHER SCHOOL ACTIVITIES

The bulk of this chapter has been devoted to the development of a foundation for preventive drug education. This section will deal briefly with the issues of detection of users, relationships with law enforcement officers, and the emergency and continuing treatment of users.

Detection. A variety of rather simple and inexpensive tests are available to detect the presence of drugs or the products of their metabolism in the bodies of users. Some people have advocated that these tests be used to detect users in school populations for law enforcement or treatment follow-up. Others have advocated, and some schools have practiced, searches of students' lockers and persons for drugs, drug-use parapher-

nalia, or for such physical evidence of drug use as needle marks or pupil dilation.

We disagree vigorously with such practices on several grounds. First, they are abhorrent to democratic principles and violate the Constitutional right of privacy. Second, they are bound to create student distrust of the school professionals involved and to close student communication with them. Third, many students use one or another drug experimentally at some time or other, and such experimentation should in no way be taken to mean that a student has a drug problem. Fourth, as we have pointed out, the narcotics laws are not based on rational thinking. In addition, too many law enforcement agents deal with youthful offenders in inappropriate and abusive ways, especially if the youth happens to be poor or black. Finally, most schoolage users who are in fact having problems reveal those problems in other ways. In some instances they may confide in a trusted adult; in others those with problems will manifest them in the form of truancy, lower academic performance, delinquency, obvious emotional disturbance, and the like.

Relationship with police. In any school, instances will arise where police intervention is necessary and desirable whether or not school officials actively seek to find such circumstances. In many cases they will come to attention through effective police work. In other cases they may be brought to attention by means of student or parent complaints or by observation of illegal behavior by school staff members. Each school jurisdiction must develop cooperatively with the police both a policy for handling such situations and a good working relationship with police officials.

Most such instances are not of the kind that require active physical police intervention. Most arise from suspected legal violations that police officers must pursue by questioning students. The generally recommended policy guideline is that no student should be subjected to police interrogation on school premises except in the presence of his or her parents. Such a policy is protective of the right of students and parents and of the relationship of the school with students and parents also.

A new breed of police is emerging in many localities. These professionals view crime prevention through close and trusting relationships with those they serve as their primary objective. In some cities, such policemen cover large high schools in which they are known as officers to the students, with whom they take the time to mingle and converse. They attempt to abort problems before they arise and to avoid booking any youngster if at all possible.

Emergency treatment. Students occasionally appear at school in a condition they themselves would describe as stoned. Most of them are aware of the cause of their intoxication and are likely to indicate what it is if an open and trusting relationship has been developed and if confidentiality is ensured.

First aid for both alcohol and marijuana intoxication is quite simple: time, rest, and reassurance. There is always the possibility, however, that these drugs may have been contaminated or used in combination with others, knowingly or unknowingly, and victims should therefore be carefully observed for coma or signs of shock.

Acute narcotic (heroin) intoxication results in lethargy that may be close to stupor. Hospitalization may be required if signs of shock or respiratory tract distress are apparent. Unfortunately, few community emergency systems are well equipped to deal with acute drug emergencies,* but most hospital emergency wards should have present opiate antagonists and should be equipped to handle emergencies that may result from overdoses of narcotics or other drugs.

Victims of LSD highs are best "talked down" by a knowledgeable friend. They need careful and close supervision because of the possibility that they may injure themselves in the course of a bad trip. In some extreme cases, counteracting drugs may be helpful.

Continuing treatment. There are many modalities of continuing treatment of alcohol and opiate dependence, of which two, methadone maintenance of heroin dependent persons and Alcoholics Anonymous, have been mentioned. Other methods include prolonged hospitalization, ambulatory treatment of persons rendered drug free by some means, therapeutic communities of various kinds, and multimode programs. Since the multimodality programs offer a variety of approaches and are thus able to move patients from one mode to another (such as detoxification, methadone maintenance, therapeutic community, in- or outpatient treatment), these have apparently been more successful than the other approaches.*

The relative effectiveness of these and other approaches is under continuing investigation. Probation-parole programs for selected criminal offenders appear to be very much worthwhile if high-quality supervision is provided. Behavioral therapy appears to hold some promise, particularly in the treatment of nicotine dependence. Crisis centers (crash pads, rap centers, hot lines, and storefront clinics) appear to be primarily useful in helping socially alienated young people, many of whom are not necessarily drug dependent but who are struggling with drug-related problems.†

Relatively few school-age youngsters are drug dependent, but many are in the experimental or social-recreational drug use stages, and many of these have related social-emotional problems for which they need help of a kind that may be provided by generalized community mental health resources rather than those specializing in drug use therapy.

Thus, school health professionals should become well acquainted with the full range

*National Commission on Marihuana and Drug Abuse, pp. 342-346.

*National Commission on Marihuana and Drug Abuse, pp. 314-325.
†Phillipson, R.: Drug abuse treatment, J. Sch. Health **42:**625-628, Dec. 1972.

of continuing treatment services available in their specific communities and should attempt to refer any youngster to the service that seems best equipped to meet his or her specific needs.

QUESTIONS FOR STUDY AND DISCUSSION

1. Which are the four psychoactive drugs most commonly used by adults and young persons in the U.S.? Which of these is the single most commonly used drug?
2. Attempt to rank order these four drugs in terms of (a) legality and (b) social acceptability.
3. Name and describe each of the five patterns of drug use identified by the National Commission on Marihuana and Drug Abuse. Which patterns are associated with high risk of dependency and which with relatively low risk?
4. What forces tend to reinforce drug use, and how?
5. What is the meaning of the concept drug dependence?
6. What benefits and risks are associated with use of caffeine, cigarette smoking, alcohol, marijuana, or heroin?
7. What are some common myths about each of these drugs?
8. Attempt to rank order these drugs in terms of risk of (a) dependency and (b) other health hazards. How does this ranking compare with your ranking for legal and social acceptability?
9. What ineffective or counterproductive approaches to the control of drugs have been attempted? Why have these approaches not worked?
10. What are the characteristics of a sensible national drug policy as recommended by the National Commission on Marihuana and Drug Abuse? With which of these do you agree and disagree, and why?
11. What recommendation with respect to drug education was made by the National Commission, and why?
12. What goals for drug education are recommended by the Commission? What additional goal is recommended by the authors? With which of these goals do you agree and disagree, and why?
13. Come to class prepared to lead a small group through one of the drug education strategies proposed either in this text or some other source. (The instructor may divide the class into small groups for rotating conduct of the strategies.)
14. What cautions are offered relative to the selection of teaching strategies and resource materials?
15. By whom and by what pattern of organization should drug education be taught?
16. By what means can school professionals detect drug users? Which of these means should and should not be used?
17. What policy is recommended for the guidance of schools relative to police interrogations of students? Do you agree or disagree with this policy, and why?
18. What school first-aid measures are appropriate for students suffering from alcohol or marijuana intoxication, for heroin emergencies, and for LSD trips?
19. How can schools best help students in need of continuing treatment of drug-related problems?

REFERENCES

American Association for Health, Physical Education and Recreation: *What education can do about cigarette smoking,* Washington, D.C., 1971, The Association.

Brecker, E. M., and editors of Consumer Reports: *Licit and illicit drugs,* Mt. Vernon, N.Y., 1972, Consumers Union.

Cornacchia, H. J., Bentel, D. A., and Smith, D. E.: *Drugs in the classroom: a conceptual model for school programs,* St. Louis, 1973, The C. V. Mosby Co.

Edwards, G.: *Reaching out: the prevention of drug abuse through increased human interaction,* Garden City, N.Y., 1972, Innovative Designs for Educational Action, Inc.

Henderson, J.: *Emergency medical guide,* ed. 3, New York, 1973, McGraw-Hill, Inc.

Miles, S. A., editor: *Learning about alcohol: a resource book for teachers,* Washington, D.C., 1974, American Alliance for Health, Physical Education, and Recreation.

National Commission on Marihuana and Drug Abuse: *Drug use in America: problem in perspective,* second report, Washington, D.C., 1973, U.S. Government Printing Office.

Winn, M.: *The drug alternative,* Washington, D.C., 1974, American Alliance for Health, Physical Education, and Recreation.

PART SEVEN

Appraising school health and health education

CHAPTER 20 ❦ Evaluation

To evaluate school health and health education programs or activities is to appraise them against a set of goals or standards that have been adopted or established for the purpose. Measurement is not evaluation, but it is an essential part of the process. Once the school health and health education programs are measured, we must then ask whether we have satisfactorily achieved or made progress toward the goal, standard, or value we set in the first place. If the answer is yes, we may then try to determine whether we can do as well in the future by expending less in the way of time, effort, and money. If the answer is no, we must then ask how the program or activity can best be changed so that goals or standards will be achieved in the future. It is this process of asking questions, trying to answer them on a more or less objective basis, and drawing implications for the future that is properly called evaluation.

Evaluation is not only essential to planning for the future but may have a number of beneficial side effects as well. It can be educational for those involved. For example, teachers may find that a film they thought would stimulate student interest actually turns them off the subject. Teachers may then develop better criteria for selecting films in the future. Evaluation results may be useful in convincing the board of health or school board that the immunization program is worthwhile and that support for it should be continued or expanded. Discovery that the sanitation program has achieved the goal of no foodborne disease outbreaks in the schools during the year may serve to cement or improve relationships between the sanitarian and food service staff members. Finally, an effective and systematic program of evaluation provides the answer, "we have one," to those citizens and groups who clamor for an accountability system.

Evaluation and accountability are threatening words to many school professionals. If evaluation is viewed and used by administrators as a means of improving professional competence rather than of eliminating supposedly incompetent individuals, then much of the threat will be removed. If all involved recognize the variety and complexity of the many factors in addition to professional competence that influence goal achievement, then professional performance becomes only one of a number of factors subject to evaluation. Finally, it must also be recognized that the long-term goals of school health and health education are largely intangible and difficult if not impossible to measure.

SYSTEMS ANALYSIS: A MODEL FOR EVALUATION

The complexities cited in the preceding paragraph may be summarized and most easily dealt with by use of a model based on systems theory (Fig. 20-1). Elements peculiar to the school health and health education system under study are built into the flow chart or presented in a separate, written description. The resulting diagram or description then becomes an analogous model of the real-life situation *if* the diagram or description is true to life.

The *system aims* description includes statements (elements) that describe the general purpose of school health and health education in a given district or school. It need not be highly detailed; it should emerge as a series of statements consistent with the philosophy of the school system, but it need not explain how the aims are to be achieved or how they are to be evaluated. The importance of the description of system aims is that all the other parts of

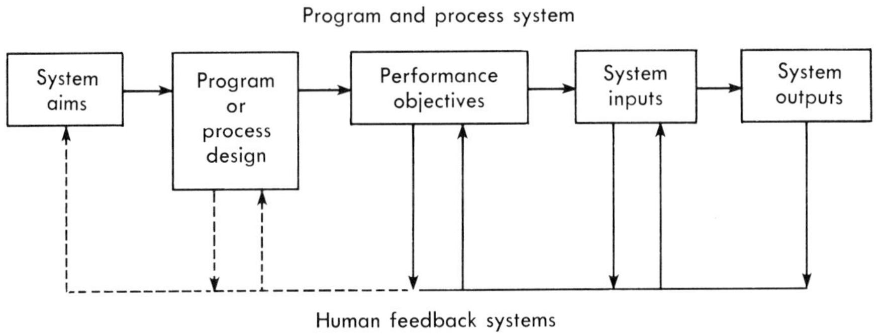

Program and process system

Human feedback systems

Fig. 20-1. Analog model of systems analysis for school health and health education. (Adapted from Hill, J. E.: *How school can apply systems analysis,* Bloomington, Ind., 1972, Phi Delta Kappa Educational Foundation, p. 15.)

the system must logically contribute to them. Such statements as the following might be included:

1. Health problems of children should be identified.
2. School-community programs should be provided to deal with these problems.

Note in Fig. 20-1 that the human feedback system is connected with both the system aims and program or process design description by means of dotted lines to indicate that professionals and others do not easily affect these two sets of elements. If change is necessary and does occur in either of these two sets, then all other parts of the system may require change.

The *program and process design* statements also need not be highly specific but should indicate the general nature and intent of those aspects of program and process that have been created specifically to contribute to the achievement of system aims. For example, the following kinds of statements might be included:

1. The health education program formulates, coordinates, and evaluates, with input from the school health council, a K-12 curriculum designed to prevent health problems and to assist students in identifying and dealing with health problems.
2. The school health services program assesses the health status of individual students and works cooperatively with others in the school, home, and community to prevent, correct, or alleviate any health problems discovered. It formulates, coordinates, and evaluates school-community programs designed to meet these ends with the advice of the school health council.
3. The school environmental health program, with the advice of the school health council, formulates environmental standards designed to protect and promote the health and safety of all school members, conducts periodic inspections, and reports to administrative authorities situations where specific standards have not been achieved.

Note that these statements, unlike the aim statements that can be evaluated only in terms of their logical consistency with other parts of the model, are capable of limited evaluation. We can ask and answer such questions as:

1. Is there a K-12 health curriculum?
2. Was the school health council consulted in its design?
3. Is there a health appraisal program?
4. Is there a set of environmental health and safety standards? Are periodic environmental inspections conducted?

There are no guidelines stated for directly evaluating the effectiveness of any of the program or process design elements, but we can tell whether the elements are or are not in place.

The statements of *performance objectives,* however, are much more specific than the preceding statements and lend themselves to direct evaluation. Each of these objectives should be written so that it succinctly and accurately describes:

1. The task to be accomplished.
2. The conditions under which the task is to be accomplished.
3. The minimum criteria for the successful completion of the task.

This is the standard definition of a behavioral objective. In addition, each performance objective stated must be logically consistent with both the program and process design and system aims statements.

The difficulties with such statements are that they tend to become so numerous that it is next to impossible to state and measure all of those we have in mind, that some important objectives do not lend themselves to objective measurement, and that the criteria for successful completion may be set at a level that is unrealistically high or low. The first difficulty may be overcome by writing a rather complete set of objectives and then discarding those that group judgment deems to be either of relatively low importance or essentially duplicated by others. If an objective can be measured only subjectively and is of high importance, it should be retained, but less confidence can be placed in its evaluation than with those that are objectively measurable. If criteria prove to be too high or too low in practice, they may be readjusted.

Examples of possible performance objective statements are:

1. At the close of the school year, 95% of the health education classes will achieve mean scores exceeding class pretest means by at least one-half standard deviation, as measured by the standard tests developed for each grade level by the faculty.
2. By the end of February, 90% of all students will be currently immunized against diphtheria, polio, rubella, and rubeola.
3. All substandard cafeteria and kitchen equipment will be repaired or replaced in all schools by Labor Day.

System inputs are designed to make pos-

sible the achievement of all performance objectives. Inputs include staff personnel, materials, supplies, and physical facilities. If systems analysis is utilized in performance budgeting, then the amounts or costs of inputs need to be closely estimated. In any event, the personnel involved are usually the most costly and essential input. Innovative persons can often discover ways of achieving goals when other inputs are inadequate, but no amount of extra supplies can make up for inadequacies in the staff time required to achieve a performance objective. Input statements may include target dates for the completion of certain tasks in recognition of the importance of time budgeting.

Input descriptions may thus assume a variety of forms; for example:

1. Each nurse serves a student population ranging in size from 900 to 1,200, with lesser numbers assigned to those serving schools in low socioeconomic areas and to those serving several small schools.
2. Approximately 90% of the health education teachers meet state certification standards, and the others are all enrolled in course work required for certification.
3. Portable equipment and required supplies for prophylaxis and topical fluoride applications are provided to each dental hygienist.
4. Laboratory service is provided at no charge by the health department to the nurses for pregnancy testing and to the sanitarian for analysis of specimens obtained in the course of sanitation inspections.
5. Completion date for staff tuberculin tests to be administered and read is November 1.

Statements should be sufficiently clear and detailed to be useful in the identification of input deficiencies by reference to authoritative standards and in the event that outputs fall below the standards set by the performance objectives.

System outputs, of course, cannot be

stated until evaluative data have been collected, processed, and interpreted. Properly written performance objectives specify the kinds of data to be collected, and they may even specify the data collection instrument to be used. For example, one of the performance objectives cited above specifies that a staff-developed knowledge test be used to measure student achievement in health education classes.

Once evaluative data have been collected and analyzed by the persons (usually professional staff) included in the *human feedback system,* actions may be taken by them or recommended to the administration for modifying system inputs, performance objectives, or, more rarely, program design or system aims in ways that are likely to facilitate improved outputs in future years.

Some simpler forms of evaluation. Not all schools have available the staff time and energy required to construct a model for systems analysis and follow through with an elaborate evaluation enterprise. Simpler, less time-consuming, and useful evaluations can still be conducted.

Health knowledge, attitude, and behavior gains that occur coincidentally with health instruction can be determined by pre- and posttesting students either with carefully constructed and tested teacher-made instruments or by use of commercially available tests. A questionnaire may be constructed and administered anonymously to students to ascertain how they feel about the present health curriculum and to obtain their recommendations for change. Books, films, and other resource materials can be reviewed by a panel of experts for factual and conceptual accuracy. Descriptive reports of unusual health education projects can be compiled.

Health service professionals can use data from their work records to compute immunization levels. They can also use work record data to determine the percentages of student referrals from the various health appraisal programs and the percentage of those referred for whom evidence of follow-up completion has been obtained. These percentages can be compared from year to year; hopefully, progress will be shown. Simple numbers of services performed are often impressive to administrators and school board members. These might include the number of students counseled with respect to obesity, drug use, suspected pregnancy, and the like, as well as the number to whom emergency care of injuries or illness was provided.

In the environmental area, school accident rates may be computed and compared from year to year. The results of health and safety inspections can be reported in the form of problems identified and the percentages of these corrected. If attention has been directed toward improvement of the school's social and emotional climate, attendance or truancy records can be compared before and after improvement occurred.

Thus, evaluation need not be elaborate to be useful. However, use of a systems analysis model is likely to result in more thorough, logical, and credible evaluations.

SOME GUIDING PRINCIPLES

It is neither essential nor desirable that output data related to every performance objective be collected every year. To do so would consume much staff time and thus detract from the ability of professionals to perform direct services. Instead, a different set of performance objectives can be selected for evaluation each year.

Nor should evaluation be limited to outputs specified by the performance objectives. New knowledge and technologies are constantly being developed that carry with them implications for change in system inputs, in program and process design, and in performance objectives. Thus, the elements in the model itself require continuing reevaluation and revision.

If data are to be used to assess progress over time toward objectives, then it is not sufficient to collect them only at the end of the year. Base line, or starting point, data are required for comparison with end-of-the-year output data. Base line data need not be collected at the start of every year.

Once collected, they will serve the purpose for as long as performance objectives, system inputs, and the nature of the student population remain constant. New base line data are required when any one of these variables changes.

A further caution is also in order. Neither improvement nor retrogression from base line to later output data *proves* that a program of school health and health education deserves credit or blame, as the case may be. This caution is especially relevant when dealing with pupil health status indicators. Pupil health status is powerfully affected by forces and circumstances beyond the influence of the school. For example, improvement in the economy can be expected to result in increase in the number of health defects corrected regardless of anything the school health program does or does not do.

If it is deemed necessary to prove the effectiveness of the program or any portion of it, a controlled experiment is required. Individual schools are assigned to control and experimental groups, either randomly or by matching them on the basis of a number of relevant characteristics such as pupil-socioeconomic status and school size. The health and other relevant programs in each pair of matched schools must be as similar as possible, except that the portion of the program under study is present in the experimental group and is replaced by an irrelevant innovative activity in the control group. The effectiveness of the experimental program in achieving its objectives can then be assessed. But such experiments, while relevant to program and process design, are not required for ongoing evaluation.

Another principle is that ultimate objectives should be stated and used in evaluation where possible; but if this is not possible, then intervening objectives as close as possible to the ultimate goal should be stated and used. For example, the ultimate goal of rubella (3-day measles) immunization is not to prevent the infection in children but to prevent birth defects by preventing it in pregnant women and girls. Measurement of the extent to which this goal is achieved is difficult if not impossible for school health professionals. They would have to collect data from hospital case records to do so. Since rubella is a mild disease, its actual occurrence is often unreported and may be unnoticed. Since rubella immunization has been experimentally shown to be highly effective, we settle for the percent of children immunized against rubella as our measure.

One of the ultimate goals of the hearing conservation program is to improve auditory acuity in those persons where improvement is possible and to preserve present levels in persons where improvement is not possible. We refer children for treatment on the basis of pure tone audiometric tests, and it is possible to retest them periodically following referral and treatment. We usually do not separate them into groups labeled "treatable" and "untreatable," but we can determine the percent of those referred and treated whose acuity improved, remained stable, or deteriorated, and even compare these percentages with those among children who were referred but not treated.

DATA COLLECTION TECHNIQUES

Data for evaluation are collected from existing records or by use of a wide variety of survey instruments. Instruments used include objective tests, inspection forms or check lists, questionnaires, and attitude and behavior survey forms. Both records and instruments may produce data that are reliable and valid or unreliable and invalid. In addition, those who collect data may deliberately distort it to make themselves and their pet programs look good, they may report it honestly and correctly, or they may make honest clerical errors. Obviously, bad data serve to invalidate the whole evaluation process.

It is possible to check the validity and reliability of record data in several ways. For example, if reporters make monthly reports, then totals from these should equal the final report totals. In addition, while one cannot expect rates and percentages from all schools to be precisely equal, rates and percentages for similar schools with similar populations and programs should fall within the same general range. Such checks may be conducted of randomly selected reports; checks of all reports are likely to be too time-consuming. If suspicious reports are received, an administrator may audit the original records from which they were compiled. Since this involves contact with the reporter, the stated assumption should be that either the report in question is in fact correct or that an honest clerical error has been made. No prior assumption of dishonesty is tenable.

Bad instruments or good ones that have been incorrectly administered also produce bad data. All instruments used should be pretested for validity and reliability, and standard instructions for their administration should be provided to users. A simple way of checking instrument quality involves two steps. First, a panel of professionals is provided with copies of the instrument together with a list of the objectives the achievement of which is expected to be measured by the instrument. The panel is asked to determine whether the instrument can logically be expected to produce data consistent with the objectives and, if not, to suggest ways in which the instrument can be improved. Second, the expert-approved instrument is submitted to pretest. For a questionnaire or test, pretesting may involve two separate administrations to the same small group of respondents, perhaps a week apart, to determine whether the two sets of responses or test scores are reasonably consistent. An environmental checklist might be pretested by having several different, equally qualified observers use it to assess a given environment. Again, the judgments thus attained should be reasonably consistent.

These procedures are costly in terms of time and effort but less costly than the collection and use of vast amounts of bad data. If instruments are available either commercially or through such agencies as state education or health departments, the validity and reliability of which have already been established, it is necessary only to determine

if they are consistent with local objectives. However, old instruments may be rather quickly outdated and should also be checked for currency. For example, until recently the correct response to a test item concerning desirable oral hygiene practices would have been "brush after every meal or snack." It is now "brush and floss at least once a day."

Since different data collection techniques lend themselves more appropriately to one or another phase of the school health program, procedures useful in the evaluation of health education, services, and environmental health will be discussed briefly below.

Health education. The expected outcomes of health education are improvements in health knowledge, attitudes, and behavior. A rather commonly held and now questioned assumption in the field has been that knowledge and attitudes are predictive of behavior, but behavior is apparently the result of more complex interactions of forces. Nevertheless, it is of value to pursue attempts to evaluate the traditional outcomes. Increase in knowledge can be considered valuable not only for its own sake but also in the interest of producing a citizenry capable of making informed decisions as parents and voters, if not always with respect to their own health. For example, health-educated citizens may be more likely than others to vote in favor of water fluoridation and to have their own children immunized against diseases. An enlightened attitude toward acne may lead future adults to be more sympathetic in their relationships with adolescents.

Health knowledge. Of knowledge, attitudes, and behavior, knowledge is the most commonly and easily evaluated. One reason for the common use of knowledge tests is the expectation that teachers will assign grades to students that hopefully represent gains in knowledge. Unfortunately, despite this, knowledge evaluation is not always well done.

One common flaw is the use of test items that are not based on clearly stated objectives. This difficulty may be overcome by preparing a complete set of behavioral objectives for each course and by including only test items that are clearly based on the stated objectives. Another criticism is that items included in a test may call for information that is irrelevant to the needs and interests of the students. This is unlikely to be a valid criticism if objectives are based on careful assessment of student needs and interests.

Many teacher-made tests are unreliable; they fail to distinguish successful learners from poor ones. Items within an objective test can be rather easily checked for reliability in schools where facilities are available for machine scoring and computer analysis of item responses. In other schools, teachers can make a simple hand analysis. The corrected answer sheets of those in the upper and lower quartiles are separated. Correct responses for each item are counted for each of the two quartiles. Those items that elicited more correct responses from those in the upper quartile than from those in the lower are most likely to be reliable.

Unreliable items may be so because they are invalid. As we indicated previously, health information is subject to fairly rapid change. Teachers need to assure themselves that the response they have chosen as correct is, in fact, correct. They can do this either by consulting a knowledgeable person, such as the nurse, or by referring to recent reference material from sources other than the text.

Multiple choice tests have qualities that cause them to be generally preferred over other types of tests. For example, they are objectively scored and provide higher opportunity for student error than do true-false tests. Although student reading ability is required, writing ability is not, as it is for essay tests. Nevertheless, other types of tests have their place. Essay tests, for example, may reveal that a student is able to regurgitate bits of factual information but has no conception of the implications of the facts for behavior in a given situation.

Attitudes. Attitudes have been variously

defined by different writers. One common definition is that an attitude is a predisposition to behave in some specified way. Another holds that it is how one feels about a specified object, such as spinach, the President of the United States, or premarital intercourse. However they are defined, they are usually measured by asking respondents their opinion about something.

When Thomas E. Dewey (who wore a mustache) ran for the Presidency against Harry S. Truman, Jimmy the Greek recalls that he hired some interviewers to ask women their opinions of men who wear mustaches. The responses indicated that very few women would trust a man with a mustache. Jimmy bet accordingly and won. The story suggests that it is indeed worthwhile to find out what opinions or attitudes prevail and that the best way to find out is to ask people.

The difficulty with this approach in schoolwork is that students learn early that it is wise to tell teachers what they wish to hear. This inhibition may be partially overcome by use of anonymous questionnaires, with the added assurance that the opinions expressed will in no way influence grades.

One common way of constructing an attitude item is to present a statement (attitude object) and to ask the respondent to check the response provided that most closely approximates his or her belief. For example:

If someone offers a person a cigarette, that person should be polite and smoke it even though he/she does not want it.

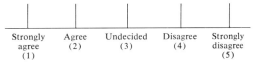

| Strongly agree (1) | Agree (2) | Undecided (3) | Disagree (4) | Strongly disagree (5) |

The same item in somewhat different form may be presented a second time later on in the questionnaire as a means of checking its reliability.

If course objectives specify certain attitudes to be developed as desirable or undesirable, it is possible to score attitude instruments. For example, the most desirable attitude might be 5 for the above statement, with 4 the next most desirable, and so on. Response 5 might thus be awarded five points, and 4 given four points. By pretesting, posttesting, and scoring, one can determine whether or not the class average has moved in the desired direction during the course. But to incorporate these scores into the course grade without letting the students know in advance that this is to be done constitutes unethical teacher behavior. To let them know would spoil the game; most intelligent students would give the "right" answers, whether they believed them or not. For this reason, attitude measurements are best reserved for evaluation of course effectiveness and to determine attitudes held by students when they enter the course. They should not be used for grading student achievement.

Practices. Although improved health practices may legitimately be considered to be the primary goal of health education, they, like attitudes, should be used as an indicator of course effectiveness rather than student achievement. The reasoning is much the same. Self-reports or even parent reports of student behavior are likely to be what the teacher wishes to hear. In addition, much behavior is determined by environmental influences. Students eat what food is available in the house, for example. Also, collecting reports of highly personal behavior, such as whether or not boys wear condoms when they have intercourse, could rightly be considered an invasion of privacy.

The point is illustrated by the response one man gave to a sociologist's question concerning a childhood experience that upset him. He said, "The teacher asked us what we had for breakfast, and I told true. Black-eyed peas and cornbread. And I was ashamed, and I cried." He did not know, and apparently never learned, that this was a far better breakfast than those eaten by many children from affluent families.

There are two basic methods of assessing behavior. One is by self-report as in the example cited above. The other is by direct observation. It is perhaps possible to secure honest self- or parent reports of behavior if these are obtained by means of anonymous questionnaires accompanied by assurance that the information will not be used for grading purposes.

Our ability to secure information about health practices is essentially limited to what can be seen in and around school. This can be informative, however. One may observe street-crossing behavior before and after safety instructions. This writer once observed and recorded what students ordered for lunch at a restaurant across the street from a high school; every one of them ordered french fries and a cola only.

Health services. Much of what can be said with respect to health services program evaluation has already been stated or implied. Simple summaries of the kinds and numbers of services provided to students may measure many of the outputs called for by performance objectives. Percentages of students referred for diagnosis and indicated care of health defects can be used to assess the effectiveness of referral procedures. Comparisons of such percentages from year to year will hopefully indicate progress as well as achievement of objectives. Most of the evaluations of health service effectiveness will be based on service statistics of one sort or another.

One of the goals of school health services must be to achieve any standards mandated by state laws or regulations. Some of these are accountable by use of service statistics. Others, however, may require that certain educational standards be met by school nurses and dental hygienists. The best evidence that these requirements have been or are being met is obtained by requiring staff members to have college or university transcripts sent to the district office.

Another objective may be of an affective nature: that students and parents who have contact with the health services will state that the experience proved helpful to them and that they were treated courteously by staff members. The information required to evaluate achievement of objectives of this kind may best be obtained by anonymous questionnaires completed by parents and students. Anonymity is important because those who have criticisms may fear retaliation if they voice them. If a questionnaire is used, items may be added that give respondents an opportunity to suggest additions to service offerings or other improvements.

Environmental services. Much of the evaluative data required for environmental services will be derived from inspection checklists and records of environmental health and safety hazard corrections. Additional valuable data may be derived from accident reports. As in the case of health services, many performance objectives may be mandated by the state, and relevant inspection or other data collection instruments may be provided by state offices.

Locally determined objectives, including standards for acceptable performance, must be developed with special situations in mind. For example, schools in localities that are noisy or subject to heavy air pollution will require plant modifications not needed by those in more favorable environments. Small schools will require less elaborate facilities than large ones.

As we previously stated, one measure of a good school social and emotional climate is improved attendance records by both students and staff. In addition, climate improvement should also be accompanied by less vandalism and instances of delinquent behavior. Administrative records data can be used to document improvement in this area.

QUESTIONS FOR STUDY AND DISCUSSION

1. What is meant by evaluation?
2. What are the benefits of evaluation?
3. Why is evaluation viewed by some professionals as a personal threat? How can the threat be alleviated?
4. What are the components of the systems analysis analog proposed in the text?
5. What is the nature and purpose of the descriptive statements used to specify system aims, program or process design, performance objectives, system inputs, and system outputs?
6. What is the human feedback system? Who is involved in it? Upon which of the system components does human feedback have the most and least corrective influence, and why?
7. What are some ways of evaluating school health and health education that are simpler than systems analysis?
8. If simple methods are available, why use systems analysis?
9. What guiding principles for evaluation are proposed in the text? What other principles can you cite from experience or what you have learned in other courses?
10. What are some of the techniques that may be used to collect evaluative data?
11. How can the validity and reliability of the data collected be improved?
12. How can data to evaluate the achievement of health education objectives best be obtained? What cautions should be observed in collecting such data?
13. In your opinion should student grades reflect attitudes and/or behavior as well as knowledge achievement? Support and defend your answer.
14. What kinds of data collection techniques are more useful in evaluating health service objectives? Environmental service objectives?
15. In what way can you use data from one aspect of the school health program to assess achievement in another aspect (health education and health services, for example)?

REFERENCES

Anderson, C. L.: *School health practice,* ed. 5, St. Louis, 1972, The C. V. Mosby Co.

Bryan, D. S.: *School nursing in transition,* St. Louis, 1973, The C. V. Mosby Co.

Eisner, V., and Callan, L. B.: *Dimensions of school health,* Springfield, Ill., 1974, Charles C Thomas, Publisher.

Hill, J. E.: *How schools can apply systems analysis,* Bloomington, Ill., 1972, Phi Delta Kappa Educational Foundation.

Kaplan, L., and Stoughton, R. W.: *Pupil personnel services guidance for introducing and developing a program of accountability,* Princeton, N.J., 1974, National Association of Pupil Personnel Administrators.

Nemir, A., and Schaller, W. E.: *The school health program,* ed. 4, Philadelphia, 1975, W. B. Saunders Co.

APPENDIX A ❧ Instructions for the control of the more common communicable diseases in the school

DEFINITION OF TERMS

Carrier. A person who harbors a specific infectious agent in the absence of discernible clinical disease and serves as a potential source or reservoir of infection for man.

Cleansing. The removal by scrubbing and washing, as with hot water, soap, detergent or washing soda, of organic matter on which and in which bacteria may find favorable conditions for prolonging life and virulence; also the removal by the same means of bacteria adherent to surfaces.

Teach all students the necessity of:

1. Keeping the body clean by sufficiently frequent soap and water baths.
2. Washing hands in soap and water after emptying bowel or bladder and always before eating.
3. Keeping hands and unclean articles, or articles that have been used by others, away from mouth, nose, eyes, and ears.
4. Avoiding the use of common or unclean eating, drinking, or toilet articles of any kind, such as towels, handkerchiefs, hair brushes, and drinking cups.
5. Avoiding close exposure of persons to spray from the nose and mouth, as in coughing, sneezing, laughing, or talking.

Communicable. Capable of being transmitted from one person or animal to another.

Contact. Any person or animal known to have been in such association with an infected person or animal as to have been presumably exposed to transfer of infectious material directly or by articles freshly soiled with such material.

Disinfection. The killing of pathogenic microorganisms by chemical or physical means.

When "concurrent" is used as qualifying disinfection, it indicates the application of disinfectant immediately after the discharge of infectious material from the body of an infected person or after soiling of articles with such infectious discharges, all personal contacts with such discharges or articles being prevented prior to their disinfection.

When the word "terminal" is used as qualifying disinfection, it indicates the process of rendering the personal clothing and immediate physical environment of the patient free from the possibility of conveying the infection to others at the time when the patient is no longer a source of infection.

Endemic. Occurring more or less constantly in a given locality.

Epidemic. Occurring in unusually large numbers in a given locality.

Immune. Protection from a communicable disease by natural or acquired means.

Incubation period. The time between the implanting of the infecting organism and the development of symptoms.

Infection. State of being infected; the state produced by pathogenic microorganisms upon their entrance into and multiplication within the body; communication of a disease from one organism to another.

Infectious. Capable of being transmitted by infection with or without actual contact; producing an infection.

Isolation. Separation of infected persons from other persons for the period of communicability in such places and under such conditions as will prevent the transmission of the infectious agent. Isolation is applied in accordance with state and local policy, which may vary from the recommendations below.

IMMUNIZATION

Importance of immunization. In the control and prevention of communicable disease immunizations should be stressed by teachers as well as by health branch personnel whenever opportunity for this type of education presents itself. Immunizations against diphtheria, pertussis (whooping cough), tetanus, and poliomyelitis are recommended for all children (with few medical exceptions) within the first year of life and against rubeola, rubella, and mumps after age 12 months. Initial immunizations must be followed by boosters at the appropriate ages in order to maintain immunity for diphtheria; pertussis, tetanus, and for poliomyelitis when killed (Salk) vaccine is used. Under certain conditions immunizations against influenza, infectious hepatitis, or typhoid are indicated.

THE COMMUNICABLE DISEASES
Chickenpox (varicella)
Nonreportable disease

Description of the disease. An acute disease, with a slight fever, mild constitutional symptoms, and an eruption that is maculopapular for a few hours and vesicular for 3 or 4 days and that leaves a granular scab.

Infectious agent. The virus of chickenpox.

Source of infection. Secretions of the respiratory tract of infected persons; lesions of the skin are of little consequence, and scabs of themselves are not infective.

Mode of transmission. Directly from person to person; indirectly through articles freshly soiled by discharges from the skin and mucous membranes of infected persons.

Incubation period. Two to 3 weeks; commonly 13 to 17 days.

Period of communicability. Probably not more than 1 day prior to and not more than 6 days after the appearance of the first crop of vesicles. Especially communicable in the early stages of the eruption. One of the most readily communicable diseases.

Susceptibility and resistance. Susceptibility is apparently universal. An attack confers permanent immunity, with possibly rare exceptions.

Prevalence. Universal. Probably 70% of persons have had the disease by the time they are 15 years of age.

METHODS OF CONTROL

Prevention. No preventive measures.

Exclusion. For a minimum of 7 days after appearance of first crop of vesicles and until all crusts are dry.

Isolation. Isolate patient. Bed rest advised.

Contacts. When the case is properly isolated, there need be no restrictions of contacts.

Readmission. Readmit the pupil providing it has been at least 7 days since appearance of first crop of vesicles and all the crusts are dry.

Note: Unusually severe cases, or cases occurring in persons over 15 years of age or at any age during a smallpox epidemic should be carefully investigated to rule out smallpox.

Common cold
Nonreportable disease

Description of the disease. A highly infectious acute catarrhal infection of the upper respiratory tract, rarely accompanied by a slight rise in temperature on the first day, chilly sensations with nasal discharge (coryza) and general indisposition or lassitude lasting 2 to 7 days. The nasal discharge may become mucopurulent due to secondary bacterial invasion, and it is not uncommon for it to spread to the lower respiratory tract and to the middle ear.

Infectious agent. Many separate viruses have been identified.

Source of infection. Discharges from nose and mouth of infected persons and possibly by the intestinal route in some cases.

Mode of transmission. Usually directly by coughing and sneezing, with droplets passing in the air from the infected person to susceptible persons, especially those within short range; indirectly by handkerchiefs, eating utensils, or other articles freshly soiled by discharges of the infected person.

Incubation period. Probably between 12 and 72 hours, usually 24 hours.

Period of communicability. Nasal washings taken 24 hours before onset and for 5 days after onset produce symptoms experimentally in man.

Susceptibility and resistance. Susceptibility is universal. A short period of increased resistance to the specific virus may follow an attack.

Prevalence. Most persons, except those living in small isolated communities, have one or more colds each year. The incidence is higher in children and becomes less with age.

Methods of control

Prevention. Preventive measures through education. All persons should be instructed in the niceties of personal hygiene, as in covering the mouth when coughing or sneezing and in disposal of nose and mouth secretions. It is advisable to have patient use disposable tissues that can be burned or put in the toilet.

On recognition of the premonitory or early stage of a common cold, the infected persons should be urged to avoid direct and indirect exposure of others.

Isolation. Such modified isolation as can be accomplished in the school until the illness is differentiated from the prodrome of another disease is to be advised.

Readmission. By school principal.

Conjunctivitis (infectious)
Nonreportable disease

Infectious conjunctivitis, "pink-eye"

Description of the disease. A very contagious eye infection characterized by a marked inflammation and redness of the conjunctivas with a mucopurulent or purulent discharge. There may also be itching and smarting of the eyes, some swelling of these tissues, and abnormal sensitivity to light.

Infectious agent. Various bacteria and some viruses.

Source of infection. Direct contact with infected persons, and indirectly by contact with articles freshly soiled with the infectious discharge of such persons. Articles used for eye makeup and passed from person to person may carry the infection.

Incubation period. Usually 24 to 72 hours.

Prevalence. Seen frequently in both elementary and secondary schools.

Methods of control

Prevention. Strict personal hygiene, careful handwashing, separate towels, and prompt treatment of infected eyes.

Exclusion. Until recovery. Immediate medical care advised.

Readmission. May be readmitted providing patient has no symptoms.

Allergic conjunctivitis

Description of the disease. Sudden onset of redness of the conjunctiva (particularly in the spring or early summer) accompanied by itching, watery discharge, and redness or inflammation (excoriation) of the cheek in chronic cases. Usually a history of multiple allergies. Noninfectious. Allergy to eye makeup is a frequent factor here.

Exclusion. None.

Diphtheria
Quarantinable disease (Report immediately by telephone)

Description of the disease. An acute infectious disease of the tonsils, pharynx, larynx, or nose, occasionally of other mucous membranes or skin. Lesions are marked by a patch of grayish membrane with surrounding dull, red, inflammatory zone.

Case fatality rate is from 5% to 10%.

Infectious agent. Klebs-Löffler bacillus *(Corynebacterium diphtheriae)*

Mode of transmission. The bacillus is transmitted by contact with patient or healthy carrier or with articles soiled by the discharges from nose, throat, and lesions. Milk can serve as a vehicle.

Incubation period. From 2 to 7 days.

Prevalence. Diphtheria is endemic and epidemic, a disease of autumn and the winter months. In communities where active immunization has been neglected, approximately one fourth of the cases and one half of the deaths occur in children under 5 years of age. In communities where childhood immunization has been adequate but reinforcing of toxoid was not continued, age distribution tends toward older persons.

Complications. Myocarditis, neuritis, bronchopneumonia, rarely nephritis.

Methods of control

Prevention. Adequate immunization. Early diagnosis and isolation of cases.

Exclusion. Immediate. Call local public health office before child is moved.

Isolation. Strict isolation of patient.

Readmission to school. For both patient and contacts, only by written permission of the county health officer.

Dysentery, amebic
Reportable disease

Description of disease. Sudden onset of mild to moderate diarrhea which lasts about 1 week. May recur if not treated. Fever not significant.

Infectious agent. *Entamoeba histolytica.*

Method of transmission. It is transmitted in cyst form through fecal contamination of food or water.

Methods of control

Prevention. Cleanliness and hygiene. Proper controls of food and water supplies.

Exclusion. Until clinical recovery; except for food handlers and contacts who are food handlers, who must be released by the county health officer.

Readmission. By a school physician or nurse, the county health department, or other licensed physician.

Dysentery, bacillary (shigellosis)
Reportable disease (Report by telephone)

Description of disease. Symptoms vary greatly in intensity. Fever, vomiting, diarrhea.

Infectious agent. *Shigella* bacilli (several groups).

Source of infection. Feces from infected person.

Mode of transmission. By eating contaminated foods or by drinking contaminated water or milk, and by hand-to-mouth transfer of contaminated material; by flies, by objects soiled with feces of a patient or carrier.

Incubation period. From 1 to 7 days.

Methods of control

Prevention. Cleanliness and hygiene. Proper supervision of food and water supplies. Fly control.

Exclusion. Each case should be considered individually. In general, exclusion continues until asymptomatic.

Readmission. By the school physician or nurse, the county health department, or other licensed physician.

Food poisoning
Reportable diseases (Report by telephone)

Description of diseases. Food poisoning is characterized by illness of sudden onset acquired through food, with a characteristic grouping of cases. It occurs either from poisoning or from infection.

A. Staphylococcus intoxication. A poisoning of abrupt and sometimes violent onset with severe nausea, cramps, vomiting, prostration, and at times severe diarrhea.

Incubation period. Interval between taking food and onset is ½ to 6 hours, usually 2 to 4.

Source of infection. The ingestion of food that has become contaminated. Organism grows when foods such as chopped or sliced meats, custard, cream fillings, salads, and salad dressing sandwiches are poorly refrigerated. People handling foods should be free of pyogenic skin infections, especially of the hands. Food handlers should pay strict attention to sanitation and cleanliness of kitchens, refrigeration, and handwashing.

B. Botulinus intoxication. A highly fatal, afebrile poisoning, characterized by headache, weakness, constipation, paralysis, and the absence of diarrhea. Initial symptoms often include visual disturbances and hoarseness.

Incubation period. Symptoms usually appear within 12 to 36 hours, possibly longer, after food containing toxin is eaten—the interval being determined by the amount of contaminated food taken and the content of botulin toxin.

Source of infection. Food, most often home-canned vegetables (including olives and peppers), meat, or fish, inadequately processed with resultant toxic formation, and often without subsequent adequate cooking.

Report suspected cases immediately by telephone to the local health officer.

C. Salmonella infection. Most commonly characterized by acute gastroenteritis with diarrhea and abdominal cramps. Fever, nausea, and vomiting are frequently present.

Infectious agent. Salmonellas of the group pathogenic for both animals and man, excluding the salmonellas of typhoid and paratyphoid that are primary human pathogens.

Mode of transmission. Epidemics are usually traced to foods such as meat, pies, poultry or poultry products, raw sausages, lightly cooked foods containing egg or egg products, unpasteur-ized milk or dairy products, food contaminated with rodent feces or by an infected food handler, or to utensils, working surfaces, or tables pre-viously used for contaminated foods such as egg products. Sporadic cases often originate through direct contact with an infected person or animal.

Incubation period. 6 to 48 hours, usually about 12 hours.

Methods of control

Prevention. Thorough cooking of all foodstuffs derived from animal sources, with particular at-tention to preparation of fowls, egg products, and meat dishes; protection of food against rodent or insect contamination; refrigeration of prepared foods.

Exclusion. Each case should be considered in-dividually. In general, exclude until asymptomatic.

Readmission (for all types of food poisoning). By school physician or nurse, health department, or other licensed physician.

German measles (rubella)
Nonreportable disease

Description of the disease. A mild febrile in-fectious disease characterized by a rash, rarely preceded by other mild nonspecific symptoms, although the rash appears the first day as discrete, fine, pink-red macules on the face; it rapidly spreads over the trunk and the extremities.

Infectious agent. The virus of rubella.

Source of infection. Secretions of the mouth, nose, and intestinal tract of an infected person.

Mode of transmission. Airborne or by direct contact with the patient, or by indirect contact with articles freshly soiled with the discharge from the nose and throat (and possibly the intestinal tract) of the patient.

Incubation period. From 14 to 21 days, usually 18 days.

Period of communicability. About 1 week before and at least 4 days after the onset of the rash. Highly communicable.

Prevalence. Worldwide. No attempt should be made to protect female children in good health from exposure to this disease (see Complications).

Complications. None usually to the school-aged child.

German measles during the first 4 months of pregnancy may result in infants with a high per-centage (25%) of congenital defects.

Methods of control

Prevention. Immunization is the only effective method.

Exclusion. The patient, only for at least 5 days from onset of rash and until clinically recovered.

Isolation. None, except to prevent contact with any woman in early pregnancy. If pregnant woman is a contact, she should see attending physician.

Readmission. When patient is clinically well.

Hepatitis, infectious and serum
Reportable diseases

Description of the disease. The two known forms of hepatitis, infectious hepatitis (IH) and

serum hepatitis (SH), produce a systemic viral in-fection in man that involves the liver and is commonly associated with jaundice and impaired liver function (see facing page).

Impetigo
Nonreportable disease

Description of the disease. Impetigo is a disease of the skin characterized by the presence of super-ficial pustules and crusts, usually on the exposed portions of the body (commonly face, ears, and around nares).

Infectious agent. Staphylococci or streptococci.

Source of infection. Skin lesions of an infected person; infected discharges from the nose and throat or ear.

Mode of transmission. Direct contact or indirect through articles recently contaminated by in-fected discharges. The infection may be readily inoculated from place to place on the patient's body by scratching. Airborne transmission may be important.

Incubation period. Usually 2 to 5 days (may be up to 14 days).

Period of communicability. Until lesions have healed, usually 1 to 2 weeks.

Asymptomatic carriers may spread the disease.

Prevalence. Very common.

Exclusions. Until healed or lesions treated and properly covered.

Readmission. When clinically well.

Influenza
Nonreportable disease

Description of the disease. An acute, highly communicable viral disease primarily affecting the respiratory tract, characterized by sudden onset of fever, chills or chilliness, headaches, sore throat, cough, prostration, and generalized muscle aches.

Infectious agent. Four types and many strains of influenza virus.

Source of infection. Discharges from the nose and throat of infected persons.

Mode of transmission. By direct contact, through droplet infection, or by articles freshly soiled by discharges of the nose and throat; pos-sibly airborne.

Incubation period. Usually from 24 to 72 hours.

Period of communicability. Probably limited to 3 days from clinical onset.

Susceptibility and resistance. Susceptibility is general. Older children and young adults are more susceptible than infants and older persons. Ac-quired immunity resulting from an attack and recovery from the disease may be of short dura-tion or may persist several years; it is effective only against specific strains of the virus. Specific resistance may be increased by vaccination with influenza virus vaccines.

Prevalence. The disease may be pandemic, epi-demic, or sporadic. Epidemics usually occur in late winter or early spring.

Methods of control

Prevention. Active immunization of persons suffering from chronic debilitating diseases or in-

	Infectious hepatitis (IH) (Catarrhal jaundice; epidemic jaundice)	**Serum hepatitis (SH)** (Transfusion jaundice, homologous serum jaundice)
Age group	Usually occurs in children and young adults.	Usually occurs in older persons.
Description	An acute infectious disease with fever, anorexia, nausea, malaise, and abdominal discomfort, followed by jaundice. Infection without jaundice is common in childhood.	Clinically indistinguishable from IH.
Infectious agent	Type A virus.	Type B virus.
Incubation period	From 2 to 6 weeks, commonly 25 days.	1½ to 6 months, usually 12 to 14 weeks.
Period of communicability	Unknown. Clinical experience suggests greater communicability is from several days before to not more than 7 days after the onset of manifest disease.	
Mode of transmission	Person to person direct fecal contamination, respiratory tract spread possible; because of close personal contact, family rates are high. Through contaminated food and water.	By direct inoculation: Transfusion of blood, serum, or plasma from infected persons, or use of contaminated needles or syringes.
Incidence	Usually epidemic.	Sporadic.
Immunity	To IH only.	To SH only.
Exclusion	Until recovery, at least 7 days from onset. No exclusion of contacts.	Until recovery.
Immunization	Gamma globulin promptly after contacts (family members only). This passive immunity lasts from 6 to 8 weeks.	
Readmission	By the school physician or nurse, the health department, or other licensed physician.	By the school physician or nurse, the health department, or other licensed physician.

dividuals in essential community service should be accomplished well before expected epidemic occurrence.

Proper disposal of articles soiled by discharges of the nose and throat of the infected individual.

Avoidance of crowds during epidemic periods.

Exclusion. Patient only until recovery.

Isolation. As directed by the attending physician. To minimize severity and to protect the patient from secondary infections, patients should go to bed at the beginning of an attack and not return to work until recovered.

Readmission. When well.

Measles (rubeola)
Reportable disease

Description of the disease. An acute, highly contagious viral disease, characterized by a prodromal stage of 3 to 5 days, during which are noted fever (101° to 104° F); coryza (watery discharge of eyes and nose); bronchitis (dry, "barking" cough), and Koplik's spots (fine white spots on the buccal mucosa that appear toward the end of the prodromal period). A dusky-red blotchy rash appears on the third to fifth day, first on the face, and then spreading to the chest, abdomen, and extremities. It usually lasts 4 to 7 days and may be followed by a branny peeling during convalescence.

Infectious agent. The virus of measles.

Source of infection. Secretions from the nose and throat of infected individuals.

Mode of transmission. By droplet spread or direct contact with an infected person; indirectly through articles freshly soiled with secretions of nose and throat; in some instances probably airborne. One of the most readily transmitted of communicable diseases.

Incubation period. Usually 10 days from exposure to onset of fever; 13 to 15 days until appearance of rash. When passive immunization is attempted but is too late to prevent infection, the incubation period may be as long as 21 days.

Period of communicability. During catarrhal symptoms; usually about 9 days, from 4 days before the appearance of the rash to 5 days after its appearance.

Susceptibility and resistance. Practically all persons are susceptible. Permanent acquired immunity is usual after having the disease. Babies born of mothers who have had the disease are ordinarily immune for the first 4 to 6 months of life.

Prevalence. Endemic in urban areas and epidemic at about 2- to 4-year intervals probably due to accumulation of large new groups of susceptible children.

Methods of control

Prevention. Immunization is the only effective method. All children who have not had the disease should be immunized starting at 12 months of age.

A protective dose of measles immune globulin should be administered to susceptible infants and children under 3 years of age in families and in institutions where measles occur.

Exclusion. During catarrhal symptoms and 7 days after appearance of rash. If exposed, nonimmune children can be inspected daily by the school nurse and they may remain in school. Immune children may remain in school.

Isolation. Patient should be isolated during period of communicability to protect him against additional infection as well as to prevent measles infection of other persons in the household, particularly of susceptible contacts of early ages.

Contacts. During an epidemic there should be daily inspection of exposed, nonimmune children and adult personnel. Schools should not be closed or classes discontinued.

Readmission. By a school physician or nurse, the health department, or other licensed physician.

Policy concerning children who have received measles vaccine. Although they may have a rash, these children may remain in school, providing they have:

1. A written statement from their licensed physician that they are not contagious and
2. Have no significant temperature.

Mononucleosis, infectious
Nonreportable disease (except in epidemic form)

Description of the disease. Infectious mononucleosis is a self-limited disease thought to be of infectious origin. It occurs in localized epidemics or sporadically, usually in children and young adults. It is characterized by a triad of symptoms: intermittent fever, sore throat, and enlarged tender cervical nodes. In more than a third of the cases, the pharynx is coated by a grayish exudate. Headache and enlargement of the spleen or liver may also be present.

Infectious agent. Unknown. Presumed to be a virus or viruses.

Source of infection. Apparently limited to man; likely source of infection, the discharge of the respiratory tract of an infected person.

Mode of transmission. Unknown; probably spread person to person by an oral-pharyngeal route that in the young adult commonly involves direct contact.

Incubation period. Seemingly varies from 4 to 42 days.

Period of communicability. Unknown, but presumably from time before symptoms appear to end of fever and clearing of the oral-pharyngeal lesions.

Susceptibility and resistance. It occurs most often in older children and young adults, although no age group is immune.

Prevalence. *Worldwide.* In U.S. most common from October through May.

Methods of control. None have been demonstrated to be effective.

Mumps (infectious parotitis)
Reportable disease

Description of the disease. An acute viral disease of sudden onset characterized by fever and by swelling and tenderness of one or more salivary glands, usually the parotid, sometimes the sublingual or submaxillary glands. Other organs may be involved (see Complications).

Infectious agent. The virus of mumps.

Source of infection. Saliva of infected persons. Sometimes the infection is inapparent in the source individual.

Mode of transmission. By droplet spread, by direct contact with an infected person, or indirectly through articles freshly soiled with saliva of such persons.

Incubation period. From 12 to 26 days, commonly 18 days.

Period of communicability. From 7 days before the appearance of symptoms and as long as 9 days thereafter, until all swelling of the salivary glands has disappeared. Principal period of communicability is, however, about the time the swelling commences.

Susceptibility and resistance. Susceptibility is general. It is seen most commonly after 3 years of age and before 40 years. An attack generally confers lifelong immunity.

Prevalence. Has its peak incidence in winter and spring, especially in school populations.

Complications. The central nervous system (meningoencephalitis) may be involved, and if past puberty, also the ovaries and testicles.

Methods of control

Prevention. Vaccination.

Exclusion. Patient only, until all swelling of glands has subsided (usually 10 days).

Isolation. Patient only, during infectious period.

Contacts. No exclusion or isolation of contacts.

Readmission. By the school physician or nurse, the health department, or other licensed physician.

Pediculosis (lice)
Nonreportable disease

Description of disease. Pediculosis is the presence of the adult louse, larva, or egg sacs (called nits) on the scalp, on hairy parts of the body, or on the clothing (especially along the seams of the inner surface). The chief symptom is itching. Lesions due to scratching often develop, with resultant purulent infections. Both lice and nits are easily seen with the naked eye.

Infesting agents. Head or body louse—*Pediculus humanus.* Crab louse—*Phthirus pubis.*

Source of infestation. Infested persons and their personal belongings, particularly clothing or bedding.

Mode of transmission. By direct contact with an infested person or indirectly by contact with infested clothing, headgear, or bedding.

Incubation period. Strictly speaking there is none, since the first adult louse to reach a new host may cause symptoms immediately. Under optimum conditions the eggs hatch in a week, and sexual maturity is reached in approximately 2 weeks.

Susceptibility. Any person may become infested if exposed.

Prevention. Direct inspection of heads of school children, especially in areas where pediculosis is prevalent.

Education in the values of using hot water and soap in the maintenance of personal cleanliness as well as cleanliness of cloths, bedding, and other possessions. Pediculosis is rare when proper cleanliness is maintained.

Treatment. The scalp and hair should be treated with one of the commercial medications (available from a druggist) that destroys both lice and nits. This should be followed by shampoo and careful removal of *all* nits from the hair with a fine-toothed steel comb.

Readmission to school. When free of infestations (lice or nits).

Pinworms (enterobiasis, oxyuriasis)
Nonreportable disease

Description of the disease. Infestation of the human intestinal tract by the pinworm usually is asymptomatic but occasionally causes a mild disease with indefinite symptoms.

Infesting agent. *Enterobius vermicularis,* an intestinal roundworm ⅛ inch to ½ inch long.

Source of infestation. Infested individuals, particularly children, and their excrements. Clothing, bedding, food, and other articles may be contaminated with eggs of the parasite.

Mode of transmission. Direct transfer of eggs by hand (especially under the fingernails) and from anal area to the mouth of the same host, or indirectly to the same host or new hosts through contaminated food and objects. Dust-borne infestation by inhalation is possible in heavily contaminated households.

Incubation period. The life cycle requires 3 to 6 weeks.

Period of communicability. Persists while worms and ova are alive. In the absence of treatment, 2 to 8 weeks unless reinfested.

Susceptibility and resistance. Pinworms are human parasites favoring the younger age group, especially school-aged children. Susceptibility is universal. No apparent resistance to repeated infestations.

Prevalence. Worldwide and exceedingly common. Crowding is an important factor.

Methods of control

Prevention. Immediate treatment of known carriers. Observance of strictest rules of hygiene. Thorough cleansing of hands and fingernails, especially after toileting and before eating.

Exclusion. None. Children who exhibit unusual scratching in the rectal area should be referred for private care or examined in school in the presence of their parents, and if evidence indicates the probability of pinworms, should be referred for further examination and treatment.

Ringworm (epidermophytosis)
Nonreportable diseases

Discription of the disease. Ringworm is a general term applied to fungus disease of the hair, skin, and nails. These fungi are known collectively as dermatophytes. For convenience, ringworm is subdivided according to sites of infection as follows: tinea capitis (ringworm of the scalp); tinea corporis (ringworm of the body); tinea pedis (athlete's foot), and tinea unguium (ringworm of the nails). The most serious school health problem is ringworm of the feet.

Ringworm of the feet (athlete's foot, tinea pedis)

Description of the disease. A scaling or cracking of the skin between the toes, and blisters containing a thin, watery fluid form can be seen. The areas between the toes are a favorable place in which the fungi may live and grow.

Infectious agents. *Epidermophyton* and various species of *Trichophyton.*

Source of infection. Skin lesions of infected persons or contaminated floors, shower stalls, towels, or other articles used by infected persons.

Methods of control

Prevention. Strict personal hygiene with careful drying of the areas between the toes after bathing.

Strict attention to the proper cleanliness and care of such areas as gymnasiums and swimming pools.

Exclusion. None. The severely infected person should not be allowed to use locker rooms, showers, or swimming pools as a protection against secondary bacterial infection.

Scabies
Nonreportable disease

Description of the disease. An infectious disease of the skin due to the itch mite, which burrows beneath the skin, forming grayish white lines housing the mite and eggs. Papules and vesicles may form; also pustules due to secondary infection caused by scratching. The webs of fingers and toes and the flexors surfaces of joints are the most common sites, although any part of the body surface may be affected. Itching is intense, especially at night and when warm.

Infectious agent. *Sarcoptes scabiei,* a mite that is rarely visible with the naked eye.

Method of infection. Transfer of parasites by direct contact with infested persons and indirectly from underclothing, gloves, or bedding of such persons.

Incubation period. Several hours are required for the itch mite to dig and burrow and become implanted in the skin. Several days or even weeks may pass before itching is noted.

Methods of control

Prevention. Public health education on the need for cleanliness of person, garments, and bedclothes.

Exclusion. Of the patient until under adequate treatment.

Contacts. Household contacts and companions should be examined.

Readmission. Upon recovery.

Smallpox (variola)

Quarantinable disease (Report immediately by telephone)

Description of the disease. A highly communicable disease characterized by sudden onset of fever, malaise, headache, backache, abdominal pain, and prostration continuing for 3 to 4 days. In children there may also be vomiting and convulsions. The temperature then falls and a rash appears that passes through successive stages of macules, papules, vesicles, pustules, and finally scabs that fall off at about the end of the third week.

Infectious agent. The virus of smallpox, variola.

Source of infection. Lesions of skin and mucous membranes and respiratory tract discharges of patients or materials contaminated therewith. Separated scabs can remain infectious for several years.

Mode of transmission. By contact with persons who have had the disease. This contact may be direct, airborne, or indirect through contaminated articles.

Incubation period. From 7 to 16 days; commonly 9 to 12 days to onset of illness and 3 to 4 more to onset of rash.

Period of communicability. From first symptoms to disappearance of all scabs and crusts, about 2 to 3 weeks. Most communicable in the early stages, shortly before and during the appearance of rash.

Susceptibility and resistance. Susceptibility is universal. Permanent immunity usually follows recovery; second attacks are rare.

Prevalence. Now rare throughout the world, but may be introduced to smallpox-free countries by international travelers.

Methods of control

Prevention. Vaccination. Smallpox is entirely preventable through proper vaccination, but routine vaccination of school children and personnel is no longer practiced in the United States.

Exclusion. Until recovery. All scabs must have disappeared and the scars must be completely healed.

Isolation. Strict isolation of patient under quarantine.

Contacts. Management is a state and local health department responsibility.

Readmission. By the health officer only.

Streptococcal infections (scarlet fever, streptococcal sore throat, and others)

Reportable disease (Report by telephone)

Description of the disease. A group of acute infectious diseases caused by Group A hemolytic streptococci, varying clinically according to the tissues affected and the presence or absence of a scarlatinal rash. Scarlet fever is streptococcal sore throat with a rash.

Distinguishing characteristics common to both of these diseases are fever, sore throat, exudative tonsilitis or pharyngitis, tender cervical lymph nodes, and strawberry tongue. The rash of scarlet fever is the result of a toxin produced by certain types of streptococci.

Other diseases produced by streptococcal infection are erysipelas, puerperal fever, cellulitis, lymphadenitis, mastoiditis, otitis media, osteomyelitis, peritonitis, septicemia, impetigo contagiosa, and other skin and wound infections.

Infectious agent. Streptococci of more than 40 distinct types.

Source of infection. Discharges from nose, throat, purulent lesions, or objects contaminated with such discharges. Nasal carriers are particularly liable to contaminate their environment. Reservoir is man: acutely ill or convalescent patients, or carriers.

Mode of transmission. By direct contact with patient or carrier, by indirect contact through objects handled, or by droplet spread. Outbreaks may occur due to contaminated milk and food.

Incubation period. Usually 1 to 3 days, rarely longer.

Period of communicability. In uncomplicated cases, during incubation and clinical illness, approximately 10 days. However, a carrier state may persist for months. Adequate treatment with antibiotic will eliminate probability of transmission from patients or carriers within 24 hours.

Susceptibility and resistance. Susceptibility is general, although many persons develop either antitoxin or type-specific antibacterial immunity, or both, through inapparent infection.

Immunity to the toxin, and hence to rash, develops within a week of the onset of scarlet fever and is usually permanent. Second attacks of scarlet fever are rare but may occur because of the two immunologic forms of toxin. Severity of the disease has been decreasing in the United States for many years.

Methods of control

Prevention. General measures include laboratory service for isolation of hemolytic streptococci and identification of serologic group and type; pasteurization of milk; and exclusion of infected persons as food or milk handlers.

Exclusion. Uncomplicated cases until clinical recovery, not less than 7 days from onset. If treated with an antibiotic, may be released on clinical recovery, provided therapy is continued for 7 to 10 days after instituting same.

Readmission. In accordance with local policy.

Tetanus
Reportable disease

Description of the disease. An acute disease induced by toxin of the tetanus bacillus growing without oxygen at site of an injury; characterized by painful muscular contractions.

Occurrence. Worldwide and at all ages.

Infectious agent. *Clostridium tetani,* tetanus bacillus.

Source of infection. Reservoir is intestinal canal of animals, especially horses, also man. The immediate source of infection is soil, street dust, or animal and human feces.

Mode of transmission. Tetanus spores enter the body through injury, usually a puncture wound, but also burns and trivial or unnoticed wounds.

Incubation period. Commonly 4 days to 3 weeks, dependent on character, extent, and location of wound.

Period of communicability. Not directly transmitted from man to man.

Susceptibility and resistance. Susceptibility is general. Active immunity is induced by tetanus toxoid, passive immunity by tetanus antitoxin.

Methods of control

Prevention. Health education.

Active immunization with tetanus toxoid starting in infancy and continuing at periodic intervals through life.

Passive immunization with tetanus antitoxin after injury, if not already immunized.

Tuberculosis
Reportable disease

Description of the diseases. Among the most common communicable diseases of man and of great importance throughout the world:

Primary tuberculosis infection (childhood-type tuberculosis). Initial pulmonary and hilar gland infection, usually with few or no symptoms, and generally healing by calcification. The tuberculin skin sensitivity test is positive and x-ray film may show typical lymph node calcification. In the early stages it may be infectious.

Pulmonary tuberculosis (adult or reinfection-type tuberculosis). May occur by reinfection from a new exposure or by direct extension of a primary-type tuberculosis. In minimal cases there may be few or no symptoms, but far advanced cases are characterized by cough, sputum, weight loss, fever, sweating, and sometimes spitting of blood. (X-ray changes commonly occur in advance of clinical manifestations.)

Infectious agent. The tubercle bacillus, *Mycobacterium tuberculosis.*

Source of infection. Respiratory secretions from open (bacillary-positive) pulmonary tuberculosis, and occasionally milk from tuberculous cattle. The reservoir is primarily man; also diseased cattle in some areas.

Mode of transmission. Direct contact with patients with open lesions; airborne; indirect through contaminated articles is less important.

Ingestion of unpasteurized milk of tuberculous cows.

Incubation period. From infection to demonstrable primary lesion, about 4 to 6 weeks; to progressive pulmonary or extrapulmonary tuberculosis may be years; the first 6 to 12 months after infection is the most hazardous period.

Period of communicability. As long as tubercle bacilli are discharged.

Susceptibility and resistance. Susceptibility is general; highest in children under 3 years, lowest 3 to 12 years. Resistance conferred by healed primary infection is limited.

Methods of control

Prevention. Public health education and control. X-ray and tuberculin-survey programs.

Isolation. Hospital treatment highly desirable. Chemotherapy commonly produces sputum conversion within 6 months.

Contacts. X-ray examination, or tuberculin testing with x-ray examination of reactors.

Readmission. In accordance with state and local policy.

Typhoid fever (Salmonella typhosa)
Reportable disease (Report by telephone)

Description of the disease. A systemic infectious disease characterized by continued fever, malaise, anorexia, slow pulse, involvement of lymphoid tissues, especially ulceration of Peyer's patches, enlargement of the spleen, rose spots on the trunk, and constipation more commonly than diarrhea. There are many mild and atypical infections.

Infectious agent. *Salmonella typhi,* the typhoid bacillus. About 50 types have been distinguished.

Source of infection. Feces and urine of patients and carriers; man is the reservoir.

Mode of transmission. Direct or indirect contact with patient or carrier. Water, milk, shellfish, raw fruit and vegetables may be contaminated directly by active cases or carriers or indirectly by flies.

Incubation period. From 7 to 21 days, average 14.

Period of communicability. As long as patients or carriers harbor organisms.

Susceptibility and resistance. Susceptibility is general although many adults acquire immunity through unrecognized infections; rates of attack decline with age after second or third decades. A high degree of resistance usually follows recovery.

Prevalence. Throughout the world; a common disease in Asia, Africa, Eastern Europe, Central and South America. In the U.S. there are about 600 to 700 cases annually, mainly in rural areas.

Methods of control

Prevention. Modern sanitation has played a major role in preventing typhoid fever, with protection and purification of food and water supplies, supervision of food handlers, and discovery and supervision of typhoid carriers. Active immunization with typhoid vaccine is valuable in areas where typhoid fever is prevalent or in the presence of an epidemic.

Exclusion. Until clinical recovery and fulfillment of the county health department regulations.

Isolation. Modified isolation of the patient is required.

Contacts. Restricted at the discretion of the health officer. Special regulations govern carriers.

Readmission to school. By the health officer only.

Venereal diseases (syphilis, gonorrhea)
Reportable diseases

Description of the diseases. Communicable diseases spread from person to person by intimate contact. VD usually refers to syphilis and gonorrhea. The germs causing syphilis and gonorrhea cannot survive for long outside the body. Therefore, contracting either syphilis or gonorrhea from door knobs, dishes, eating utensils, or public toilets is unlikely. VD can be contracted from sores on the skin or mucous membranes as well as from the genital lesions of an infected person.

Exclusion. None required.

Gonorrhea. GC, as it is more commonly called, is a local disease of the genital body parts, and occasionally it may spread to other parts of the body. In the male, the disease manifests itself as a burning upon urination and a discharge of pus. If not treated early, it may produce sterility. In the female, the early symptoms of GC are less pronounced. Progression of the disease often leads to infection of the fallopian tubes, ovaries, and lower abdomen, causing severe pain. This process often results in sterility due to scarring and closure of the tubes or to emergency surgery.

Infectious agent. *Neisseria gonorrhoeae* (bacteria). Laboratory tests will disclose the organism.

Incubation period. Within 5 days for 85% of males following exposure; 2 to 8 days for females. Reservoir is man.

Mode of transmission. Sexual contact, usually sexual intercourse.

Immunity. There is no immunizing agent (vaccine) against gonorrhea. An attack of the disease does not afford protection against reinfection.

Syphilis. The first sign of *primary syphilis* is a single, painless lesion or sore called a chancre. In a short time, which may vary from a few weeks to 6 months, *secondary syphilis* signs appear. Whitish patches in the mouth or throat, "moth eaten" or patchy falling hair, low fever, painless swelling of lymph glands, and pain in bones and joints may all be signs of secondary syphilis. While the primary and secondary manifestations persist, the disease is highly contagious.

The final category, *noninfectious late latent syphilis*, can become destructive and may eventually cause heart disease, insanity, paralysis, blindness, or death. These end results of untreated or inadequately treated syphilis may not take place until 10 or 30 years after the primary infection.

Infectious agent. *Treponema pallidum* (spirochete). Laboratory tests will disclose the organism.

Incubation period. From 10 to 90 days, usually 21 days following exposure.

Mode of transmission. Direct physical contact, usually during sexual relations.

Immunity. There is no immunizing agent (vaccine) against syphilis. Early treatment protects the body against the systemic advance of the disease process.

Whooping cough (pertussis)
Reportable disease

Description of the disease. An acute bacterial infection involving the trachea, bronchi, and bronchioles and characterized by a typical cough, usually of 1 to 2 months' duration.

Infectious agent. *Bordetella pertussis,* pertussis bacillus.

Source of infection. Discharges from the laryngeal and bronchial mucous membranes of infected persons. Man is the reservoir.

Mode of transmission. By direct contact with an infected person, by droplet spread, or indirectly by contact with articles freshly soiled with discharges of such persons.

Incubation period. Commonly 7 days, almost uniformly within 10 days, and not exceeding 21 days.

Period of communicability. Particularly communicable in the early catarrhal stage before paroxysmal cough confirms provisional clinical diagnosis. After paroxysms are established, communicability gradually decreases and becomes negligible for ordinary nonfamilial contacts in about 3 weeks even though spasmodic cough with whoop may persist. For control purposes, the communicable stage is considered to extend from 7 days after exposure to 3 weeks after onset of typical paroxysms.

Susceptibility and resistance. Susceptibility is general. One attack confers immunity.

Prevalence. A common disease among children regardless of race, climate, or geographical location. Marked decline in areas having active immunization programs and good medical care.

Methods of control

Prevention. Immunization of all preschool children.

Exclusion. Exclusion of patient from school for 21 days after onset of paroxysmal cough and until clinical recovery.

Isolation. For the recognized period of communicability.

Contacts. Exclusion of nonimmune children from school and public gatherings for 14 days after last exposure may be omitted if exposed nonimmune children are seen by a nurse on arrival at school each day for 14 days after last exposure. Hyperimmune gamma globulin may be used.

Readmission. By a school physician or nurse, the health department, or other licensed physician.

APPENDIX B ❧ First-aid procedures*

Responsibility for first-aid treatment and the nature of recommended treatment are matters of local policy. The following are offered as suggestions only.

Abdominal pain. Pain in right flank induced by exertion is not appendicitis. Pain in abdomen, irrespective of activity, with tenderness and sometimes nausea and vomiting, is *suspicious* of apendicitis. Parents should be advised to obtain professional advice and care for the child.

Burns

Slight (first or second degree). Apply sterile gauze after keeping under cold water for 10 to 15 minutes.

Severe (blisters or charred skin). Apply loose sterile dressing only. Send to receiving hospital or private physician after notifying parent.

Cinder or brush burns. Cleanse out foreign matter with warm water and soap solution. Scrub if necessary to remove dirt. Cover with sterile gauze.

Chemical burns. Immediately flush copiously with water or antidote if external, olive oil or egg white if internal. Refer for immediate medical care.

Acid burns to eye. Flush eye thoroughly with water. Refer to medical care.

Acids burns of the skin. Wash with running water, then neutralize immediately with ammonia solution, wash after. Then apply sterile gauze.

Acid burns of the mucous membrane. Rinse with water, follow with a solution of sodium bicarbonate.

Acid burns (internal)
1. Give insoluble magnesia, magnesium carbonate, or lime water.
2. Give milk.
3. Refer for medical care.

Alkali burns to eye. Flush eye thoroughly with water. Refer for immediate medical care.

Alkali burns of the skin. Wash with running water, then neutralize immediately with vinegar. Then apply sterile gauze.

Alkali burns of the mucous membrane. Rinse with water and follow with equal parts of vinegar and water.

Alkali burns (internal)
1. Give 1 pint of solution composed of equal parts of vinegar and water.
2. Refer for medical care.

Other burns of eyes. Flush eyes copiously with water. Cover with a loose nonpressure bandage. See that child gets expert care as soon as possible.

Cuts

Arteries. Evidenced by intermittent spurting of blood. If hemorrhage cannot be controlled by a firmly applied pressure bandage and serious loss of blood is threatened, a tourniquet should be used. If soft rubber tubing is not available, wrap handkerchief or towel above wound tightly enough to stop bleeding. The tourniquet should be placed close to wound but not at wound edge. The tourniquet should not be released except by a physician. Notify parents at once. Send to family physician or nearest receiving hospital.

Small cuts and abrasions. Cleanse with clean warm water and soap solution. When thoroughly dry, cover with sterile gauze and tape.

Severe cuts and abrasions. Sterile gauze is the only dressing to be used on wounds of pupils sent to the receiving hospital or private physician, as antiseptics or ointments obscure wound and make proper cleansing difficult. If bleeding, use sterile pressure bandage.

Dog bites

Animal bites, especially dogs and cats. The wound should be washed thoroughly with bar soap or liquid soap, full strength. One percent solution of Zephiran may be used if available. The deeper wounds should be thoroughly irrigated. Allow to dry and apply sterile gauze. Refer at once for further treatment to personal physician or receiving hospital.

Drowning. See Artifical respiration under Respiration.

Earache. Send child home and recommend medical care.

Electric shock. See Artificial respiration under Respiration.

Eyes

Chemical burns of eyeball. See Other burns of eyes under Burns.

Foreign body in eye. Use warm water in medicine dropper to try to flush the particle out. If not easily washed out, refer to nurse, physician, or receiving hospital.

Convulsive seizure. Let patient lie on the floor. Provide fresh air and keep crowd away. Give nothing by mouth. Loosen tight collar or

---

*This material on first-aid procedures is derived and updated from an eight-page folder distributed to its schools by the Health Services Branch of the Auxiliary Services Division of the Los Angeles City School Districts. It is used here with their permission.

clothing. Remove hard objects against which injury might occur. After patient is quiet, remove to the rest room and send for parents.

Fainting. Keep child's head down. Give nothing by mouth. Loosen clothing, and keep crowd away. If unconsciousness is prolonged, call parents or send to receiving hospital.

Fractures. Do not move child from place of injury until emergency splints are applied. Keep child lying down. Notify parents. In minor fracture cases with little or no shock, child may be taken to receiving hospital unless parents desire to make other arrangements. In fractures with severe pain and shock, call receiving hospital.

Suspected spine fracture. Usually caused by fall from great height or a crushing blow. Child may be paralyzed. *Do not move child from place of injury.* Send for ambulance.

Headache. Apply covered ice cap with child in reclining position. Look for signs of contagious disease. If child has rash, fever, cough, sore throat, or nasal discharge, isolate until he or she can be sent home.

Head injuries. Do not move from place of injury unless imperative, then move as carefully as possible. Keep child lying down, even if injury appears to be minor. Cover with blanket. Treat for shock.

If mucus is collecting in nose or throat and difficulty in breathing is observed, turn patient on side.

Bleeding from scalp wounds may be controlled by sterile pressure bandages.

If patient is conscious and thoroughly warm, covered ice cap to head may be used if it makes him/her comfortable.

If unable to locate parents, call for ambulance. Never allow child to walk home, go by the bus, or ride bicycle if there has been shock, disorientation, or convulsion. Notify parent to call for child even if he or she appears to have recovered.

Head injuries severe enough to cause even momentary unconsciousness should be observed carefully for several days.

Insect bites and stings

Bee stings. Remove stinger. Immediate application of ice or ice water gives relief. If marked swelling occurs, refer for medical care.

Insulin shock. Sudden pallor, weakness, sweating, mental confusion, convulsions, or unconsciousness. Give sugar, candy, orange juice, or Karo syrup if conscious. If unconscious, call emergency hospital at once.

Nosebleed. Place child in sitting position with head erect. Apply gauze with pressure to anterior portion of nostrils for at least 15 minutes, by the clock.

Poisoning—by chemicals. See Chemical burns under Burns.

Respiration

Stopping of respiration—by electric shock, immersion, etc. Give artificial respiration and send for emergency medical aid at once.

Artificial respiration. The mouth-to-mouth (or mouth-to-nose) technique is considered the most practical method for emergency ventilation of a victim of any age who has stopped breathing. This technique is basically the same for both adults and children.

Mouth-to-mouth technique

Clean out the mouth.

With victim on his or her back, *tilt* the head as far back as possible (one hand pushing the crown of the head down with the other hand lifting the jaw up).

Open your mouth wide and place it over the mouth of the victim, with your cheek against his/her nose. Blow into mouth. (With infant or small child it is possible to cover *both* mouth and nose with your mouth.)

Remove your mouth, gasp in fresh air, and repeat.

"Huff and puff," blowing into victim's mouth about 12 times per minute, 20 times per minute for children or infants (think of the lungs as paper bags—small puffs to fill small bags, big puffs to fill big bags).

If you have a blanket, pillow, coat, or towel, fold it and place it under shoulders. This will further help extend head. Do not delay in this. Breath into your victim first, then do this if it can be done without delay.

Splinters. Do not remove if deeply imbedded, or if there is possibility of splinter breaking off.

Notify family to seek necessary care, or if serious, send to receiving hospital.

Sprains or bruises. If seen early, use cold compresses. Follow with supporting bandaging. If seen late, hot compresses give more relief. Rest. Notify family to seek necessary care.

Note: Apply ice only in covered ice bag or with a layer of heavy cloth between ice and skin.

Wounds. Wash with soap and scrub away from the wound. (Remember that any "sterile" bandage is no longer sterile once it is opened.) When thoroughly dry, apply sterile dressing. If wound is deep or dirty, refer patient to physician or receiving hospital. See Cuts.

Thermometer technique

Use clean thermometer. After use, clean immediately by washing thoroughly with soap solution and water. Rinse in cold water and place in container of alcohol. Rinse with water again. Put in clean container.

For additional information, see the *American Red Cross Manual of First Aid Instructions.*

Index